SEXUALITY *and* INTIMACY

An Occupational Therapy Approach

Edited by Kathryn Ellis, OTD, OTR/L, AASECT–SC,
and Joseph Christian Ungco, OTD, OTR/L

American
Occupational Therapy
Association

AOTA Vision 2025
As an inclusive profession, occupational therapy maximizes health, well-being, and quality of life for all people, populations, and communities through effective solutions that facilitate participation in everyday living.

Mission Statement
The American Occupational Therapy Association advances occupational therapy practice, education, and research through standard-setting and advocacy on behalf of its members, the profession, and the public.

AOTA Staff
Sherry Keramidas, *Executive Director*
Matthew Clark, *Chief Officer, Innovation & Engagement*

Elizabeth Dooley, *Vice President, Strategic Marketing & Communications*
Laura Collins, *Director, Communications & Publications*
Ashley Hofmann, *Acquisitions & Development Manager, AOTA Press*
Amy Ricci, *Product Manager & Business Analyst, AOTA Press*

Rebecca Rutberg, *Director, Marketing*
Amanda Goldman, *Marketing Manager*
Jennifer Folden, *Brand Designer*

American Occupational Therapy Association, Inc.
6116 Executive Boulevard, Suite 200
North Bethesda, MD 20852-4929
www.aota.org
To order: 1-800-729-AOTA (2682) or store.aota.org

Printed and bound by CPI Group (UK) Ltd, Croydon, CR0 4YY

ISBN: 978-1-56900-608-5
eBOOK ISBN: 978-1-56900-609-2
Library of Congress Control Number: 2023933070

Cover design by Steve Parrish, AOTA, North Bethesda, MD
Composition by Manila Typesetting Company, Manila, Philippines
Printed by Gasch Printing, Odenton, MD

Suggested citation: Ellis, K., & Ungco, J. C. (Eds.). (2023). *Sexuality and intimacy: An occupational therapy approach.* AOTA Press.

Dedication

The editors dedicate this textbook to the real people whose stories were deidentified and shared throughout the textbook for the purpose of learning. The editors would like to specifically thank the Network for LGBTQIA+ Concerns in OT as well as military service members and their families who have contributed by sharing their stories and lived experiences that inspired and influenced us.

—K.E. and J.C.U.

Contents

Figures, Tables, Exhibits, Case Examples, and Reflection Prompts

Figure

Table

Exhibits

Case Examples

Reflection Prompts

About the Editors

Kathryn Ellis, OTD, OTR/L, AASECT–SC (she/her), is the founder/CEO of the Institute for Sex, Intimacy & Occupational Therapy, an education and consulting company with the mission to dismantle restrictive sexuality norms that limit occupational therapy clients as well as occupational therapy professionals, both as clinicians and sexual beings. She developed the Occupational Therapy Sexuality and Intimacy Clinic at Walter Reed National Military Medical Center in Bethesda, Maryland, and is the co-author of *Sex and Intimacy for Wounded Veterans: A Guide to Embracing Change.* She is an American Association of Sexuality Educators, Counselors, and Therapists Certified Sexuality Counselor and a consultant on sexuality and intimacy projects and initiatives. Her private practice, Dr. Kathryn Ellis Sexual Wellness Counseling, is based in Delaware.

Joseph Christian Ungco, OTD, OTR/L (they/them), is the associate director for diversity, equity, and inclusion (DEI) education, client services, and data analytics for the Fred Hutchinson Cancer Center in Seattle, Washington. They lead several organization-wide DEI initiatives, including the bias mitigation education program and gender-inclusive and accessible spaces initiative. They also continue to serve in DEI roles in occupational therapy, including serving as co-chair of the national Network for LGBTQIA+ Concerns in Occupational Therapy and sitting on the executive council for the Occupational Therapy Multicultural, Diversity and Inclusion National Network. Dr. Ungco's work is centered on amplifying the voices of those most affected by systems of oppression and actualizing structural change.

Introduction

Joseph Christian Ungco, *OTD, OTR/L, and* **Kathryn Ellis,** *OTD, OTR/L, AASECT–SC*

Sex is an ADL (American Occupational Therapy Association [AOTA], 2020b). Sexuality and intimacy contain so much more than the *act* of sexual activity. *Occupations* are the "everyday personalized activities that people do as individuals, in families, and with communities to occupy time and bring meaning and purpose to life" (AOTA, 2020b, p. 79). Beyond the physical mechanics of "sexual activity," sexual and intimate occupations encompass a broad range of personally meaningful activities for building intimate partnerships, developing a sense of self, actualizing desire, and experiencing pleasure.

Although sex and intimacy are mentioned in occupational therapy professional documents (i.e., *Occupational Therapy Practice Framework;* AOTA, 2020b), we have heard from many occupational therapy practitioners, students, and colleagues who continue to face many barriers when it comes to addressing sexual and intimate occupations. Barriers include lack of theoretical framework, lack of foundational knowledge, limited practical experience, harmful stigma and clinician bias, institutional barriers, or simple "embarrassment." Despite these seemingly insurmountable personal and institutional barriers, we've helped occupational therapy professionals dismantle these restrictions to address this meaningful and titillating area of practice for their clients. In this text, authors share key knowledge and lessons we've learned from well over 230 years of combined experience addressing the sexual health needs and goals of our clients.

This textbook presents a comprehensive and holistic scope of occupational therapy that is intended to broaden readers' perspective on our profession's role. Conversations around sexuality have been silenced for far too long in the occupational therapy profession. However, as discussions about power and oppression continue to be highlighted in public discourse, the topic of sexuality requires intentional evaluation and occupational therapy professionals need to consider co-existing perspectives, practices, and realities related to sexual occupations and the human experience.

Moving through this text, readers will learn the foundational knowledge to be competent and comfortable integrating sexual and intimate occupations into practice, academia, policy, and research.

A Note About the Authors and Editors

Kathryn "Kates" Ellis was first attracted to sexuality in occupational therapy practice because she saw it as a practice gap. Her love and passion for the topic itself quickly followed. She noted that health care providers did not feel prepared to address sexuality and often felt uncomfortable by the topic, resulting in a gap in the occupational therapy profession that aspired to provide holistic care. For this reason, Kates had an educational mission in parallel to developing her skills as a clinician. Her first AOTA Annual Conference & Expo presentation was in 2015, co-led with Caitlin Dennison, "Engaging in Sexual Activity and Intimacy Post-Polytrauma Combat Injury: An Occupational Therapy Perspective" (Ellis & Dennison, 2015). The session was so widely attended that the conference organizers asked them to present the presentation for a second time that day to allow for more people to attend. This experience solidified for Kates the need for widespread institutional change at the professional level to equip occupational therapy professionals at the individual level with the skills and comfort to address sexuality and uphold the occupational therapy values of being holistic and client-lead practitioners.

Joseph Christian "Joe" Ungco's start in sexual and intimate occupational therapy came from a very personal place. As an occupational therapy student and queer person of color, they rarely saw themselves represented within the profession; people like them were missing in its research, education, and practice. They became interested in sex and intimacy as they noticed that not only were sexual and intimate occupations rarely discussed, even more rare was any information on LGBTQIA+ sex and intimacy. Thus began Joe's professional interest in both LGBTQIA+ health and sexual and intimate occupations. In 2019, they co-developed and presented the workshop "Queering & Cripping[1] Sex: Sexuality as an Activity of Daily Living Moving Beyond Heteronormative Ableist Perspectives" at AOTA's Annual Conference & Expo (Kingsley et al., 2017). This session, co-led with Karrie Kingsley and Liz Schmidt, was well-received for its intersectional look at LGBTQIA+ identities and disability in the context of sex and intimacy. It was at this workshop that Joe and Kates first met and immediately started comparing notes on the ways we had supported the sexual and intimate needs of our communities.

During our initial conversations, we took great pleasure in finding unexpected similarities in our work. For example, talking about adaptive equipment and modified techniques for anal play that Joe described for queer, disabled folks were similar to Kates's approach in supporting straight, cisgender men curious to explore anal erogenous zones. We also found commonalties across our differences in gender, sexuality, and racial experiences about the roles of gender self-view, sexual self-view, and the environment in building intimate partnerships. When it came to talking through our challenges in the occupational therapy field, we quickly found common ground in the perspective that "functional independence" wasn't enough—we wanted the profession to incorporate a focus on joy and pleasure. Our years of collaboration since have been full of joy and pleasure in pushing the scope of occupational therapy. We have worked on continuing education courses,

[1] The word *cipping* comes from "crip theory" as a form of reclaiming the word *cripple*. It means to apply a disability justice lens to something. "Cripping" in the context of this session was taken from Robert McRuer's (2006) work on intersecting communities around disability and queerness.

conference presentations, graduate coursework, professional panels, external reviews, blogs, consultation, and various projects to challenge our profession to be more inclusive, pleasurable, and sexy.

In 2017, Kates started discussion with AOTA Press about this textbook. Kates contemplated how the text would be lacking without diverse voices, specifically of underrepresented voices, to show the expansive co-existing sexual perspectives and realties. Readers would benefit from hearing a variety of perspectives to better see the shared human experiences on a topic that often focuses on difference, stigma, taboo, and exclusion. She knew that with Joe, they could achieve this together.

We are acutely aware that the occupational therapy profession is not representative of the United States as a whole and have taken care to develop a textbook that resists reinforcing heteronormative, cisnormative, and White-centered narratives dominating our professional literature. For this reason, we intentionally curated authors who could contribute to our goal for centering and amplifying voices that have been historically marginalized and underrepresented in the occupational therapy profession. This approach also serves to bring greater alignment with U.S. demographics and the communities that occupational therapy practitioners serve. Seventy-six percent of the authors in this text are members of underrepresented groups in occupational therapy, including Black, people of color, disabled, LGBTQIA+,[2] Muslim, Indian, Middle Eastern, or immigrant communities. Additionally, many of our authors hold intersecting identities and membership in multiple, diverse communities. All of the authors specialize in sexuality, and a few work outside of the occupational therapy profession. Through this text's authors' identities and experiences, this book will offer perspectives of more universal significance that are more representative of the communities and individuals occupational therapy practitioners serve.

By decentering of whiteness, maleness, and straightness, some readers may feel like certain groups are not represented in this text. The authors encourage readers to consider how information can be generalized to other populations and consider challenging their preference for certain groups to be centered.

What to Expect

This textbook is organized to guide readers through a developmental process that starts with a broad understanding of sexual and intimate concepts and one's own positionality in these areas of occupation. Chapter 1, "Pleasure, Eroticism, and

[2] The term *LGBTQIA+ communities* refers to the diverse and unique communities formed by lesbian, gay, bisexual, transgender, queer, intersex, asexual, and additional sexual and gender minoritized people. As greater awareness, social acceptance, and safety improve for these individuals and communities, new terms may emerge as language evolves to describe identities that exist outside of societal recognition and acceptance.

Occupational Therapy," presents an overview of the topic. It is followed by three chapters that include critical reflection, beginning with sexual identity in Chapter 2, "Understanding Sexual Identity." Readers can engage in a process of self-reflection on their own comfort and connection to sexuality in Chapter 3, "Guided Self-Reflection of Self as a Sexual Being." In Chapter 4, "Sexuality, Bias, and Impact: Preventing Clinician Harm," readers will learn how unconscious bias affects clinical decision making. Chapter 5, "Sexual and Intimate Occupations Across the Lifespan," invites occupational therapy practitioners to integrate their general knowledge of human development with key developmental aspects of sexuality and intimacy over the human lifespan, from birth through death.

After establishing this foundational knowledge, the second half of the textbook follows the occupational therapy process to provide readers with an understanding of how to address sexual and intimate occupations in their practice. The chapters supporting evaluation begin with introducing the occupational therapy Sexual Assessment Framework (OTSAF), assessment strategies, and goal writing in Chapter 6, "Sexuality and Intimacy Screening and Assessment." In-depth analysis of occupational performance for sexual activity and intimate partnerships is provided in Chapter 7, "Intimate Partnerships," and Chapter 8, "Sexual Activity as an ADL." Trauma-informed care approaches for working with clients on sexual and intimate occupations are described in Chapter 9, "Trauma-Informed Care."

In Chapter 10, "Personal Narratives of Sex, Intimacy, and Meaning," authors share their own experiences with sexual and intimate occupations; readers are encouraged to read these narratives to understand the diversity in sexual and intimate experiences and perspectives. This is also an opportunity for readers to apply what they have learned thus far to encounter real people's stories. Finally, Chapter 11, "Intervention for Sexual and Intimate Occupations," supports practitioners in holistic intervention planning and implementation for cognitive, emotional, and physical considerations.

Voyeuristic Content

By exposing participation in an occupation that is often unobserved by and unfamiliar to those not participating in it, reading this book may feel voyeuristic. ***Voyeurism*** is the "the practice of taking pleasure in observing something private, sordid, or scandalous" (Merriam-Webster, 2022). Readers may find it satisfying and exciting from an intellectual perspective to have an inside look at what is often taboo. It is also possible the content can elicit feelings of sexual pleasure or curiosity; in fact, this is likely, given an entire textbook on the topic of sex. Readers might wonder, "Is this ok?" "What does this mean?" or "What if I feel this way during a treatment session?" We posit that these feelings are normal, not uncommon, and not an ethical violation. And too often, this fear of voyeurism—of observing our clients in a sexually exposed way—is a barrier to addressing sexuality and discourages the practitioners from asking what may feel like prying questions.

Occupational therapy practitioners can normalize feelings of curiosity that feel voyeuristic. The instruction for practitioners is to sit with those feelings and begin to parse out what curiosity is truly voyeuristic and what is essential for the therapeutic process. Using the strict criterion of "need to know," practitioners can ask questions, despite the questions feeling prying, to help facilitate therapeutic decision making. Through this text, readers can begin to normalize feelings of sexual curiosity and satisfaction when engaging with sexually relevant content, prepare for those feelings when working with clients, and understand how to continue the occupational therapy process.

Selection of Authors and Content

The understanding of sexuality in mainstream American discourse is narrow and determined by those who hold positions of power: White, patriarchal, heteronormative, cisnormative, middle-class people (Collins, 2017; McGrath & Sakellariou, 2015; Mona et al., 2017; Sakellariou & Algado, 2006; Tepper, 2000). Likewise, the occupational therapy profession is founded on Western, White, heterosexual, cisgender, Christian, middle class, capitalist, patriarchal values, and those values are reflected in our profession's demographics (AOTA, 2020a; McGrath & Sakellariou, 2015). The profession is 90.6% female and 84% White (AOTA, 2020a) and is significantly different from the U.S. population, which is 50.5% female and 59.7% White (U.S. Census Bureau, 2020). Limited data have been collected on occupational therapy professionals' identities in terms of sexual orientation, gender-expansive identities, disability status, and additional identity factors.

Occupational therapy practitioners should avoid thinking about sexuality in terms of fitting their clients into niches or categories; it is not a question of being prepared for *if* they get a client who is, for example, LGBQTIA+, Muslim, and disabled. The reality is that none of our clients are served when viewing them solely through the narrow views of sexuality described earlier (i.e., White, cisgender, heterosexual). This book is intended to help the reader develop a broad lens through which all sexuality can be viewed and integrate "niches" into standard practice.

Occupational therapy practitioners are both required and encouraged to continue learning. Sexuality is expansive and fluid, changing across one's life course, so practitioners need to stay intentionally curious about themselves and others as sexual beings, how pleasure and eroticisms influence engagement, and how ways of having sex (which we call "ways of doing") might be positioned against evolving societal norms. When learning about sex, occupational therapy practitioners must pursue education and resources from educators of diverse backgrounds and identities to maintain a broad lens.

Focus on Context and Culture

Throughout the text, sexuality and intimacy are presented through cultural lenses. Understanding contextual factors, such as culture and environment, is critical for effective practice in an area that is frequently stigmatized. For example, one component of sexual and intimate occupations is attracting and selecting a potential partner. Both this process and what a person considers "attractive" is highly culturally derived. However, this text focuses primarily on the United States and similar Western societies that may share similarities in how sexual and intimate occupations are generated, understood and performed.

Cross-cultural studies have found substantial differences in perceptions of attractiveness of women based on cultural context (e.g., Boothroyd et al., 2020; Chan & Hurst, 2022; Tovee et al., 2006). One study comparing South African Zulu men with British White and Black men showed preference for women with larger body sizes; the researchers posited that this was likely a result of culture-specific values, such as thinness being associated with illness in South Africa while being associated with attractiveness in England (Tovee et al., 2006). The researchers also studied a group of South African Zulu migrants who moved to England and found that after 18 months of living in England, their perceptions of attractive bodies had shifted to be more aligned with British than with South African ideals (Tovee et al., 2006). This is just one example of how culture directs attraction and the perceptions we hold towards others. Thus, it is important for readers to carefully consider the context of their own perspectives, practice, and communities.

Lifelong Learning

This textbook is intended to provide an overarching, general education into sex and intimacy in the context of occupational therapy practice. As such, we chose to focus on generalizable factors affecting sexual and intimate participation (e.g., contexts, occupations, performance skills) and complemented this content with information on key skills occupational therapy practitioners need to be effective in this area and, indeed, in their entire practice (e.g., cultural humility, awareness of bias, trauma-informed approaches).

Although this textbook provides a solid foundation for addressing sexual and intimate occupations into occupational therapy practice, it offers a survey of the topic for generalist practitioners and does not include diagnosis- or impairment-specific content. We encourage readers to seek supplemental sources for in-depth content specific to their own practice needs, such as the short course "Sexuality and Breast Cancer: For Women and Individuals Assigned Female at Birth" (Ellis, 2020) or a course on interventions for LGBTQIA+ people who have experienced trauma.

As readers consider how to expand their knowledge on this topic, we encourage them to think critically about the sources they find, given the relatively limited availability of inclusive, educational, and nonjudgmental health care literature and its frequently narrow focus on White, cisgender, heterosexual sexual experiences. To intentionally expose themselves to information representing a range of perspectives, we encourage occupational therapy professionals to seek out community-based resources, such as the following organizations:

- Sexual Health for Muslims (https://sexualhealthformuslims.com/)
- Afrosexology (https://afrosexology.com/)
- Local LGBTQIA+ centers
- The Network for LGBTQIA+ Concerns in Occupational Therapy (https://www.otnetworkmembers.org)
- The Fenway Institute (https://fenwayhealth.org/the-fenway-institute/)
- The American Association of Sexuality Educators, Counselors, and Therapists (https://www.aasect.org/).

And, of course, practitioners should listen to stories from their clients and others to understand more about underrepresented cultures.

This intentional approach to lifelong learning is particularly critical given the social stigmas and taboos surrounding sexuality in society. To best support all our clients, occupational therapy practitioners must understand, validate, and affirm the experiences of communities frequently underrepresented in our professional resources.

References

American Occupational Therapy Association. (2020a). *2019 workforce and salary survey.*

American Occupational Therapy Association. (2020b). Occupational therapy practice framework: Domain and process (4th ed.). *American Journal of Occupational Therapy, 74*(Suppl. 2), 7412410010. https://doi.org/10.5014/ajot.2020.74S2001

Boothroyd, L. G., Jucker, J. L., Thornborrow, T., Barton, R. A., Burt, D. M., Evans, E. H., . . . & Tovée, M. J. (2020). Television consumption drives perceptions of female body attractiveness in a population undergoing technological transition. *Journal of Personality and Social Psychology, 119*(4), 839.

Chan, J., & Hurst, M. (2022). South Asian women in the United Kingdom: The role of skin colour dissatisfaction in acculturation experiences and body dissatisfaction. *Body Image, 42,* 413-418.

Collins, R., Strasburger, V., Brown, J., Donnerstein, E., Lenhart, A., & Ward, M. (2017). Sexual media and childhood well-being and health. *Pediatrics, 140,* S162–S166. https://doi.org/10.1542/peds.2016-1758X

Ellis, K. (2020). *Sexuality and breast cancer: For women and individuals assigned female at birth.* Institute for Sex, Intimacy and Occupational Therapy.

Ellis, K., & Dennison, C. (2015, April 16–19). Engaging in sexual activity and intimacy post-polytrauma combat injury: An occupational therapy perspective [Conference Presentation]. *AOTA Annual Conference & Expo, Nashville, TN, United States.*

Kingsley, K., Ungco, J. C., & Schmidt, E. (2019, April 4–7). Queering & cripping sex: Sexuality as an activity of daily living moving beyond heteronormative ableist perspectives [Conference workshop]. *AOTA Annual Conference & Expo, New Orleans, LA, United States.*

McGrath, M., & Sakellariou, D. (2016). The Issue Is—Why has so little progress been made in the practice of occupational therapy in relation to sexuality? *American Journal of Occupational Therapy, 70,* 7001360010. http://dx.doi.org/10.5014/ajot.2016.017707

McRuer, R. (2006). *Crip theory: Cultural signs of queerness and disability.* New York University Press.

Merriam-Webster. (2022, June 7). *Voyeurism.* https://www.merriam-webster.com/dictionary/voyeurism

Mona, L. R., Cameron, R. P., & Clemency Cordes, C. (2017). Disability culturally competent sexual healthcare. *American Psychologist, 72,* 1000–1010. https://doi.org/10.1037/amp0000283

Tepper, M. S. (2000). Sexuality and disability: The missing discourse of pleasure. *Sexuality and Disability, 18,* 283–290. https://doi.org/10.1023/A:1005698311392

Tovee, M., Swami, V., Furnham, A., & Mangalparsad, R. (2006). Changing perceptions of attractiveness as observers are exposed to a different culture. *Evolution and Human Behavior, 27,* 443–456. https://doi.org/10.1016/j.evolhumbehav.2006.05.004

U.S. Census Bureau. (2020). *American community survey public use microdata sample.* https://datausa.io/about/background

1

Pleasure, Eroticism, and Occupational Therapy

Kathryn Ellis, *OTD, OTR/L, AASECT–SC;* **Joseph Christian Ungco,** *OTD, OTR/L; and* **Jenn Soros,** *PhD, OTR/L*

CHAPTER HIGHLIGHTS

- Introduction to occupational therapy's role in sexual and intimate occupations
- Pleasure and eroticism
- Foundational guiding framework
- Putting the erotic in occupational therapy

KEY TERMS AND CONCEPTS

Becoming
Being
Belonging
Doing
Empowerment
Enablement
Eroticism
Inclusion
Inclusive classification
Occupational justice
Occupational Perspective of Health model
Occupational science
Occupations
Sexual activity
Sexuality

> *Sex is the most common behavior among humans after birth, breathing, sleeping, and death.*
>
> —adrienne marie brown, social justice facilitator, doula and healer, pleasure activist (2019, p. 122)[1]

[1] See also Brown (2017).

Sexuality is a complex human experience. It is a state of mind that represents how individuals feel about themselves, relate to other people,[2] establish relationships, and express themselves (AOTA, 2013). Although sexuality involves biological, psychological, cognitive, emotional, physical, social, erotic, and spiritual factors that vary from person to person, it also is embedded in environmental, political, cultural, and historical context. Sexuality relates to every part of the occupational therapy domain in some way: occupations, contexts, performance patterns, performance skills, and client factors. This chapter introduces key concepts to build a foundation for exploring a variety of sexual and intimate occupations and how they apply to occupational therapy practice, education, and research.

Sexuality as an occupation differs from most other occupations, because sexuality is both highly personal and involves huge variation in sexual values and beliefs, sexual expression, and how people engage in sex. This expansiveness of possibility around sexuality is poorly understood in part because of the restricted view of sexuality and silence that surrounds it in modern U.S. society. Although sexual and intimate occupations may be highly meaningful for individuals, social norms and stigma limit how sexuality is shared with others, compared with other shared occupations. For example, participation in a community of running enthusiasts or in a religious community is freely discussed. Fellow runners might share the latest shoe technology with each other in a group chat, or churchgoers might get together for Bible study. In both contexts, discussion of the occupation takes place without hesitation. Meanwhile, highly valued, intimate occupations may be regulated with norms and policies such as "don't ask, don't tell" or through other forms of social stigma, such as a "TMI" rejoinder when a person shares about a sexual experience.

Sexuality is different from other occupations. It has little socially acceptable space for ease of discussion, joy, and acceptance. People generally are private about their sexuality and, even in a supportive environment, are hesitant to discuss it. Discussion of sexuality in contemporary, mainstream U.S. society tends to occur in the context of policy (e.g., abortion, anti-trans laws) or be idealized by inaccurate media portrayals of sexual activity, such as Hollywood films, perfectly curated Instagram posts, and pornography. With such limited narrative space, it can be challenging for any occupational therapy professional to discuss sexuality with their clients.

This chapter positions sexual pleasure and eroticism firmly in occupational therapy's purview and scope, discusses occupational therapy frameworks for understanding sexuality and intimacy occupations, and orients readers to the remaining chapters in this text. The sections that follow introduce key concepts for sexuality and occupation, describe how existing occupational therapy frameworks are a suitable foundation for sexual and intimate occupational therapy

[2] The original text of this document stated "how they relate to others from the same and opposite gender." The original statement reinforces binary notions of gender and excludes the wide-ranging spectrum of gender identities.

assessment and intervention, and offer considerations for further professional development.

Pleasure and Eroticism

Pleasure is a measure of freedom.

—adrienne maree brown (2019, p. 3)

Eroticism has its own moral justification because it says that pleasure is enough for me; it is a statement of the individual's sovereignty.

—Mario Vargas Llosa[3] (1991, p. 7)

Sexual and intimate occupations are foundational to being human. In fact, the existence and survival of our species rely on our ability to engage in sexual and intimate occupations. These occupations serve many functions, but most uniquely, they provide avenues for people to experience pleasure, eroticism, and joy.

When asked, "What are the 'functions' of sex," occupational therapy students in Joseph Ungco's *Sexuality, Gender and Intimacy* graduate course at Ithaca College often identify social bonding, expression of love, maintaining relationships, stress reduction, and procreation. With a bit of prompting, they also eventually identify meaningfulness, pleasure, and overall fulfillment. What makes identifying pleasure as a goal of sex in a professional health setting seemingly secondary to those other functions? Shouldn't it feel good to participate in occupations of our choosing?

Although pleasure and eroticism may at first glance appear unrelated to occupational therapy's role in supporting autonomy in occupational engagement, we assert that pleasure and eroticism are actually at the core of what we strive for as occupational therapy practitioners. As described in the quotes above, pleasure can be experienced as a measure of one's freedom. It has the potential to provide a sensory, cognitive, and emotional experience that shows us what true independence and freedom *feels* like. ***Eroticism*** is more than feeling sexual; it is also a perspective on meaning and beauty related to sexual desire, sensuality, and romantic love. The writer Mario Vargas Llosa (2015) asserted that eroticism and pleasure demonstrate an individual's sovereignty, or authority to manage themselves. What matters more: that a client is engaging in a sexual activity as "independently" as they can, or that the client feels a sense of freedom and sovereignty through that occupation? Consider a client who requires minimal assistance for bed mobility. In this scenario, what affects quality of life more is whether

[3] Mario Vargas Llosa is a Peruvian novelist, journalist, essayist, and former politician. He won the Nobel Prize in Literature in 2010 "for his cartography of structures of power and his trenchant images of the individual's resistance, revolt, and defeat" (The Nobel Prize, n.d.).

they enjoy the experiences they have in the bed regardless of need for assistance. Occupational therapy is *the* profession that supports clients in achieving sovereignty in how they engage in the places they live, learn, work, or play, including sexual and intimate occupations.

This text is not strictly about sexual activity as an ADL (AOTA, 2020). Conducting an activity analysis of a sexual activity in a certain context, while considering the client factors and activity demands, is a valuable occupational therapy skill. Such skills are not about sexuality as much as they are about the occupational therapy process. For example, prescribing energy conservation will require the same occupational therapy process whether the client is engaging in playing sports or sex play. What is required from the occupational therapy professional in this case is a holistic understanding of sexuality, a comfort discussing it, and a dedication to celebrating sex versus a bias toward relegating this occupation to secondary status.

This text moves beyond the mechanics of sex and instead focuses on the skills needed to celebrate sex and eroticisms for the joy they can contribute to our existence. "The 'function' of eroticism is that it brings pleasure, satisfaction, and purpose together and encourages us to pursue change to become more authentic and find more joy in our daily lives" (Ungco, 2022). Occupational therapy practitioners have to talk about pleasure and eroticism because they are factors that make meaning out of sexual activity occupations. Just as competition and camaraderie make playing sports meaningful beyond the activity of kicking a soccer ball, so pleasure and eroticism elevate sex beyond the mere physicality of the experience. Without a focus on rituals, roles, uniqueness, creativity, cognitive arousal, and togetherness, the mechanics of sex become the center focus of "sexual function" and leave a physical activity to be analyzed (Vargas Llosa, 2015).

Foundational Guiding Framework

The framework for this book relies on concepts articulated by AOTA and other nongovernmental organizations as well as various models of occupation.

Sexual Activity as an ADL

Occupations are "everyday activities that people do as individuals, in families and with communities to occupy time and bring meaning and purpose to life. Occupations include things people need to, want to and are expected to do" (World Federation of Occupational Therapists [WFOT], 2022). Sexual activity is an occupation and, more specifically, an ADL (AOTA, 2020). The *Occupational Therapy Practice Framework: Domain and Process* (4th ed.; *OTPF–4*) defines ***sexual activity*** as "engaging in the broad possibilities for sexual expression and experiences with self or others (e.g., hugging, kissing, foreplay, masturbation, oral sex, intercourse)" (AOTA, 2020, p. 30).

World Health Organization Sexual Rights

The World Health Organization (WHO; n.d.) outlines that sexual rights are human rights, including the right to sexuality education; to be sexually active; to have consensual sexual relationships; and to have a safe, satisfying, and pleasurable sex life. Similarly, according to the WFOT (2019), people have the right to engage in occupations—specifically, the right to participate in various occupations, choose occupations, and freely participate in occupations, including sexuality and intimacy.

Occupational Science

Occupational science is the scientific study of people as occupational beings and the human need to participate in daily occupations across the life course in various environments (Yerxa, 1990). According to Yerxa (1990), *occupation* is a complex and multidimensional concept that includes both playful and productive activities. The context in which an occupation occurs may fulfill one's physical, psychological, social, cultural, and spiritual needs. Engagement in occupation is incredibly personal, and through fulfilling their desired occupational roles, people may achieve a sense of value in life. To completely understand occupation, one must recognize a person's experience with the occupation and the meaning, or lack thereof, of the occupation.

Occupational Perspective of Sexual Health

Ann Wilcock developed the ***Occupational Perspective of Health model***, which revolves around four key constructs: *doing, being, belonging,* and *becoming* (Wilcock, 1998; Wilcock & Hocking, 2015). Occupational participation is a determinant of health and quality of life, and the balance of these factors in the context of occupation is essential to health and wellness.

Wilcock's (1998) theory states that people engage in occupations to fulfill physiological and psychological needs. A person's choice of occupations is influenced by several factors, including culture, skill level, available resources, social and environmental constraints, political context, gender expectations, and historical contexts (Wilcock & Hocking, 2015). These principles can also apply to sexual activity. People engage in occupations to fulfill physiological and psychological needs that can be described in terms of doing, being, belonging, and becoming.

Doing

The ***doing*** aspect of occupation is the performance of the occupation. *Doing* includes both things that people feel they have to do and things that they want to do (Wilcock, 1998; Wilcock & Hocking, 2015). What people do shapes societies and cultural environments (Wilcock, 1998; Wilcock & Hocking, 2015). Through the act of doing, the physical and mental state is engaged, thereby affecting overall health (Wilcock, 1998; Wilcock & Hocking, 2015). Concerning sexual activity, the act of doing relates to the occupation of and engagement in sexual activity.

Being

The ***being*** aspect of occupation is a more personal component of occupation and relates to a person's sense of occupational identity (Wilcock, 1998; Wilcock & Hocking, 2015). *Being* is about being true to oneself (Wilcock, 1998); this is a critical concept relating to one's understanding of their sexual identity and being true to it. The concept of *being* related to sexuality involves role validation, affection, intimacy, and sexual gratification as their authentic selves (Lynch & Fortune, 2019). Being and doing are often interrelated in sexual activity, because one's sexual identity (being) may inform the sexual activity (doing; Lynch & Fortune, 2019).

Belonging

Belonging relates to being a part of a group or community and feeling associated or connected with others (Wilcock & Hocking, 2015). Occupational belonging can provide people with a feeling of acceptance, security, and happiness and may extend to provide them with a sense of meaning (Wilcock & Hocking, 2015). In terms of sexual activity, it may evolve that the belonging within a relationship is more important than the act of sexual activity (Lynch & Fortune, 2019). The sense of belonging may also include the sense of being part of a community, such as LGBTQIA+ communities,[4] one's geographical community, social communities, spiritual communities, or kink communities. As with being and doing, the sense of belonging in one's sexuality is important to a person's health and well-being (Lynch & Fortune, 2019).

Becoming

Becoming is a state of development, transformation, maturity, and self-realization; it includes the creation of a self-image through engagement in occupation (Wilcock, 1998; Wilcock & Hocking, 2015). Concerning sexuality, the concept of becoming is critical, because the process allows a person to become who they want to be sexually (Lynch & Fortune, 2019). *Becoming* is an evolving process, because a person continues to develop their sense of sexual self-image and sexual expression over

---

[4] The term *LGBTQIA+ communities* refers to the diverse and unique communities formed by lesbian, gay, bisexual, transgender, queer, intersex, asexual, and other sexual and gender minoritized people. As greater awareness, social acceptance, and safety improve for these individuals and communities, new terms may emerge as language evolves to describe identities that exist outside of societal recognition and acceptance.

the course of their life (Lynch & Fortune, 2019; Wilcock, 1998; Wilcock & Hocking, 2015).

Occupational Justice

The theory of occupational justice emerged from the field of occupational science. The basis of ***occupational justice*** is that people should have equity and equal access to occupations, including where the occupation occurs, resources, and the benefits and challenges that arise from engagement in the occupation (Wilcock & Hocking, 2015). Underpinning the theory of occupational justice is Wilcock's (1998) Occupational Perspective of Health model. Deprivation of access to desired occupations is an occupational injustice, which can have a negative impact on individual health, well-being, and quality of life. Engagement in occupation has the power to both promote and impair health (Townsend & Wilcock, 2004), and it is critical to be aware of both sides of engagement in occupation.

Core ideas

Occupational justice maintains that people are independent occupational beings who have the right to choose and participate in occupations according to their individual and autonomous preferences (Stadnyk et al., 2009; Townsend & Wilcock, 2004). Through this lens, sexual activity is an occupation, and participation is therefore important for health and quality of life. People who value engagement in sexual activities, therefore, have the right to participate in those meaningful occupations.

As with other models of occupation, a foundational tenet of occupational justice is that people are occupational beings who need to engage in various occupations to fulfill various needs (Townsend & Wilcock, 2004). Participation in occupations helps a person develop their identity, including a sense of self and community identity (Townsend & Wilcock, 2004). Within the context of occupations related to sexual activity, the need to engage in such occupations may fulfill various personal needs, such as health, reproductive, personal fulfillment, and social needs. It is thus imperative for occupational therapy practitioners to treat sexual activity as an occupation.

As noted, occupational justice sees participation in occupations as interdependent with the societal context in which the occupation takes place and the resources needed to engage in the occupation (Townsend & Wilcock, 2004). The social context influences the meaning, value, opportunity, and resources required to engage in desired occupations (Townsend & Wilcock, 2004). Contexts and resources determine both the possibilities and the limitations of the desired occupation (Townsend & Wilcock, 2004). For people who want to engage in sexual activities, the physical, social, and cultural contexts can significantly enhance or limit the engagement in the occupation of sexual activity.

For example, consider a woman with cerebral palsy who was sexually assaulted. For about 2 years after the assault, she felt uninterested in sex, which was distressing to her because it was previously one of her favorite occupations. She lived in a city where she was able to access trauma-focused psychotherapy, because treatment was covered by her insurance and the building was ADA compliant. The sex education she received growing up was fear based and abstinence only, and it was not inclusive of topics relevant to people with physical disabilities. The curriculum did not include different ways people can experience sexual pleasure. She worked with an occupational therapist specifically on ways she prefers to experience pleasure during sex and how to communicate this to partners. In this way, she was able to reclaim her pleasure during sexual activity. During the 2016 election she felt specifically troubled by learning the newly elected president had said, "Grab her by the pussy," and a few months of low desire for sexual activity followed. Her partner at the time made casual jokes during sex about "grabbing her," so she broke up with him. She felt validated when she was able to speak with her female friends about her feelings, which they also shared. Eventually, she implemented the strategies she learned in therapy and was able to desire and enjoy sex again.

Principles

The principles of occupational justice involve individuals' rights, responsibilities, and freedoms related to occupational engagement (Stadnyk et al., 2009; Townsend & Wilcock, 2004). The first principle, ***empowerment*** through occupation, encourages feelings of personal drive, motivation, purpose, confidence, identity, and joy through engagement in occupation. The next principle of occupational justice is the ***inclusive classification*** of occupations. Accepting inclusive classification acknowledges that not all occupations are the same (Stadnyk et al., 2009). Inclusive classification is a critical element when discussing sexual occupations beyond heteronormative, partnered sexual activity (McGrath & Sakellariou, 2016; Tellier, 2017). To have an inclusive classification for sexual activity, one must recognize partnered and nonpartnered activity, various sexual orientations and gender identities, and the expansiveness of human sexual activities.

Another principle of occupational justice is the enablement of occupational potential (Stadnyk et al., 2009; Townsend & Wilcock, 2004). The principle of ***enablement*** builds upon the principles of empowerment and inclusive classification. Policies, laws, and economic practices affect the enablement of occupations. The Americans with Disabilities Act of 1990 (P. L. 101-336) is an example of a policy that enables occupational engagement by prohibiting discrimination based on disability and includes equal access to sex education for individuals with disabilities.

The final principle of occupational justice is diversity, inclusion, and shared advantage in occupational participation (Stadnyk et al., 2009; Townsend & Wilcock, 2004). ***Inclusion*** is an essential construct of occupational justice—everyone is entitled to participate in their wanted and needed occupations (Townsend & Wilcock, 2004). The principle of diversity and inclusion covers not only sexual activity but also sexual orientations, gender identities, and relationship statuses.

Occupations related to sexual activity can provide tremendous meaning to people. Occupational justice builds on the concepts of empowerment through occupation and inclusive classification of occupations to view how policies, laws, and economic practices affect engagement in occupations. By looking at the interconnection of occupational justice principles as they relate to specific occupations, we obtain a broad picture of the effects of societal, personal, environmental, historical, and other contexts on engagement in sexual activity (Townsend & Wilcock, 2004). Occupational justice looks not just at the right to engage in sexual activity but at what engagement in occupation provides for individuals' health and well-being (Stadnyk et al., 2009; Townsend & Wilcock, 2004).

Putting the Erotic in Occupational Therapy

Theoretical frameworks discuss sexuality but offer little inclusion and celebration of eroticism and pleasure. They lack a holistic approach to addressing sexuality in clinical practice. Therefore, occupational therapy practitioners should consider how pleasure motivates sexual engagement and infuse their clinical decision-making process with eroticism. This process, however, is not modeled in mainstream academia, research, or health care, let alone the occupational therapy profession. Jones (2019) reviewed 300 articles from the *Journal of Sex Research* that were published between 2010 and 2015 and found that disease and pathology were the main focuses of the articles. For example, many articles focused on high-risk behaviors of gay men rather than examine the roles that seeking pleasure and a sense of belonging, as well as a distrust of health care systems, play in their decision making. Similarly, articles focused on the dysfunction of low desire or inorgasmia in women, rather than explore what sexual experiences women actually find pleasurable and whether they are engaging in the sex they find most pleasurable.

Occupational therapy practitioners' holistic understanding of the factors that facilitate engagement in occupations offers a distinct opportunity to advocate for the inclusion of pleasure and eroticism as a starting point for discussing sexuality. Eroticism can be infused into occupational therapy education and practice in the following ways:

- Understand the discussion of pleasure as being in alignment with ethical and professional behavior standards. The *OTPF–4* already includes pleasure, meaning, and value; it is the occupational therapy practitioner's responsibility to ensure that their practice setting supports incorporation of occupational therapy's full scope and domain, including sexual and intimate occupations.
- Put policies and procedures into place to enhance service delivery. Assessment, intervention planning, goals, and outcome measures should

include pleasure and satisfaction among the positive outcomes of treatment in alignment with traditional outcome measures for independence, autonomy, and function.

- Focus treatment related to sexuality on the end goal of pleasure rather than the attainment of a skill that reduces a barrier to pleasure. For example, treatment focusing on pain management techniques to reduce pain during sex will be less effective if the goal is merely to reduce pain. The measurement of success for the intervention using this approach should include whether the client's sexual experiences are pleasurable. The practitioner who positions pleasure as central to occupational engagement will continue to assess whether pain management strategies have made the sexual experience more pleasurable and, if not, what interventions will enable pleasure.
- Become comfortable with asking clients how they feel pleasure, who their partners are for erotic activities, and what sexual activities they prefer and enjoy. Occupational therapy practitioners should approach sex in a nuanced way and use curiosity, not assumption, to guide questioning that informs clinical decisions. A curious practitioner asks about how their client engages in sexual occupations and what is meaningful to the client. They seek clarification without judgment, of themselves or the client, if the client provides information they do not understand or the practitioner needs more information to make clinical decisions.
- View clients not as they present—for example, in a coma—but instead be prepared to advocate for their sexual rights throughout their life course. A man in a medically induced coma who has burns over his body, including the genitals, is likely to have excruciatingly painful erections. The occupational therapy practitioner can advocate for a multidisciplinary discussion of how penile skin integrity and flexibility must be considered in treatment while the person is in a coma.
- Acknowledge that clients' sexual activities and the meaning sex holds for them is likely to differ from that of the occupational therapy practitioner. Only then can practitioners begin to see the nuance in sexual occupations, not make assumptions about their clients, and accurately apply the occupational therapy process. For example, assuming that the client has sex with one person at a time would lead to an inaccurate activity analysis if the client actually has sex with two people at a given time. Assuming that a client has sex with their body, when the client prefers sex in the virtual space, will also lead to a problematic activity analysis.

Consider how these examples position pleasure as paramount to the client's quality of life. Readers should keep these principles in mind as they progress through the book. Doing so will enhance comprehension of the information throughout the text and begin the incorporation of the erotic and pleasurable into the occupational therapy process.

Summary

This chapter provided an orientation to occupational therapy's role in sexual and intimate occupations, pleasure, and eroticism and a guiding framework for learning about sexuality in a professional context. Pleasure and eroticism are ways in which individuals can exercise their sovereignty over their body and choices. Engaging in sexual and intimate occupations is vital to enhancing quality of life through bringing pleasure, eroticism, and joy into everyday living. Occupational therapy practitioners are perfectly situated to address sexuality and intimacy in clinical practice, yet social norms, exacerbated by professional culture and academic curricula, have not supported practitioners in doing so. To fully serve our clients, practitioners must move beyond independence as the only measure of occupational engagement. Centering pleasure and eroticism in occupational therapy practice requires the practitioner to build self-awareness and a critical understanding of historical and cultural contexts that influence the ways in which people engage in sexual and intimate occupations.

Kathryn Ellis, OTD, OTR/L, AASECT–SC (she/her), developed the Occupational Therapy Sexuality and Intimacy Clinic at Walter Reed National Military Medical Center in Washington, DC, and is the co-author of *Sex and Intimacy for Wounded Veterans: A Guide to Embracing Change.* She is the founder and CEO of a continuing education company, the Institute for Sex, Intimacy & Occupational Therapy. She is an American Association of Sexuality Educators, Counselors, and Therapists Certified Sexuality Counselor and a consultant on sexuality and intimacy projects and initiatives. Her private practice, Dr. Kathryn Ellis Sexual Wellness Counseling, is based in Delaware.

Joseph Christian Ungco, OTD, OTR/L (they/them), is the associate director for diversity, equity, and inclusion (DEI) education, client services, and data analytics for the Fred Hutchinson Cancer Center in Seattle. They lead several organization-wide DEI initiatives, including the bias mitigation education program and gender-inclusive and accessible spaces initiative. They also continue to serve in DEI roles in occupational therapy, including serving as co-chair of the national Network for LGBTQIA+ Concerns in Occupational Therapy and sitting on the executive council for the Occupational Therapy Multicultural, Diversity and Inclusion National Network. Dr. Ungco's work is centered on amplifying the voices of those most affected by systems of oppression and actualizing structural change.

Jenn Soros, PhD, OTR/L (she/her), is an assistant professor at Cleveland State University in the Department of Occupational Therapy in Cleveland, Ohio. Dr. Soros's area of research focuses on sexuality and intimacy from an occupational perspective.

References

American Occupational Therapy Association. (2013). *Fact sheet: Occupational therapy's role with sexuality.* https://www.aota.org/-/media/Corporate/Files/AboutOT/Professionals/WhatIsOT/RDP/Facts/Sexuality.pdf

American Occupational Therapy Association. (2020). Occupational therapy practice framework: Domain and process (4th ed.). *American Journal of Occupational Therapy, 74*(Suppl. 2), 7412410010. https://doi.org/10.5014/ajot.2020.74S2001

Americans With Disabilities Act of 1990, Pub. L. 101-336, 42 U.S.C. § 12101.
Brown, A. M. (2017). *Emergent strategy: Shaping change, changing worlds.* AK Press.
Brown, A. M. (2019). *Pleasure activism.* AK Press.
Jones, A. (2019). Sex is not a problem: The erasure of pleasure in sexual science research. *Sexualities, 22,* 643–668. https://doi.org/10.1177/1363460718760210
Lynch, C., & Fortune, T. (2019). Applying an occupational lens to thinking about and addressing sexuality. *Sexuality and Disability, 37,* 145–159. https://doi.org/10.1007/s11195-019-09566-7
McGrath, M., & Sakellariou, D. (2016). Why has so little progress been made in the practice of occupational therapy in relation to sexuality? *American Journal of Occupational Therapy, 70,* 7001360010. https://doi.org/10.5014/ajot.2016.017707.
The Nobel Prize. (n.d.). *The Nobel Prize in Literature 2010.* https://www.nobelprize.org/prizes/literature/2010/summary
Stadnyk, R., Townsend, E., & Wilcock, A. (2009). Occupational justice. In C. H. Christiansen & E. A. Townsend (Eds.), *Introduction to occupation: The art and science of living* (2nd ed., pp. 329–358). Pearson Education.
Tellier, S. (2017). Advancing the discourse: Disability and BDSM. *Sexuality and Disability, 35,* 485–493. https://doi.org/10.1007/s11195-017-9504-x
Townsend, E., & Wilcock, A. (2004). Occupational justice and client-centred practice: A dialogue in progress. *Canadian Journal of Occupational Therapy, 71,* 75–87. https://doi.org/10.1177/000841740407100203
Ungco, J. C. (2022, January 6). *Let's talk about sex: Intro to class* [Unpublished lecture]. Ithaca College. https://canvas.ithaca.edu/courses/17271/pages/lets-talk-about-sex-intro-to-course?module_item_id=352303
Vargas Llosa, M. (1991). *In praise of the stepmother.* Faber.
Vargas Llosa, M. (2015, July). Ars erotica. *Harpers.* https://harpers.org/archive/2015/07/ars-erotica
Wilcock, A. A. (1998). Reflections on doing, being and becoming. *Canadian Journal of Occupational Therapy, 65,* 248–256. https://doi.org/10.1046/j.1440-1630.1999.00174.x
Wilcock, A., & Hocking, C. (2015). *An occupational perspective of health* (3rd ed.). Slack.
World Federation of Occupational Therapists. (2019). *Occupational therapy and human rights* [Position statement]. https://wfot.org/resources/occupational-therapy-and-human-rights
World Federation of Occupational Therapists. (2022). *About occupational therapy.* https://wfot.org/about/about-occupational-therapy
World Health Organization. (n.d.). *Sexual health.* https://www.who.int/health-topics/sexual-health#tab=tab_1
Yerxa, E. J. (1990). An introduction to occupational science, a foundation for occupational therapy in the 21st century. *Occupational Therapy in Health Care, 6*(4), 1–17. https://doi.org/10.1080/J003v06n04_04

2

Understanding Sexual Identity

M. Nicole Horsley, *PhD;* **Kathryn Ellis,** *OTD, OTR/L;*
and **Wade Robinson,** *OTD, OTR/L*

CHAPTER HIGHLIGHTS

- Sexual identity terminology
- Where does the idea of "normal" come from?
- Difference and intersectionality
- Queerness
- LGBTQIA+ health
- The sex-positive occupational therapy practitioner

KEY TERMS AND CONCEPTS

Aromantic
Asexuality
Bisexual
Cisgender
Difference
Erotic
Femininity
Gay
Gender
Gender-affirming care
Heteronormative
Intersectionality
Intersex
Lesbian
LGBTQIA+
Masculinity
Nonbinary
Pansexual
Polysexual
Pronouns
Queer
Sex
Sex positivity
Sexual identity
Sexual liberation
Sexual orientation
Sexual pleasure
Sexuality
Social determinants of health
Transgender

This chapter aims to challenge ideals of the default "norms" around sexuality and encourage readers to rethink aspects of sexuality within the field of occupational therapy. ***Sexuality*** is a broad, multidimensional concept that "encompasses sex, gender identities and roles, sexual orientation, eroticism, pleasure, intimacy, and reproduction. Sexuality is experienced and expressed in thoughts, fantasies, desires, beliefs, attitudes, values, behaviors, practices, roles, and relationships" (World Health Organization [WHO], 2006, p. 5). ***Sexual identity*** is the internal sense of self and preferences related to the sexuality concepts mentioned above. Everyone has a sexual identity that follows a developmental sequence throughout the life course (Dillon et al., 2011). ***Sexual orientation,*** which is related to sexual identity, describes the way in which people experience and express attraction sexually, romantically, and emotionally.

Sexuality is interwoven across all aspects of the domain of occupational therapy, including occupations, contexts, performance patterns, performance skills, and client factors (American Occupational Therapy Association, 2020; see Reflection Prompt 2.1). Often omitted in our understanding of sexuality is the importance of expression and joy to achieve sexual liberation in many facets of our clients' lives. ***Sexual liberation*** is the state of being free from sexual standards, rules, or laws that are restrictive; it occurs without coercion or harm.

This chapter defines common terms regarding sexuality identity while disrupting the cultural construction of norms around difference, intersectionality, and queerness. It provides a critical understanding of sexual identity and positions pleasure within the scope of occupational therapy. Discussion then centers on the infusion of the erotic into occupational therapy and strategies for occupational therapy practitioners to work with clients in a sex-positive way.

Sexual Identity Terminology

Language is both a product and form of culture, so it is a powerful tool for expressing sexual identity. Gender and sexual orientation are simultaneously different and entangled. There is broad variety in how people identify their gender and sexual identities and their sexual preferences. The terms people use to describe themselves are personal and deliberate and for each person to decide and assert. Exhibit 2.1

REFLECTION PROMPT 2.1

Which Clients Receive Sex and Intimacy Occupational Therapy, and Why?

It is rare for occupational therapy educators to discuss sexuality as a broad client factor that is relevant to all clients. Instead, they usually discuss this topic only as it concerns specific instances and diagnoses, a common one being people with spinal cord injury (SCI). Consider why the discussion of sexuality is limited in occupational therapy. For example, why is sexuality more frequently discussed when learning about SCI versus multiple sclerosis or intellectual and developmental disabilities? Using a critical lens, we could consider whether it is because more men than women experience SCI. Is it hard to imagine how someone would be sexual without an erect penis? Or perhaps we have a difficult time talking about sexuality with people who have had disabilities their whole life instead of with those who acquired their disability. Is it easier to think of someone who was previously not disabled as sexual? What might make it difficult for an occupational therapy practitioner to discuss sexuality with someone with intellectual and developmental disabilities? Why might some instances or diagnoses be much less likely to be discussed in the occupational therapy curriculum (e.g., sex during or after menopause)? For each of these questions, consider the social norms that could be influencing occupational therapy practitioners, researchers, and professors. Consider how ableism, ageism, or sexism might influence an occupational therapy educator's or professional's decision to address sex with specific clients.

EXHIBIT 2.1
Common Terminology

- ***Cisgender*** (or *cis*) describes a person whose gender identity aligns with the one usually associated with the sex assigned to them. The word comes from the Latin word for "on this side"; in contrast, the *trans* prefix means "on the other side" or "beyond." The prefixes have been used in chemistry and other sciences for many years (Jarry, 2021). The term *cis* is preferable to *nontrans* or *biological*.
- ***Femininity*** and ***masculinity*** are socially constructed in numerous ways and have been expressed in many different ways throughout history. Although femininity and masculinity have no universal meaning, in U.S. society the concepts are constructed upon a set of attributes, behaviors, and roles that are alleged to be based on biology. Historically, themes of femininity in the United States centered on idealized White femininity from the Victorian era: pale and genteel. This narrow lens of femininity has continued to position traditional notions of femininity as White, heterosexual, middle class, and cisgender. Western culture frames masculinity as dominant, defined in opposition to femininity, which is centered on passive attributes.
- ***Gender-affirming care*** refers to a spectrum of social, psychological, behavioral, or medical (including hormonal or surgical) services and resources designed to support and affirm someone's gender identity.
- ***Intersex*** describes a person whose biological sex is ambiguous. Genetic, hormonal, or anatomical distinctions can make a person's sex ambiguous (e.g., adrenal hyperplasia, Klinefelter syndrome).
- ***LGBTQIA+*** refers to people who are lesbian, gay, bisexual, transgender, queer, intersex, or asexual, among other diverse sexual and gender identities.
- ***Nonbinary*** refers to someone whose gender exists beyond the socially constructed man–woman binary system. Neither *woman* nor *man* appropriately represents the person. Nonbinary is one of many gender-expansive identities, such as genderqueer or genderfluid, that describe gender identities that transcend exclusionary views of masculinity and femininity. Nonbinary people may express themselves in any way and are not expected to appear androgynous.
- ***Polysexual*** or ***pansexual*** describes attraction to multiple genders and sexual identities.
- ***Transgender*** (or *trans*) is an umbrella term that may be used to describe people whose gender identity differs from their sex assigned at birth or exists beyond cisnormative notions of gender within their culture. Additional terms or labels used to denote gender identity and expression include *transgender man, transgender woman, man, woman, genderqueer,* and *gender expansive*. A person who is transgender may or may not decide to alter their bodies hormonally or surgically.

describes common terminology related to sexual identity, and readers can consider their personal experience with identity terms in Reflection Prompt 2.2.

For example, for many people, pronouns are an important part of identity; pronouns are how they refer to themselves and how others should refer to them as well. ***Pronouns*** are parts of speech that replace nouns, including names. Singular, first-person pronouns (I, me, my) and second-person pronouns (you, yours) are used for everyone. Singular third-person pronouns (he/him, she/her, they/them[1])

[1] The 7th edition of the American Psychological Association style guide (APA, 2020), which many occupational therapy professionals refer to for guidance when writing, endorses the use of "they/them" pronouns when referring to a singular third person (e.g., "The client values his or her occupations") or when uncertain of someone's personal pronouns (e.g., "Alex went to their therapy session").

REFLECTION PROMPT 2.2
Identity Terms

The terms that people use to label themselves differ based on region, culture, and personal experience. They are also influenced by temporal context. Consider the following questions:

- What meaningful terms do you use to identify yourself? (These terms can be related to sexuality or not.)
- How do you feel when people disregard these terms, do not find them important, disagree with those terms, or refer to you in other ways?
- If you have not experienced these terms being discounted, consider why not.

are used as appropriate, based on the pronouns the person being referred to uses. Regardless of gender identity or expression, proper use of someone's name and pronouns is important, and asking what they prefer is appropriate.

A person's pronouns are not necessarily indicative of their gender. For example, ze/hir are gender-neutral pronouns. Ze is usually pronounced with a long e, and hir and its forms are typically pronounced like the word *here.* Examples of their use are as follows: "Ze is working." "It's just hirself." "Those belong to hirs." "Hir pens are on the table." Additional sets of pronouns can also be used, such as per/pers, ey/em, xe/xem, and so forth. When someone does not use pronouns, refer to them by name. Gender-neutral titles can be used in place of Mr. or Ms., such as Mx., which is pronounced like *mix.*

Where Does the Idea of "Normal" Come From?

People's sexual behaviors, preferences, and expression are often judged against what is considered "normal," but what is more important is where ideas of normal come from. In Western cultural traditions, the policies, power structures, and social norms tend to normalize straight and cisgender sexuality, thereby rejecting anything else and creating adversity for those outside such norms. Because of heteronormative and cisnormative expectations, people, including straight and cis people, may engage in activities that they feel they should engage in or enjoy regardless of whether they enjoy or prefer those activities and, conversely, abstain from certain activities that they feel they should not do or not enjoy.

Sexuality is shaped by social constructions established by communities, nations, and societies. It is sustained through collective and individual ideals and participation, which influence our sense of our sexual lives and identities. We learn what is normal, acceptable, or desirable from what we are taught instead of what we enjoy, which, in turn, aids in developing our own sexual identity. When we can learn what we like and who we are, free of external or internal judgment, we can strengthen our authentic sexual identities and preferences.

Social determinants of health are environmental factors that influence health outcomes and quality of life. They include the physical, social, and economic conditions into which people are born (WHO, 2017). Social determinants of health include exclusion or erasure of sexuality outside of straight or cisgender identities, which leads to discrimination and creates myths of "abnormal" or "deviant" sexual identities and preferences. Sexual identity, sexual practices, and sexuality that fall outside of the accepted norm result in disadvantages that appear in forms of racism, sexism, fatphobia, transphobia, homophobia, and social economic class and gender inequalities. "Invalidation and inequity" of sexual identities, sexualities, and sexual expression negatively affect physical and mental health (Neumann et al., 2021, p. 195).

The repression of sexuality produces tropes and narratives of domination and oppression, which generate socioeconomic inequalities and discriminatory practices. Laws and policies discriminating against or even criminalizing particular sexual behaviors or expression reinforce a norm that is upheld by tradition, habit, religion, and fear. See Table 2.1 for examples of anti-LGBTQIA+ policies. Sexual repression can be culturally reinforced, such as distilling a woman's worth to her status as a "pure" virgin, which represses and denies her sexual desire, makes her vulnerable to assault and exploitation, and reinforces patriarchal power dynamics.

TABLE 2.1

Anti-LGBTQIA+ Policies: Contextual Factors, Examples, and Potential Occupational Implications

Contextual Factor	Example	Potential Occupational Implications (and Affected Occupations)
Obstruction of occupational participation: State and federal lawmakers frequently introduce legislation targeting LGBTQIA+ people and legalizing discrimination, such as preventing adoption by same-sex parents or barring transgender people's access to bathrooms (Cahill, 2009; White Hughto et al., 2015). The fear and anxiety around using and accessing public bathrooms, either because of discrimination or state and institutional laws, lead to chronic stress and harmful health outcomes, such as lower urinary tract, kidney, and bladder infections (Hardacker et al., 2019).	In North Carolina, bathroom bills HB 2 and HB 142 restricted use of bathrooms, changing rooms, and showers in state-run buildings to a person's sex assigned at birth.	• Transgender people are unsafe using bathrooms consistent with their identity (IADLs: community mobility; social participation). • Gender nonbinary and transgender people's concentration, attention, and performance of tasks may be hindered by discomfort and stress (education and work).

(Continued)

TABLE 2.1

Anti-LGBTQIA+ Policies: Contextual Factors, Examples, and Potential Occupational Implications (*Cont.*)

Contextual Factor	Example	Potential Occupational Implications (and Affected Occupations)
Disproportionate increase in health disparities as a result of widespread toxic stress events: The HIV/AIDS epidemic of the 1980s and COVID-19 global public health crisis starting in 2020 have amplified the legal and health risks affecting LGBTQIA+ people's lives. They also have exacerbated the inequities and disparities faced by the community, including poverty, access to care, housing insecurity, overall poor health, and discrimination (Goldberg, 2020; Human Rights Campaign Staff, 2020).	• Goldberg (2020) noted that converging risk factors for the LGBTQIA+ population made contracting COVID-19 more likely and dangerous (e.g., increased likelihood of living in poverty, experiencing housing insecurity, having higher smoking and asthma rates). • Access to medical care is less likely (because of discrimination from care providers and decreased access).	• LGBTQIA+ people are less likely to have health insurance coverage and access to medical care and protective devices, such as masks, soap, and sanitizer (IADL: health management; ADLs: personal hygiene and self-care). • LGBTQIA+ people are more likely to work in economically affected industries, experience a loss of jobs and pay cuts, and struggle to pay bills and obtain basic necessities (IADL: financial management; work).
Cisnormative and heteronormative environments with the expectation of binary gender identities: Environments influence how and whether a person engages in an occupation. Places that are overtly or purposefully gendered may be traumatic environments for members of the LGBTQIA+ community. Transgender and gender nonbinary people may altogether avoid certain environments that are known to be unsafe or unwelcoming. Clothing stores, places of work, hair salons, and other people's homes have been identified as some of the avoided and triggering environments because of the oppression of the gender binary and other factors.	• A cisgender lesbian woman who wears men's clothing and presents as "androgynous" is able to ignore the comments and stares she receives in women's public bathrooms. However, with time, her discomfort grows, and the stress and anticipation of being yelled at or told to "get out" reaches the point to which she chooses to not even try using public restrooms unless there is a single stall. • A genderqueer person is held up in airport security because the TSA agent selects "male" on the scanning machine, which then reads the person's body as hiding contraband.	• A person is less likely to go to a gym or pool for physical fitness out of fear of changing in the locker room and accessing the bathroom (IADL: health management). • A person experiences both increased stress around choice of clothing incongruent with one's identity and bullying as a result of gender expression (ADLs: dressing and grooming). • A person has discomfort and anxiety when shopping for clothes because of judgment from salespeople and patrons while browsing, selecting, and purchasing items in the "men's" section versus the "women's" section. The person is challenged with

(Continued)

TABLE 2.1

Anti-LGBTQIA+ Policies: Contextual Factors, Examples, and Potential Occupational Implications (*Cont.*)

Contextual Factor	Example	Potential Occupational Implications (and Affected Occupations)
		finding the right fit of clothing and deciding which changing room to use (IADL: shopping). • A person fears invasive searches and additional screening because of binary technology, thus potentially reducing the likelihood of travel (IADL: community mobility; leisure: traveling for vacation; work: job performance if required to travel for work).
Hypervigilance as a way of ensuring community safety: Hypervigilance is a common behavior of people who have experienced trauma. A conscious or subconscious decision, it results in a continual "scan" of the environment and other people for safety. LGBTQIA+ people may engage in *code switching* as a means of self-protecting one's identity or oneself; that is, for safety, they suppress or "switch" how they present by making a shift in gender expression, vocal tone, mannerisms, or language use. They do so consciously or subconsciously, depending on the environment.	• A bisexual Latina woman expects to face stigma at an upcoming job interview, leading to hypervigilance and not performing her best. She feels like she has to monitor her behaviors and speech as well as conceal her identities to assimilate to the job's culture and environment. She is continually aware of how others are judging her personally as well as questioning the quality of her work. • A transgender teenager working in a convenience store changes her tone of voice based on assessment of safety in relation to the customer in front of her. She feels exhausted from this daily emotional burden.	• A person has decreased comfort making eye contact and challenges with effective interpersonal communication, resulting from past negative experiences, and fear for safety (social participation: workplace and peer interactions; work: job performance). • A person has increased stress because of an inability to present authentically at work or with family. They also fear rejection and isolation as well as losing housing and financial support (IADL: health management—social and emotional health; work: job performance and maintenance; social participation: community and family participation).

Note. ADL = activity of daily living; IADL = instrumental activity of daily living; LGBTQIA+ = lesbian, gay, bisexual, transgender, queer, intersex, asexual, and other sexual and gender minority; TSA = Transportation Security Administration.

Source. Adapted from "Addressing LGBTQIA+ Trauma: Your Role and Your Responsibility," by N. Neumann, D. Neu, D., and J. C. Ungco, 2021, in A. Lynch, R. Ashcraft, and L. Tekell (Eds.), *Trauma, Occupation, and Participation: Foundations and Population Considerations in Occupational Therapy* (pp. 203–204). AOTA Press. Copyright © 2021 by the American Occupational Therapy Association. Adapted with permission.

Unless occupational therapy practitioners consciously self-reflect on the norms they believe to be true or consider normal, they run the high risk of harming clients by expecting such norms from their clients (see Chapter 4, "Sexuality, Bias, and Impact: Preventing Clinician Harm," for more information). For example, a practitioner who says, "I'm surprised you're having sex. Shouldn't you be saving sex for marriage?" to a 26-year-old unmarried female client with cerebral palsy who expresses the need to have a goal related to sexuality, reflects bias and can cause harm. Practitioners who make a client feel uncomfortable in a health care setting can affect the client's willingness to seek medical care and thereby affect their overall health and well-being. Clients who receive support from health care providers and can safely share aspects of their sexuality have better health outcomes and satisfaction with their experience and are more likely to use health care services (Ruben & Fullerton, 2018).

Occupational therapy practitioners are obligated to disregard their view of normal when it comes to sexuality, sexual identity, and expression. Consideration of how sexuality contributes to the sense of self, social determinants of health, and occupational engagement is essential for practitioners to develop a holistic understanding of each client. Sexuality encompasses many occupations of daily living and aspects of identity and is an extremely important part of quality of life. Engaging in sexual activities and expressing oneself sexually can enhance the emotional, mental, spiritual, and physical well-being of clients. There is a persistent need for developing pleasure-centered practices in occupational therapy interventions to treat concerns about sexuality, sexual desire, and enjoyment.

Difference and Intersectionality

Understanding the social dynamics of difference is central to shifting perspectives about sexual identity. ***Difference*** is broadly conceptualized as the ways in which people differ from one another along the lines of socially substantial identities and characteristics. It involves social identities related to race, gender, class, sexuality, ability, and national origin. Difference also includes individual characteristics, such as education level, family type, and health conditions.

An important aspect of difference is the concept of intersectionality, which embraces various identities that intersect or overlap with each other, shaping social and structural experiences in ways that are intertwined with privilege and disadvantage. ***Intersectionality*** refers to how social categories such as race, gender, class, and sexuality are interlocking systems of oppression and privilege. An intersectional lens helps occupational therapy practitioners understand, for example, how a poor, disabled, elderly, lesbian, Black woman's experiences within the health care system differ from those of a young, able-bodied, wealthy, White, heterosexual man. This concept was initially used, in a legal proceeding, to bring awareness to the inequitable conditions experienced by women of color in and outside of the work environment (Crenshaw, 1989).

Differences in racial and gender identities historically have been constructed as deviant compared with what is considered the default: White, able bodied, cisgender, heterosexual, and middle to upper class. Social constructs assimilate, reject, and ultimately control certain sexual identities or sexual scripts that assist with constructing personal attraction to or preference for certain sexual behaviors, activities, and people. In a ***heteronormative*** point of view, the default sexual identity is heterosexuality, a sexual identity constructed between people of the "opposite sex." This preference is strongly reinforced through sex education, religion, pop culture, family systems, political policies, and economic structures. Homosexuality is constructed in opposition, describing sexual attraction between people of the "same sex." These polarized binaries assume everyone is cisgender while stigmatizing homosexuality.

Sex refers to anatomical and physiological differences between beings based on external genitals, internal gonads, chromosomes, and hormone composition. ***Gender*** is a socially constructed category based on sex assigned at birth. Gender includes a sense of masculinity, femininity, a combination of both, or an absence of either. Because gender is a social construct, expected norms based on gender are assigned by society and fluctuate across different time periods and cultures. For example, at one time in Western culture, it was the norm for wealthy men to wear powdered wigs and heeled shoes. Although sex and gender have separate meanings, with sex being a biological category and gender socially constructed, they are intertwined.

Ideas of femininity and masculinity shift over time in response to sociocultural changes. In women's studies, traditional conceptions of femininity were at times dismissed by some activists as fragile and weak, and some advocates went so far as to declare that women who embraced their femininity were unfeminist (Boxer, 1998). The conversation eventually shifted to acknowledge the distinction between a White patriarchal idealized view of femininity as weak and other perceptions of femininity that acknowledge the values and strengths of femininity (e.g., Gilligan, 1982; Scott, 1988).

As early as the 17th century, Western views of femininity idealized White women as models of self-respect, self-control, modesty, and sexual purity and stereotyped Black women as tempting, seductive, and lewd (Pilgrim, 2012). This White-idealized version of femininity values pale, genteel, passive, heterosexual, middle-class, nondisabled, and cisgender women who needed male protection and is dictated by patriarchal constructs (Frankenberg, 2020). This version is at its nature exclusive, barring those who are non-White, queer, nonbinary, fat, and disabled, among many other characteristics.

No universal way in which femininity—or masculinity—is constructed and embodied exists (see Chapter 5, "Sexual and Intimate Occupations Across the Lifespan," for discussion of the impact of toxic masculinity). On the contrary, femininity can be expressed in many possible ways. Two such examples are Chicana femininity and Indigenous feminism, which differ from the default White idealized femininity and offer more inclusive and intersectional ways for femininity to be expressed and understood (Carrillo & Dean, 2020; Dorries & Harjo, 2020).

Queerness

Historically, the term *queer* meant strange or abnormal (Case Example 2.1). When used in the context of sexuality, the word *queer* was often used in a derogatory

CASE EXAMPLE 2.1. SAARTJIE BAARTMAN: THE BLACK BODY AS INHERENTLY QUEER

In the early 18th century, *queer* was synonymous with strange, odd, peculiar, or abnormal. The classification in the West of people being either homosexual or heterosexual happened at the same time as differentiating the Black body from the White because of 19th-century discourse on racial differences. Arguably, the Black body is inherently queer because as a non-White body, it is considered unusual and out of place (Somerville, 2000). Whereas the White or European body serves as the default, the Black or African body serves as a "master text" denoting racial difference.

An example of historical perspectives that influence perspectives today is the story of **Saartjie Baartman**. Baartman was an indigenous southern African Khoikhoi woman who, along with other women from her community, was put on display in Europe as a freak show attraction in the early 1800s. Their bodies were perceived as a curiosity and of scientific interest as well as eroticized. Baartman and others were referred to as a "Hottentot Venus," which is now regarded as a prime example of racial colonial exploitation and dehumanization of Black people.[2]

Additionally, Black people were routinely sold as "specimens" to ambitious White doctors to sustain the myth of deviance, hypersexualizing the Black body. This myth was the justification for sexual exploitation, forced breeding, and rape. To prove racial differences between women of African and European descent, gynecologists focused on the size and visibility of the clitoris. They developed iconography extending both to women of African descent and to lesbians, marking them as symbols of deviance and hypersexuality. Establishing these sexual differences as inherent to Blackness and homosexuality provided powerful stereotypes, contributing to myths of non-White and nonheterosexual identities as unnatural and overtly sexual that still persist to this day.

[2] To learn more about Saartjie Baartman, see Ashley (2021). An example of the iconography is available at https://tinyurl.com/ykka3ckd. See also Friar (2021) for more on the eroticization of the Black female body.

manner to mean effeminate or gay boys and men (Somerville, 2000). ***Queer*** has been refashioned during the late 20th and early 21st century as another understanding or category for gay, lesbian, bisexual, and transgender people (Somerville, 2000). The term becomes another way to discuss sexuality and gender presentations that differ from heterosexuality and cisgender. Its reclamation is a marker of difference and a refusal of heterosexuality as the construct that controls the narrative.

Queer is not a synonym for LGBT identities; rather, it is a critique of all things oppressively normal. As a perspective, it rejects fixed identities, recognizing that people and sexuality can and do change over time. The term ***gay*** is inclusive of gender and biological sex; however, it is primarily used to describe men whose sexual orientation is toward other men. ***Lesbian*** refers to women who are sexually attracted to other women. ***Bisexual*** implies a sexual orientation toward both women and men (see also polysexual and pansexual in Exhibit 2.1). Often stigmatized as social pariahs, people who are bisexual may experience invalidation of their sexual identity by both the straight and the LGBTQ+ community (Friedman et al., 2014).

Although LGBTQ+ identities are experienced and enjoyed by many people and are therefore practical for our understanding of sexuality, such definitions rely on fixed notions of woman or man. In rejection of these fixed notions, the term ***polysexual,*** defined as the attraction to multiple genders and sexual identities, is used intentionally to disrupt the binary implied in the above definitions. Polysexual people are attracted to people from the full spectrum of sexual identities. Significantly, the gendering of people is broader than the classification and meaning of woman or man used previously. People who are polysexual[3] are attracted to various sexual identities performed by an inclusive range of gender identities. This term rejects the heterosexual–homosexual binary hidden in the term *bisexual.*

Asexuality is characterized by a lack of sexual attraction or low interest in sexual activity. Although it may include a total absence of sexual interest or desire for sexual activity, asexual people may have strong romantic or emotional attraction to others. A lack of or limited interest in romantic attraction is referred to as ***aromantic.*** These terms may be considered sexual orientations. Asexuality is often pathologized and medicalized and is seen as a deviance or a psychological deficit. It may be regarded as a "queer" orientation because it illuminates normative expectations for a person to want to experience sexual desire. A misconception is that asexuality includes people who experience a decrease in sex drive and are troubled by it. Asexual people are not troubled by the absence of or low interest in sexual activity, and asexuality is not considered a disorder (Brotto & Yule, 2017). Moreover, it is distinct from abstinence or celibacy.

---

[3] Polysexual is not to be confused with polyamorous. *Polyamory,* or *poly,* is the practice, desire, or acceptance of having more than one intimate or sexual connection at a time with the knowledge and consent of everyone involved. It is described as consensual, ethical, and responsible nonmonogamy. The practice of polyamory stresses ethics, honesty, and transparency.

LGBTQIA+ Health

The study of LGBTQIA+ health has historically had many institutional barriers. Unique health inequities within and between different LGBTQIA+ subgroups have been identified only recently by researchers (Cicero et al., 2020; Institute of Medicine, 2011). Information related to sexual orientation and gender identity (SOGI) is usually not entered into electronic health records (EHRs) or collected during national surveys, and these data remain unavailable and unaccounted for during statistical analyses of patient demographics. However, the Centers for Disease Control and Prevention (CDC; 2020), along with other national and federal organizations, have recommended collecting SOGI information and entering it into EHRs so that LGBTQIA+ health disparities can be better understood.

Occupational therapy practitioners can collect and enter SOGI information by ensuring that they ask about each client's sexual identity during sessions and updating the client's chart. Best practice recommendations are to ask about sexual orientation, gender, and assigned sex as three separate questions (CDC, 2020).

The Sex-Positive Occupational Therapy Practitioner

Sexual desires and activities are fluid, broad, and diverse. ***Sex positivity*** is broadly conceptualized as affirming human sexuality, health, and pleasure that are consensual and free of coercion, shame, and stigma. Being sex positive means embracing the varieties of sexual identities and preferences that exist as well as each person's right to decide how to express their gender and sexuality. Being sex positive also means promoting body positivity, safe(r) sex, reproductive justice, and sexual exploration of fantasies and bodily sensations; prioritizing a healthy sex life; and advocating for consensual sexual freedom rather than sexual repression. A sex-positive occupational therapy practitioner is one who affirms their clients' sexual identity, centers pleasure, and supports their sexual health (see Reflection Prompt 2.3). Case Examples 2.2 and 2.3 outline sex-positive scenarios in occupational therapy practice.

Sexual Pleasure

WHO (2006) identified sexual pleasure as a fundamental component of sexual health. The World Association of Sexual Health stated that ***sexual pleasure*** "is the physical and/or psychological satisfaction and enjoyment derived from shared or solitary erotic experiences, including thoughts, fantasies, dreams, emotions, and feelings" (Ford et al., 2021, p. 614). Occupational therapy practitioners can embrace

REFLECTION PROMPT 2.3
Creating a Norm of Sex Positivity

Engage in a brainstorming activity that imagines a sex-positive world, that is, a world with the following norms:

- Feeling good is a part of daily living, where pleasure is a collective driving force.
- Interactions are dripping with love and care.
- Consent is paramount to the sexual experience.
- All types of bodies are recognized as deserving of pleasure.
- Ethical pornography, which pays fairly and is free of sexual exploitation, is the only pornography that exists.
- Reproductive rights are human rights.
- Sex work is decriminalized, safe for all parties, and recognized as honest work.

What would this world look like? Are there people who are made less vulnerable or more vulnerable in it? Who can thrive in this world? What else would you add?

CASE EXAMPLE 2.2. HANS: CENTERING PLEASURE

A certified occupational therapy assistant (COTA) working at a pediatric clinic has a teenage client, **Hans,** who recently got into trouble for masturbating at school multiple times in a short period. Hans's parents reported that this behavior had never been a problem before and, as far as they knew, Hans only recently discovered masturbation. They asked the COTA for strategies to discourage Hans from masturbating altogether. The COTA suggested that the parents instead try to redirect the behavior to a more appropriate time and place, such as in Hans's bedroom in the morning or evening. By working with the parents to determine what an appropriate context would be, the COTA made a Social Story™ to delineate that "private time" was okay as long as it took place while Hans was alone in his room and took the time to clean up properly afterward.

WHO's pleasure-centered philosophy of sexual health[4] and sexual wellness that rejects rigid notions of a normal or abnormal way to experience pleasure.

Essential to sexual empowerment is gratification through sexual exploration, producing sexual experiences that are emotionally and mentally enjoyable as well as physically pleasurable. Occupational therapy practitioners can use their knowledge of the sensory system during interventions with clients to help clients understand and explore what sensory inputs give them pleasure. Assessment and intervention should include questions and activities that encourage clients to use

[4] WHO (2006), in addition to identifying pleasure as a fundamental component, stated that sexual health must be free of coercion, discrimination, and violence. It is also dependent on access to comprehensive, good-quality information about sex and sexuality. In addition, people must acknowledge the risks they may face and their vulnerability to the adverse consequences of unprotected sexual activity, have access to sexual health care, and live in an environment that affirms and promotes sexual health.

CASE EXAMPLE 2.3. THOMAS: ADVOCATING FOR PRIVACY, DIGNITY, AND RESPECT

At a skilled nursing facility, a multidisciplinary meeting is called to discuss a patient with end-stage dementia, **Thomas,** who has been putting the handle end of his utensils into his anus, which is causing perforations to his skin. Thomas remains in his bed and is able to eat independently, but the facility is unable to provide him 1:1 supervision during mealtime. Upon hearing about this situation, many of the staff laugh, but the occupational therapist does not. The staff is tasked with determining what to do.

The physical therapist speaks first and suggests calling Thomas's son to ask whether the patient is gay. The sex-positive occupational therapist speaks up and informs staff that sexual activity and preferences do not denote sexual orientation. Moreover, determining whether the patient is gay would not provide relevant information for the issue at hand. She then advocates for Thomas's right to privacy, dignity, and respect, asserting his right to privacy about his preferred sexual practices or sexual orientation, even to the exclusion of his children. Finally, the therapist tells the staff that the patient is likely seeking sensory input and stimulation through putting the utensil in his anus. She suggests adapting a sex toy that would be safe for anal insertion and leaving it easily accessible at the bedside for the patient.

their senses to explore their preferences or dislikes with curiosity. For example, practitioners can ask questions such as, "In an ideal sexual scenario, what is present in your environment, for example, what smells or sounds?" or "Touch is an important aspect of sexual activity, but people have widely varying preferences for touch. Do you know whether you prefer light touch or deep pressure when you are being touched?"

Occupational therapy practitioners can facilitate people making sexual decisions based on their preferences and desires and then accessing these decisions through modifications, adaptations, and strategies. For example, using the assessment of sensory preferences, consider a client who says being on vacation and smelling the ocean would help facilitate their desire. The practitioner may suggest lighting a candle that smells like the ocean in preparation for sexual activity to help the client transition into a sexual mood.

Using the assessment of touch preference, consider the client who prefers deep pressure. They report that their partner affectionately places their hand on their low back at times they are not expecting it, and it "makes them squirm." This situation causes friction because the client's partner does not understand why the client dislikes this type of touching. The practitioner can help the client script how to communicate their touch preferences to their partner. For example, the client can say, "Don't touch me lightly on my low back. Instead, tell me you're going to hug me and wrap your arms around me in a tight hug."

Sexual pleasure is complex, riddled with uncertainties and barriers that produce feelings of shame, guilt, and disgust. Everyone develops a language and relationship to pleasure. It is formed through various experiences, which may be connected to trauma, religious beliefs, social conditioning, or systematic barriers preventing people from centering pleasure as a possibility. Audre Lorde (2007), an academic, thought leader, and social justice advocate, gave guidance to strip the experiences of trauma and social conditioning that are influential to our sexual self-view by teaching us that we have been taught "to fear the yes within ourselves, our deepest cravings. But, once recognized, those which do not enhance our future lose their power and can be altered" (p. 56).

Infusing the Erotic Into Occupational Therapy Practice

Applying an erotic lens to occupational therapy intervention reinforces the profession's commitment to helping clients live life to its fullest. The profession already embraces the belief that people thrive through their engagement in occupation. Although *eroticism* might feel like a new word or concept in the sphere of occupational therapy, it is deeply connected to occupational satisfaction, client autonomy, and living life fully. Although an occupational therapy practitioner might be very comfortable affirming the passion and joy a client has for a hobby such as cooking, the practitioner might feel unsure about how to support passion and joy in a sexual occupation through determining goals and intervention.

As discussed in Chapter 1, "Pleasure, Eroticism, and Occupational Therapy," the ***erotic*** is a positive conceptualization of sexuality that acknowledges the philosophical meaning and beauty of sexual desire, excitement, sensuality, and romantic love. Audre Lorde, in a 1978 lecture, offered one powerful perspective on the erotic:

> The erotic is a resource within each of us that lies in a deeply female and spiritual plane, firmly rooted in the power of our unexpressed or unrecognized feeling . . . a measure between the beginnings of our sense of self and the chaos of our strongest feelings. It is an internal sense of satisfaction to which, once we have experienced it, we know we can aspire. (Lorde, 1978, cited in brown, 2019, pp. 27–28)

Lorde derived a spiritually affirming power centering the erotic as a source of fruitfulness and power. Sexuality is not fixed; it is fluid, and ever changing—there is no rhyme nor reason. The erotic, Lorde asserted, speaks to a person's "capacity for joy" (Lorde, 1978, cited in brown, 2019, p. 31). Moreover, Lorde's description of the erotic is influenced by the perspective that each person has both masculine and feminine energy,[5] separate from gender identity, gender expression, and

[5] Masculine energy can be thought of as logical, procedural, intellect, rule following, controlling, and competitive; feminine energy can be thought of as creative, sensual, intuitive, nurturing, collaborative, and expressive. Using this perspective, eroticism is in alignment with feminine energy because it is fueled by creativity, curiosity, sensuality, and trusting one's intuition.

sex assigned at birth. Lorde posited that eroticism is more in line with feminine energy, but her assertion is yet another example of how various constructs of masculinity and femininity exist (Tibebwa, 2022).

bell hooks (2015), a Black feminist activist, poet, and cultural critic, described a universal understanding of "common passions, sentiments shared by folks across race, class, gender, and sexual practice" (p. 12). Yearning sustains the joy in saying yes to exploration and feeling good and to "shared space and feeling" that "open up the possibility of common ground where our differences may be disrupted through a shared longing for liberation" from restrictive politics, which do not honor our desires (p. 13). Sexual intimacy and expression can be a powerful occupation, one deeply valued by clients, and occupational therapy practitioners need to be prepared to support and validate their clients' sexual identities, their need and desire for sex, and the role the erotic has in sexual occupations. hooks asserted that through sexuality, we can fulfill the yearning we have to feel pleasure and engage in erotic occupations or other occupations we feel passionately about.

A pleasure-centered framework advocates for sexual liberation that is inclusive of personal desires. Centering pleasure within sexual education to explore and change occupational therapy practitioners' outlook on sexual health and wellness, interpersonal relationships, and self-care helps to recognize and embrace our—and our clients'—most authentic selves.

The authors dare you, the reader, to explore the erotic and use it to guide your thinking about sexuality (see Chapter 3, "Guided Self-Reflection of Self as a Sexual Being," to assist with this process). Pleasure, eroticism, and joy expand one's view of sexuality, sexual desire, and sexual acts. Occupational therapy practitioners can rethink sexuality by replacing the urge to categorize sexual expressions, activities, and preferences as normal or sexually deviant with intentionally centering pleasure. Centering pleasure can provide a path for practitioners to understand how sex, gender, and sexuality have varied radically through history and use love, care, kindness, service, creativity, imagination, and justice in the therapeutic interaction.

Summary

Consider how sexuality begins within each person as a personal factor, is then expressed through engagement in ADLs and IADLs, and extends beyond each person to intertwine with social determinants of health and the social environment. As holistic clinicians, we need to consider these facets of sexuality and ensure that, through our interactions and treatments, we are facilitating participation in occupations that are affirming of sexual identity and sexual liberation and inclusive of pleasure and medically accurate sexual health information. Occupational therapy practitioners can best serve their clients through a commitment to dismantling systems of oppression and celebrating new narratives that position variation in sexual identities and preferences as the norm.

M. Nicole Horsley, PhD, is an assistant professor of African Diaspora Studies and affiliate faculty in Women's, Gender, and Sexuality Studies and Screen Cultures at Ithaca College in Ithaca, New York. Her work interrogates the discourse on Black women's bodies, disease, organs, and sexual pleasure.

Kathryn Ellis, OTD, OTR/L, AASECT–SC (she/her/hers), developed the Occupational Therapy Sexuality and Intimacy Clinic at Walter Reed National Military Medical Center in Bethesda, Maryland, and is the coauthor of *Sex and Intimacy for Wounded Veterans: A Guide to Embracing Change.* She is the founder and CEO of a continuing education company, the Institute for Sex, Intimacy & Occupational Therapy. She is an American Association of Sexuality Educators, Counselors, and Therapists Certified Sexuality Counselor and a consultant on sexuality and intimacy projects and initiatives. Her private practice, Dr. Kathryn Ellis Sexual Wellness Counseling, is based in Delaware.

Wade Robinson, OTD, OTR/L (he/him, they/them), has worked in sexual health since 2014. He educates other medical providers about sexuality-affirming practice and treating patients with concerns related to sex and intimacy at Walter Reed National Military Medical Center in Bethesda, Maryland. He holds an OTD from the University of South Dakota.

References

American Occupational Therapy Association. (2020). Occupational therapy practice framework: Domain and process (4th ed.). *American Journal of Occupational Therapy, 74*(Suppl. 2), 7412410010. https://doi.org/10.5014/ajot.2020.74S2001

American Psychological Association. (2020). *Publication manual of the American Psychological Association* (7th ed.).

Ashley, R. R. (2021, July 15). How Sarah Baartman's hips went from a symbol of exploitation to a source of empowerment for Black women. *The Conversation.* https://theconversation.com/how-sarah-baartmans-hips-went-from-a-symbol-of-exploitation-to-a-source-of-empowerment-for-black-women-160063

Boxer, M. J. (1998). *When women ask the questions: Creating women's studies in America.* Johns Hopkins University Press.

Brotto, L. A., & Yule, M. (2017). Asexuality: Sexual orientation, paraphilia, sexual dysfunction, or none of the above? *Archives of Sexual Behavior, 46,* 619–627. https://doi.org/10.1007/s10508-016-0802-7

brown, A. M. (2019). *Pleasure activism: The politics of feeling good.* AK Press.

Cahill, S. (2009). The disproportionate impact of antigay family policies on Black and Latino same-sex couple households. *Journal of African American Studies, 13,* 219–250. https://doi.org/10.1007/s12111-008-9060-7

Carrillo, V. G., & Dean, S. R. (2020). Understanding the impact of Chicana feminism on college success: A literature review. *Journal of Hispanic Higher Education, 19,* 99–110. https://doi.org/10.1177/1538192718795256

Centers for Disease Control and Prevention. (2020). *Collecting sexual orientation and gender identity information.* https://www.cdc.gov/hiv/clinicians/transforming-health/health-care-providers/collecting-sexual-orientation.html

Cicero, E. C., Reisner, S. L., Merwin, E. I., Humphreys, J. C., & Silva, S. G. (2020). The health status of transgender and gender nonbinary adults in the United States. *PlOS One, 15*(2). https://doi.org/10.1371/journal.pone.0228765

Crenshaw, K. (1989). Demarginalizing the intersection of race and sex: A Black feminist critique of anti-discrimination doctrine, feminist theory and anti-racist politics. *University of Chicago Legal Forum, 1989,* 139–167. https://chicagounbound.uchicago.edu/uclf/vol1989/iss1/8

Dillon, F. R., Worthington, R. L., & Moradi, B. (2011). Sexual identity as a universal process (pp. 649–670). In S. J. Schwartz, K. Luyckx, & V. L. Vignoles (Eds.), *Handbook of identity theory and research.* Springer. https://doi.org/10.1007/978-1-4419-7988-9_27

Dorries, H., & Harjo, L. (2020). Beyond safety: Refusing colonial violence through indigenous feminist planning. *Journal of Planning Education and Research, 40,* 210–219. https://doi.org/10.1177/0739456X19894382

Ford, J. V., Corona-Vargas, E., Cruz, M., Fortenberry, J. D., Kismodi, E., Philpott, A., . . . Coleman, E. (2021). The World Association for Sexual Health's declaration on sexual pleasure: A technical guide. *International Journal of Sexual Health, 33,* 612–642. https://doi.org/10.1080/19317611.2021.2023718

Frankenberg, R. (2020). White women, race matters: The social construction of whiteness. In L. Black & J. Solomos (Eds.), *Theories of race and racism* (pp. 519–533). Routledge.

Friar, T. (2021). The black female body: Representation of the erotic in contemporary visual art in Africa. *E-REA: Revue Électronique d'Études sur le Monde Anglophone, 19*(1). https://doi.org/10.4000/erea.13034

Friedman, M. R., Dodge, B., Schick, V., Herbenick, D., Hubach, R. D., Bowling, J., . . . Reece, M. (2014). From bias to bisexual health disparities: Attitudes toward bisexual men and women in the United States. *LGBT Health, 1,* 309–318. https://doi.org/10.1089/lgbt.2014.0005

Gilligan, C. (1982). *In a difference voice: Psychological theory and women's development.* Harvard University Press.

Goldberg, S. B. (2020). COVID-19 and LGBT rights. In K. Pistor (Ed.), *Law in the time of COVID-19* (pp. 98–108). Columbia Law School. https://scholarship.law.columbia.edu/cgi/viewcontent.cgi?article=3691&context=faculty_scholarship

Hardacker, C. T., Baccellieri, A., Mueller, E. R., Brubaker, L., Hutchins, G., Zhang, J. L. Y., & Hebert-Beirne, J. (2019). Bladder health experiences, perceptions and knowledge of sexual and gender minorities. *International Journal of Environmental Research and Public Health, 16,* 3170. https://doi.org/10.3390/ijerph16173170

hooks, B. (2015). *Yearning: Race, gender, and cultural politics.* Routledge.

Human Rights Campaign Staff. (2020, July 1). *HRC observes Black, Indigenous, People of Color Mental Health Month 2020.* Human Rights Campaign. https://www.hrc.org/news/hrc-observes-black-indigenous-people-of-color-mental-health-month-2020

Institute of Medicine. (2011). *The health of lesbian, gay, bisexual, and transgender people: Building a foundation for better understanding.* National Academies Press.

Jarry, J. (2021). The *word "cisgender" has scientific roots.* McGill Office for Science and Society. https://www.mcgill.ca/oss/article/history-general-science/word-cisgender-has-scientific-roots

Lorde, A. (1978). *Uses of the erotic: The erotic as power.* Out & Out Books.

Lorde, A. (2007). *Sister outsider: Essays and speeches* (Rev. ed.). Crossing Press.

Neumann, N., Neu, D., & Ungco, J. C. (2021). Addressing LGBTQIA+ trauma: Your role and your responsibility. In A. Lynch, R. Ashcraft, & L. Tekell (Eds.), *Trauma, occupation, and participation: Foundations and population considerations in occupational therapy* (pp. 195–221). AOTA Press.

Pilgrim, D. (2012). *The Jezebel stereotype* [Exhibit]. Jim Crow Museum, Ferris State University, Big Rapids, MI. https://www.ferris.edu/HTMLS/news/jimcrow/jezebel/index.htm

Ruben, M. A., & Fullerton, M. (2018). Proportion of patients who disclose their sexual orientation to healthcare providers and its relationship to patient outcomes: A meta-analysis and review. *Patient Education and Counseling, 101,* 1549–1560. https://doi.org/10.1016/j.pec.2018.05.001

Scott, J. (1988). Deconstructing equality-versus-difference: Or, the uses of poststructuralist theory for feminism. *Feminist Studies, 14*(1), 33–50. https://doi.org/10.2307/3177997

Somerville, S. B. (2000). Queering the color line: *Race and the invention of homosexuality in American culture.* Duke University Press. https://doi.org/10.1515/9780822378761

Tibebwa, S. (2022). Restoring the balance: The sacred union of our divine feminine and masculine energies. In K. Tobin & K. Alexakos (Eds.), *Contemplative practices for sustaining wellness* (pp. 102–118). Brill.

White Hughto, J. M., Reisner, S. L., & Pachankis, J. E. (2015). Transgender stigma and health: A critical review of stigma determinants, mechanisms, and interventions. *Social Science and Medicine, 147,* 222–231. https://doi.org/10.1016/j.socscimed.2015.11.010

World Health Organization. (2006). *Defining sexual health: Report of a technical consultation on sexual health, 28–31 January 2002, Geneva.* Author.

World Health Organization. (2017). *Determinants of health.* https://www.who.int/news-room/questions-and-answers/item/determinants-of-health

3

Guided Self-Reflection of Self as a Sexual Being

Sameera Qureshi, *MS, OTR, and* **Kathryn Ellis,** *OTD, OTR/L, AASECT–SC*

CHAPTER HIGHLIGHTS

- Honoring oneself as a sexual being
- Background of sexual health education in the United States
- Cultural competence and cultural humility
- Strategies for sexual self-reflection
- Intrapersonal self-reflection: knowing the self and knowing yourself with clients
- Creating a positive client experience

KEY TERMS AND CONCEPTS

Attunement
Belief
Bias
Community agreements
Cultural competence
Cultural humility
Direct messages
Ecological model
Experience of self and time
Grounding
Indirect messages
Intersectionality
Intimacy
Journaling
Mindful somatic exploration
Reframing
Responsive desire
Self-compassion
Self-disclosure
Self-intimacy
Self-love
Self-reflection
Sexual activities
Sexual arousal
Sexual desire or interest
Sexual expression
Sexual health
Sexual health and family planning
Sexual health education
Sexual response
Sexual self-view
Shame
Simultaneity
Spontaneous desire
Therapeutic use of self
Thought experiments
Trigger
Unconditional positive regard
Values

We occupational therapy practitioners have values, beliefs, biases, identities, and novel life experiences that are influenced by our environment and cultures (Hammell, 2013; West et al., 2012). We are cultural beings, just like our clients. It is imperative for us to be conscious of the self-schema that generates our individual uniqueness and establishes our individual norms. Only by being mindful of and evaluating our own norms can we prevent our own understanding and biases from infiltrating the therapeutic relationship (Hammell, 2013; Stayton, 1998).

For this reason, the first step in preparing to address sexuality with clients is to establish a strong self-reflection practice of understanding oneself as a sexual being. ***Self-reflection*** is listed in the *Occupational Therapy Practice Framework: Domain and Process* (4th ed.; *OTPF–4;* American Occupational Therapy Association [AOTA], 2020) as a cornerstone of occupational therapy practice that uniquely influences the occupational therapy process and distinguishes occupational therapy practitioners from other professionals. The *OTPF–4* defines ***experience of self and time*** as "awareness of one's identity (including gender identity), body, and position in the reality of one's environment and of time" (AOTA, 2020, p. 52). In essence, it is the act of thinking about oneself to gain self-awareness of one's thoughts, behaviors, values, beliefs, and biases.

Our ***sexual self-view***—how we have awareness about, understand, and define ourselves as sexual beings—is complex, ever changing, and influential, even when we are in the role of a practitioner working with clients. So much of how we have learned and continue to learn about our sexual selves takes place indirectly, and we often have not been given the time, space, and grounding to gain greater awareness about this critical part of ourselves. This chapter provides occupational therapy practitioners with information and prompts for self-reflection, and it provides activities aimed at diving into our sexual self-view—both *intrapersonally,* or within ourselves, and *interpersonally,* or with clients and other practitioners with whom we will interact.

To model the process of acknowledging that the authors' own identities and experiences influence their work and the lens through which this material is presented, the authors share their positionality to the material in this chapter:

- I, Sameera Qureshi, am a Muslim-Canadian immigrant who currently lives in the United States. I am of Pakistani-Iranian ethnicity and am a straight, cisgendered, married woman who received limited formal sexual health education growing up. My identity is frequently not represented in sex education. I am self-employed as a sexual health educator focused on Muslim communities and practitioners who serve them.
- I, Kathryn Ellis, am straight and White. I was raised as and am attributed as a cisgender woman in the Northeast United States. I do not have a disability and have never been admitted into a hospital. I have dated people with physical and cognitive disabilities. I hold a terminal degree for my profession and am now self-employed as an educator and clinician. I am very comfortable talking about sex now, both personally and as a practitioner, but this was not always the case. My Catholic grade school offered just abstinence-only sex education, and at my public high school, I did not receive formal sexual health education.

This chapter aims to educate readers on the necessity of self-reflection for occupational therapy assessment and intervention related to sexuality and to guide readers through a self-reflection of themselves as sexual beings and of their relationships with others when discussing sexuality in various contexts. Readers can use this process to critically analyze their own identity and positionality and how they influence their clinical work.

The focus on self makes this chapter different from the other chapters; for this reason, "we" as used in the remainder of this chapter generally encompasses all of us—you, the readers; we, the authors; and occupational therapy practitioners in general. The chapter uses "you" when addressing readers in order to be therapeutic and to highlight the personal work that is encouraged with this chapter.

Honoring Oneself as a Sexual Being

As we explore our sexual self-view, it is important to consider that this exploration can bring to the surface many mixed feelings. Reflecting on our sexual health and exploring our experiences with it can be uncomfortable or unfamiliar. ***Sexual health*** is

> a state of physical, emotional, mental and social well-being in relation to sexuality; it is not merely the absence of disease, dysfunction or infirmity. Sexual health requires a positive and respectful approach to sexuality and sexual relationships, as well as the possibility of having pleasurable and safe sexual experiences, free of coercion, discrimination and violence. (World Health Organization [WHO], 2006, cited in WHO, n.d.)

Even with this definition in mind, there can be uncertainty with what we know or do not know about sexual health, or what we think we "should" know. We also may be challenged when our sexual self-view seems to conflict with known societal expectations or when we have difficulty placing into words what we are feeling because we have not had previous space to process this or heard language that we feel describes us.

Sexual health education (or sex education) means learning about a broad variety of topics related to sex and sexuality. It ideally explores values and beliefs about those topics and helps people gain the skills that are needed to navigate relationships with oneself, one's partners, and one's community and to manage one's own sexual health. Sex education may take place in schools, at home, in community settings, or online (Planned Parenthood, n.d.). Many of us who did not receive sex education that met our needs as sexual beings have feelings of internalized guilt or shame about our lack of knowledge (e.g., medically accurate sexual health information) or our own sexual preferences and dislikes. ***Shame*** can be much more damaging than guilt, because shame is a painful feeling of being unworthy and deeply wrong; it is a belief that we do not deserve to feel whole, complete, and grounded.

It is important to take time to establish an understanding of our sexual self-view, knowing that it is fluid and affected by our environment, life experiences, attitudes, and beliefs (Whitney & Fox, 2017). For this reason, what we believed about sex and relationships as children and adolescents is often going to be different from what we believe and value as adults, and new versions of beliefs and values will continue throughout life. Readers whose identities and experience closely align with dominant American paradigms of White, able-bodied, monogamous, straight, and cisgender as "the standard" may find themselves challenged to reflect deeply and critically on themselves as sexual beings; their reality matches the standard, which can facilitate a lack of awareness. Conversely, readers who have been historically marginalized and "othered" by these paradigms may be more likely to have engaged in deep self-reflection, because their reality contrasts with the standard, which can facilitate awareness. That said, lack of awareness and deep reflection on the self as a sexual person is widespread for many of us, again due to reinforcing social messages that discourage this contemplation.

Wherever you find yourself, your awareness as a sexual person is deepened through critically reflecting on implicit assumptions and beliefs that are socially directed. Additionally, even if you feel you have previously engaged in significant self-reflection, you are encouraged to work through the self-reflection process just the same. Note the changes and new iterations of beliefs and values that you have adopted during your life.

Background of Sexual Health Education in the United States

Before we dive into self-reflection, we must consider factors that may have affected our sexual self-view. When we examine these factors, an ecological model is ideal. Initially posited by developmental psychologist Urie Bronfenbrenner in the mid-20th century, an ***ecological model*** recognizes that multiple factors and the interplay among them influence our sexual self-view, including systems, societies, communities, families, and intrapersonal factors (Bronfenbrenner, 1979; Dahlberg & Krug, 2002). One ecological factor that may have influenced your sexual view is the sexual health education you received.

Sexual health education in public schools has a long, arduous history in the United States. Beginning in 1912, public schools used handouts and pamphlets to educate their students on reproduction and pregnancy. Much of the information was vague and deliberately limited (Planned Parenthood, 2016). From the 1960s on, support for sex education in schools began to gain widespread support. Beginning in the 1980s, however, in large part because of legislative policies and opposition to the availability of birth control and abortions among certain segments of society, a debate began pitting abstinence-only education against a more comprehensive approach to sex education, which provided information about sexual health, including information about contraception.

Education about sex and sexuality in U.S. schools thus progressed in the two divergent directions of abstinence only or comprehensive (Planned Parenthood,

2016). The comprehensive direction was based on the belief that medically accurate and comprehensive information about sexual health would decrease risk-taking behaviors among young people. The abstinence-only direction was based on the belief that medically accurate, comprehensive information would increase risk-taking behaviors among young people. Significant evidence now shows that a comprehensive approach to sex education promotes sexual health among young people by reducing sexual risk-taking behavior. The abstinence-only approach has not shown these results (Bordogna et al., 2023).

Unfortunately, a great lack of consensus exists among the entities that control school curricula about sexual health education, and no national oversight is in place to ensure that all young people in the United States are receiving comprehensive and medically accurate sexual health education. As of July 2022, only 29 states and the District of Columbia required public schools to teach sex education, and 16 states provided abstinence-only sex education. Thirteen states required that consent be a part of the curriculum, nine states had policies to include LGBTQIA+ inclusive education, and 5 states required comprehensive sex education (Sexuality Information and Education Council of the United States, 2022).

In addition, sexual health education curricula are often developed by heterosexual, cisgender, White people. Programs typically do not reflect diverse identities related to cultures, religions, ethnicities, abilities, gender, and sexual orientation. There is also a lack of opportunity to consider our own values as they relate to our sexual self because much of sex education continues to emphasize teaching facts and information, leaving less room for a nuanced and tailored approach for diverse identities. Although the accessibility of sexual health information for young people has improved—mainly because of social media and the surge of online sex education platforms led by diverse sexuality educators—that was not the case when many of us were growing up.

The way in which we received—or did not receive—sexual health education was predominantly out of our control. For example, our parents or guardians might not have consented to our attending sex education classes at school, and they might not have been educated themselves. In addition, some of our caregivers might not have educated us about topics related to puberty, healthy relationships, and sexual decision making. Some of us were raised in communities in which sexual health education was embedded into religious or cultural activities in which we participated, and others did not have this experience. Perhaps we had an older sibling, cousin, or friend provide us with mostly accurate, but incomplete, sex education.

All of this is to say—and reassure you—that systemic factors may have affected your ability to access and internalize sexual health education. Our experience with sex education as children and youth was generally out of our control. These factors have been at play for decades and continue to provide barriers for delivering a healthier sex education system in the United States. At the same time, it may be reassuring to know that, as adults, we now can access the information we need in the way that best fits who we are.

Now you are ready for your first self-reflection (Reflection Prompt 3.1). For this and many of the other reflections, you will need a notebook or paper for journaling and taking notes.

REFLECTION PROMPT 3.1
Reflecting on Your Sex Education

- What was your experience with sex education? Did you attend classes at school or perhaps through your religious or cultural community? Or both?
- If you did not attend classes, what was the reason?
- How much of what you experienced or learned was in your control?
- How did your experiences with sex education—or lack thereof—affect you physically, mentally, professionally, and spiritually?

Take a few moments to journal or make notes about your sex education.

Cultural Competence and Cultural Humility

It is widely accepted that clinicians need to be sensitive to the role of culture in working with clients. This section describes two approaches to addressing the role of culture in the clinician–client relationship: cultural competence and cultural humility.

Cultural Competence

The term "cultural competence" was first used in the late 1980s by social worker Terry L. Cross and his colleagues, but it was not until almost a decade later that health care professionals began to be formally educated and trained in this concept (Betancourt et al., 2002; Cross, 1988). ***Cultural competence*** is "a set of congruent behaviors, attitudes, and policies that come together in a system, agency, or professional to work effectively in cross-cultural situations" (Cross, 1988, p. 1). In 2002, cultural competence in health care emerged as a field and has since been increasingly embedded into medical education curricula and taught in health settings around the world (Betancourt et al., 2002). Cultural competence emphasizes the idea of effectively operating in different cultural contexts and altering practices to reach different cultural groups on the basis of training that describes each group. The idea that culture can be learned by an outsider reinforces the idea that culture is experienced the same way by everyone in that culture, regardless of individual uniqueness or the influence of intersecting identities (Hammell, 2013). Ironically, this approach implies cultural homogeneity and creates and reinforces stigma.

Cultural competency also rarely includes a discussion of what one might expect when working with, for example, White people or straight people, further reinforcing whiteness and straightness as the norm, and the idea that White, straight health care providers do not need to engage in reflection or analysis of White culture or straight culture.

Hammell (2013) observed that "culture pertains not solely to ethnicity or race but to any dimension of diversity, including class, gender, sexual orientation, and ability" (p. 224). The mistreatment, poor clinical decision making, and harm resulting from "othering" occurs in all social categories of difference.

Cultural Humility

Cultural competency is about attempting to know another culture to operate as if within it, but ***cultural humility*** is about understanding your own culture and how practicing it affects your interactions with people from a culture that differs from your own. It is used to develop the skills necessary to work with a diverse client population. Cultural humility instructs the occupational therapy professional to challenge the likely unconscious assumptions that their values, beliefs, and attitudes are the norm and to accept that their culture is just one perspective among many other perspectives (Hammell, 2013). In this approach, practitioners engage in critical self-reflection to acknowledge the differences within the client–therapist relationship rather than view the client as different from oneself (Hammell, 2013; Tervalon & Murray-García, 1998). As Hammell (2013) argued,

> The starting point for working across these differences consists in developing a critical consciousness of one's own assumptions, beliefs, values, and biases; an understanding of how one's own perspectives may differ from those of other people; and an acknowledgement of the unearned advantages, privileges, and power that derive from multiple dimensions of one's own particular social position. Thus, cultural humility incorporates a commitment both to critical self-evaluation and to redressing power imbalances between therapists and clients. (p. 226)

When we can view clients' experiences and identities as coexisting among ours and recognize that we may never fully understand them, we begin to see that cultural competency is not possible and thereby learn the value of practicing cultural humility.

Occupational therapy practitioners are responsible for knowing themselves in relationship to others, not for fully understanding others. Within this relationship, we will make mistakes because of our incompetencies; learning and humility are ongoing experiences. Sexual cultural humility might be even more vital than other domains of occupation because of the "omission, silence, lack of dialogue around sexuality, which can leave us and others unconsciously convinced that our own perceptions are the norm" (Ellis, 2023). Reflecting on ourselves as sexual beings is vital to the ability to work across cultures with our diverse client populations (Hammell, 2013; Ott, 2017; Stayton, 1998; West et al., 2012).

Strategies for Sexual Self-Reflection

Self-reflection may be challenging or confusing. Readers are encouraged to consider implementing the coping strategies described in the following sections to navigate discomfort they may feel during the reflection prompts presented later in this chapter.

Reframing

Reframing is the cognitive strategy to consider alternative perspectives in response to a negative or stressful feeling or experience. You are encouraged to reframe wanting to have a concrete and unchanging understanding of yourself as a sexual being and acknowledge the natural evolution of this schema. Sexual development and identity are not fixed but change throughout life. Our sensory system is hardwired to seek pleasurable experiences for ourselves; as we develop, explore, and engage in occupations related to sexual expression, sexual activity, and intimacy, how we prefer to engage and how we feel about those occupations can change (Whitney & Fox, 2017). If this self-reflection creates a shift of awareness and new perspectives, and then a resulting frustration with older perceptions, know that this process is normal. You might experience excitement or discomfort, or you might experience both at the same time. Fluidity of beliefs, perceptions, attitudes, sexual preferences, and sexual dislikes is a normal aspect of living through life and maturation. For example, someone could enjoy oral sex and not prefer nipple play, but then after childbirth experience orgasms from nipple play and no longer enjoy oral sex. Then, in their 50s, this person could begin to prefer to have sex with women, which they had never done before or experienced.

Self-Compassion and Self-Love

As children we have only so much control over the sexual health education we receive, yet we are influenced by what we learn as we develop, and we are further expected to perform within the norms and rules of the system. For example, the ways in which we directly and indirectly learn about compassion and love affect how we understand and demonstrate self-compassion and self-love. As adults, we often have more control over the material we are exposed to, and we can autonomously seek out learning, yet our awareness of expectations for sexual performance and expression can be deeply pervasive.

As we become more aware, many of us might feel frustrated about what we did not know earlier in our lives. Despite not having control over what we learned, we might judge ourselves for our current developmental status. For this reason, self-compassion and self-love are paramount. ***Self-compassion*** is the understanding that suffering is universal; it encourages us to practice acceptance of our current state. ***Self-love*** gives us permission to understand our authentic self and to view ourselves without judgment or apology. Self-love encourages us to process through pain points and rejoice in our uniqueness (Lorde, 2020). Through developing self-love, we can begin to show the world our authentic self, which is an act of loving oneself (Lorde, 2020).

Consider that if you were a group leader for a group discussion on these topics, you would probably promote ground rules for tolerance, respect, and empathy toward others. Establish the same ground rules for yourself and offer yourself tolerance, respect, and empathy.

Journaling

Journaling is a powerful tool for self-reflection. You are encouraged to journal all self-reflection prompts. Journaling will help you slow down your thoughts and focus on those that are most important and authentic to you. In addition to journaling the self-reflection prompts, it's helpful to journal about any feelings that come up during the process. After completing a prompt, consider "How do I feel?" or "How do I feel about this reflection?" and then journal about those feelings. Calling these feelings into awareness can help you see areas for self-compassion.

Grounding

Grounding is another coping skill that can support you during self-reflection practice. ***Grounding*** first requires you to pay attention to the sensations of the body; it is particularly helpful when thoughts are both distracting and distressing. If self-reflection is causing distress, it might show up first in body sensations such as increased heart rate, stomach discomfort, or muscle tension. Grounding techniques include focusing on the sensation of breath moving in and out of your nose or on your chest rising and falling as you breathe. You can also rub your hands on your legs or wiggle your toes against the ground. As you ground, you are activating your parasympathetic nervous system, which produces a calm homeostasis for you to continue cognitive reflection on difficult topics.

Mindful Exploration

Mindful somatic exploration involves self-exploration of your body's physical sensations while practicing mindfulness techniques of curiosity, nonjudgment, and observation. Many of the prompts in this chapter encourage cognitive exploration of thoughts and feelings, yet some of the prompts might spark an interest to learn about yourself through embodiment—that is, by physically exploring your sensory system. If the desire to physically explore your sensory responses and experiences arises, you are encouraged to again incorporate grounding techniques. Grounding helps process physical sensations without the interruptions of cognitive thoughts or judgments. As you engage in sensory exploration, such as self-touch, masturbation, or touch with others, allow yourself to feel sensations without judgment or expectation of what you think you are *supposed* to feel. Simply *feel the feelings*. Techniques for enhancing awareness of body sensations are focusing on your breath sensations first, then expanding to feelings throughout your body.

Take Time and Take Care

Self-reflection can be enjoyable, insightful, and difficult all at the same time. For this reason, you are encouraged to take your time with this process so that you do not feel overwhelmed or confused. It is not expected that you answer all of these prompts at once, and you can visit this chapter over time. You are the expert on yourself. Should the process feel overwhelming, take a break from self-reflection, engage in self-care, and implement coping skills to self-soothe. Come back to the prompts only when you feel ready, and know that there is no set timeline for working through the self-reflection exercises.

Remember, You Are Learning

Understanding oneself as a sexual being is not something one innately and organically knows; most of us were not taught how to self-reflect in general, let alone on ourselves as a sexual being. We are not born with the self-reflection skills to explicitly think about our intricacies, complexities, nuances, and uniqueness. For this reason, our norm might just be thought of as "it is what is." The prompts in this chapter might be an exercise in learning both self-reflection and about yourself as a sexual being. Approach this process as you might approach any learning experience. Knowledge acquisition can feel awkward or confusing at first; practice helps with comprehension. Consider the ways in which you learn best and approach the sexual knowledge prompts in next section accordingly.

Intrapersonal Self-Reflection: Knowing the Self

Using terminology from the *OTPF–4*, the next sections provide prompts to build or deepen your self-awareness and self-concept as a sexual being. More than 60 questions are provided, and it is best not to try to answer them in one sitting. Remember to pace yourself and use the strategies for self-compassion and self-love described earlier. You are encouraged to start and stop, revisit questions later, revisit all of them again, and reflect on them while you read this text. You are the expert on you, so think about how you want to pace yourself. For example, you could

- answer five questions each day;
- answer five questions each time you read a chapter in this textbook;
- set a timer for 10 minutes each day to answer questions; or
- answer questions that feel easy first, and answer a harder one each day afterward.

Regardless of what strategies you choose, you can always stop if you start to feel overwhelmed. It is okay to be right where you are in your understanding of yourself as a sexual being; this is a continual and fluid process, so the best thing to do is frequently revisit these questions. For this reason, we recommend against educators assigning graded assignments for this chapter.

As you go through these questions, understand that there is no right answer; everyone will have a different answer and reflection. This is the beauty of the variations among humans. Take the occupation of cooking. For some people, this activity could be highly meaningful as a hobby, whereas for others, it could be highly meaningful as a way to connect with others as a ritual or as a family obligation. Some people could engage in cooking within a romantic, sexual, or erotic context—maybe by themselves, while wearing lingerie, or with a partner. Within this context, cooking could be meaningful because it is sexual for the person. Or perhaps there are people who feel cooking is sexual every single time they cook regardless of setting, reason, outfit, or context. And some people engage in cooking merely as a means to an end to get people fed, and if they can, they avoid cooking. Each association and preference is normal and possible.

Now, consider body image and sexual self-view. One person might not view their body as sexual, whereas another might feel the opposite way about their body. Both feelings are normal and have no bearing on whether either person uses their body in a sexual way, views their body positively, expresses themselves sexually, engages in sexual activity, or enjoys sex. Said simply, we cannot stress enough that you are normal just as you are!

Sexual Self-View

As described earlier, your sexual self-view is how you view yourself as a sexual being. It involves your objective understanding of your sexual identity, such as sexual preferences, sexual expression, gender identity, and sexual orientation, as well as your subjective opinion on how you feel about yourself, including self-worth, self-esteem, and body image. Reflection Prompt 3.2 is an exercise to further your understanding of yourself as a sexual being.

The next section, "Sexual Desire, Arousal, and Response," explains what sexual interest and desire are as well as the body's response to both. At the end of that section, you are asked to reflect on what interests you sexually. Reflection Prompts 3.3–3.5 will help you prepare for that reflection.

REFLECTION PROMPT 3.2
Myself as a Sexual Being

Take out a sheet of paper, draw a horizontal line, and put 0 at the left end and 10 at the right end. Then number from 1 to 9 in between the two ends. On the scale of 0 (*very uncomfortable*) to 10 (*very comfortable*), rate how you view your own comfort level with yourself as a sexual being. Then, do the following two things:

1. Write down the comfort level that correlates to the number you chose.
2. In your journal, explain why you chose this number.

REFLECTION PROMPT 3.3
Can I Have the Things That I Want?

Across an entire piece of paper, draw a two-column table. Put "Feels Okay" at the top as the heading for the first column and "Feels Not Okay" as the heading for the second column. In each column, list whether each of the following six prompts feels okay or does not feel okay, and journal your reflections for each:

1. Am I allowed to have sexual interests? Am I allowed to want the things that I want when it comes to sex and relationships?
2. Is it okay for me to facilitate pleasure for my partner(s)? Is it okay for me to receive pleasure from them?
3. Is it okay for me to not want sex?
4. If I feel neutral or indifferent about myself as a sexual being, is this okay with me?
5. Is it okay for me to want pleasure?
6. What else do I identify as "Feels Okay" and "Feels Not Okay"?

REFLECTION PROMPT 3.4
Self-Definition

Respond to the following seven questions and allow yourself to journal whatever comes up:

1. What does "sexual liberation" mean to me?
2. How would I best describe my gender identity?
3. What are my pronouns?
4. How would I best describe my sexual orientation?
5. How do I feel about my body?
6. How do I view myself as a sexual being?
7. What feels easy? What feels hard?

REFLECTION PROMPT 3.5
Views of Myself

Next, draw another two-column table with "My Views of Myself" as the heading for the first column and "Others' Views of Me" as the heading for the second column. Think about views and opinions you may have heard about you or people who are like you, and then consider whether you agree with those opinions. List some thoughts you have about what you think of yourself and what messages you have heard from others. Ask yourself, How does my authentic view of myself as a sexual being align or counter "typical" or "historical" societal expectations?

Sexual Desire, Arousal, and Response

Sexual desire or interest is the want for sex, and ***sexual arousal*** is the excitatory feeling during sex and enjoyment of pleasurable sensations during the sexual experience. More specifically, desire can be spontaneous or responsive. ***Spontaneous desire*** is when arousal does not depend on environment or context; people can feel like the desire for sex is ever present or easily accessible

(Nagoski, 2015). ***Responsive desire*** is when desire is activated in response to an appropriate context for that person (Nagoski, 2015). Responsive desire is influenced by sexual accelerators and brakes—factors that turn us on or turn us off. For example, among an exponential variety of combinations, someone may find they have more desire when they feel relaxed, are flirted with, are living their life in alignment with their authentic identities, feel positive self-worth, are educated about their sexual self, or enjoyed the last time they had sex. They may find they have less desire when they are exhausted, stressed, in pain, postpartum, disempowered, grieving, bullied, self-critical, unsupported by their partner(s), or managing multiple competing life priorities. Desire can fluctuate between spontaneous and responsive, depending on a person's life circumstances. As such, it is important to think about desire in a nuanced way, reflecting on factors, contexts, and experiences that may contribute to either an accelerated feeling of desire or one that is slowed down or paused (Nagoski, 2015).

Sexual response is the body's central nervous system's automatic response, such as an erection, increased heart rate, vaginal lubrication, or orgasm, to a sexually relevant environment, thought, or experience. Note that sexual responses do not imply arousal, enjoyment of the sexual experience, or consent. Sexual arousal is a cognitive process of integrating the somatic experience of receiving sexual stimulation, the environment, and the desire to determine whether the experience is enjoyable and pleasurable. For example, someone who is enjoying (sexual arousal) masturbation or any other sexual activity (somatic experience) may experience a sexual brake (loss of desire) if a roommate walks in on them because the environment is no longer conducive for a pleasurable sexual experience (environment) and they no longer have an erection or are lubricated (sexual response). Also, sexual response and sexual arousal are often congruent, but only about 75% of the time (Nagoski, 2015). For example, someone can be sexually aroused cognitively but they do not experience a sexual response such as erection, lubrication, or orgasm. Desire, sexual arousal, and sexual response patterns are not fixed entities and tend to change both from day to day and over the course of one's life, depending on context. Reflection Prompt 3.6 focuses on exploring your sexual desire and what you find sexually arousing.

Sexual Expression

Sexual expression is the outward expression of sexual self-view and sexual values to those around us—our partner(s), family, friends, or greater society. Sexual expression involves mannerisms, dress, behaviors, and manner of speech; overall, it is the choice of what to express and what not to, based on sexual values. Sexual expression evolves throughout our lifetime and depends on myriad factors: life stage, current context, involvement with a partner, and our internalized learning about sexuality and sex. Reflection Prompt 3.7 aims to support your reflection on how you choose to sexually express yourself.

REFLECTION PROMPT 3.6
My Desire and Arousal Preferences

1. Do I feel that I experience spontaneous desire or responsive desire more frequently? Does this change, depending on context and experience?
2. As I reflect on the conditions that support my desire, what accelerates them? Which of the following factors hinder or decrease desire?
   - mental and physical well-being (e.g., physical health, body image, mood, worry about sexual functioning)
   - partner characteristics (e.g., appearance, health, smell, mental state)
   - relationship characteristics (e.g., trust, power dynamic, emotional connection, shared values)
   - setting (e.g., public, private, distance)
   - other life circumstances (e.g., work-related or family stress, holiday or occasion)
   - things I do (e.g., self- or partner-guided fantasy, forms of sexual intimacy).
3. How might a partner accelerate my sexual desire or put the brakes on my sexual desire? (If you have a partner or partners, you can apply this reflection to any or all of them.)
4. What do I find myself interested in (desire) or enjoying (arousal), sexually, if anything—for example, dancing, self-pleasure or masturbation, strip clubs, physical intimacy with a partner, sexual intercourse, sexting, kink, breast play, kisses on the ear, exploration of erotic literature?
5. As I reflect on how I feel during times I experience sexual desire or sexual arousal, are there patterns to these feelings?
6. How do I know that I am feeling sexually aroused? Is it physical, cognitive, emotional, or spiritual in nature—or some combination of these?
7. If I think about why certain activities turn me on, what comes up for me as possible reasons? Do they feel like authentic reasons, or are they conditioned responses based on what I feel should make me sexually aroused?
8. How do I feel about feeling aroused? What thoughts come to mind as I feel myself becoming aroused?
9. Do I feel comfortable communicating my arousal and desire with my partner(s)?
10. What am I curious about further exploring—if anything—with regard to sexual arousal and desire?

REFLECTION PROMPT 3.7
My Sexual Expression

1. How do I understand sexual expression according to how I define myself as a sexual being?
2. As I reflect on where I am in my life, what does my sexual expression look like publicly and privately? Does it vary, depending on different public or private contexts?
3. What values do I hold around sexual expression? How do my values affect my sexual expression?
4. How important is it for others or the world to see my sexual expression? Is it meaningful for me to reserve this expression? Is it meaningful for me to display this expression? Do I feel neutral or indifferent about sexual expression?
5. Who am I the most comfortable showing myself to as a sexual being?
6. Drawing activity: Envision yourself in sexual expression and then draw what you see. (This activity is not just for artists. Give yourself freedom to draw out or sketch what comes to mind.)

Sexual Activity

Sexual activities, which we refer to broadly in this section as "sex," are the broad possibilities of sexual experiences and activities with self or others that are perceived as sexually relevant through the somatic sensation of pleasure in the brain or social conditioning of what is sexually relevant and permitted. Review the following prompts to explore your beliefs, preferences, and patterns related to sexual activity (see Reflection Prompt 3.8).

REFLECTION PROMPT 3.8
My Sexual Activity

1. How do I define *sex*?
2. What could pleasure look like for me?
3. Am I interested in sexual pleasure? Not interested? Feel neutral or indifferent?
4. If I am interested in self-pleasure, how could I do this?
5. What does the sex look like that I have, desire, prefer, get excited about?
6. What do I enjoy about being sexual? If I have never been sexual, what do I think I might enjoy about being sexual? What do I feel excited to do?
7. Are there specific ways I want to be touched? (Think about location, pace, and firmness or gentleness.)
8. Are there actions I want to do to someone else to facilitate pleasure for them that would also feel exciting for me?
9. Are my preferences aligned, not aligned, or both with "typical" or "historical" societal expectations"?
10. On the same 0 (*very uncomfortable*) to 10 (*very comfortable*) scale you drew earlier (see the "Sexual Self-View" section), identify the degree of importance sexual activity has in your life by labeling "Sexual activity importance" next to the corresponding number.
11. Fill in the blanks:

For me, sex are activities I do to feel __________. When I think about the activities that are relaxing to me, ____________ comes to mind. There are times when I do not feel particularly sexy or sexual, such as when I am ________ [*insert activity that is not sexually relevant to you*]. When I am not feeling particularly sexual, when I do _____________ [*list something you could do that might turn you on*] or when _________ [*list something that could happen in your environment that could turn you on*] happens, I feel more interested in sex. When I am with myself, I enjoy ___________ [*name a way you explore your sexuality*] as a way to explore myself sexually. Sometimes I think about being with another person or people, and I envision us _____________ [*name an activity, sexual or otherwise, you would find enjoyable*], which would feel good to me. I don't tolerate certain kinds of touch well, and those ways include ___________ [*name ways and places you do not like being touched*]. Some ways I love being touched are ______________ [*name ways you like being touched and where*]. I like being ________ [*insert sexual action like kissed, caressed, licked, pinched*] on my _________ [*insert body part*].

When I am being sexual, which could be dancing, sitting close with someone, or having sex, the environment matters to me. An environment that I think would be great to have sexual experiences in is the following: _____________ [*describe an environment: What is the temperature? What sounds, smells, or sights are you experiencing?*] When it comes to all activities that might be pleasurable [*sexual or otherwise*], at this moment, what I want the most is ______________ [*name pleasurable activity*].

Intimacy

Intimacy is a close, personal, trusting relationship with another person or group of people that includes giving and receiving affection and support. ***Self-intimacy*** is related to being aware of and connecting with our authentic, inner self and may include our self-concept, worth, comfort, and compassion toward ourselves. Intimacy with others is how we choose to share parts of ourselves with others and may include emotional, physical, spiritual, or sexual components or values. Reflection Prompt 3.9 is intended to assist you with exploring your beliefs, preferences, and patterns related to intimacy.

REFLECTION PROMPT 3.9

My Beliefs, Preferences, and Patterns Related to Intimacy

1. What practices do I currently use to strengthen and honor the relationship with myself—for example, taking time for self-reflection, engaging in self-care activities, having "me time," praying, journaling, taking myself out on a date, doing positive affirmations, or seeking help when I need it?
2. What does the intimacy that I desire look like?
3. Why do people have romantic relationships?
4. Am I interested in intimate relationships? Not interested? Feel neutral or indifferent? Why?
5. What activities help me emotionally connect to others?
6. How do I manage conflict in interpersonal relationships?
7. How do I show others that I love them?
8. Draw a horizontal line across a sheet of paper in a landscape orientation and label *unhealthy relationships* at one end and *healthy relationships* at the other. Reflect on signs that indicate whether the relationships could be healthy or unhealthy. Place those signs on this continuum. For example, where might you place the following: expecting quick text responses, enjoying going out on dates and planning them often, attending spiritual services together, experiencing physical or emotional abuse. Now think of some of your own.
9. Draw two overlapping circles (i.e., a Venn diagram), and label one circle "What about myself do I want to share with others?" and the other, "What about myself do I not want to share with others?" List those things in each circle. The middle section, where the circles overlap, can be either "I don't know" or "Only with some people"—your choice!
10. On the same 0 (*very uncomfortable*) to 10 (*very comfortable*) scale you drew earlier (see the "Sexual Self-View" section), identify the degree of importance intimate activities have in your life by labeling "Intimate activities: importance" next to the corresponding number.
11. Take the whole page to draw a Venn diagram. Label one circle "Sexual activities" and the other "Intimate activities." List the activities in the appropriate circle, and list the ones that feel like both to you in the section that overlaps.

Sexual Health and Family Planning

Sexual health and family planning involves understanding and practicing habits and routines that sustain health, such as communicating about birth control and sexually transmitted infection (STI) status with new partners, giving and receiving consent, and establishing a plan to try to become a parent or to try not to become a parent. Reflection Prompt 3.10 will guide you in considering what you learned about sexual health and what is important to you related to your sexual health.

REFLECTION PROMPT 3.10
My Sexual Health Education

1. What did I learn about birth control? What did I learn about STIs?
2. Could the sexual activity I engage in result in an STI? If so, how can I prevent this?
3. Am I actively trying to become a parent? How has this process been for me?
4. Could the sexual activity I engage in result in a pregnancy? If I do not want to become pregnant or do not want my partner(s) to become pregnant, how can I engage in sex without getting pregnant?
5. What is my understanding of sexual consent? Where did I learn this from?
6. How do I know I want to have sex?
7. Visual exercise: Based on your answers, write a list of what you know and where you feel there are gaps in your knowledge regarding sexual health. For each gap, consider and jot down where you could find reliable information.

Values, Beliefs, and Biases

Everyone has a unique schema and concept formation for sexuality based on their own combination of values and beliefs. Values and beliefs are unique to each person but are heavily influenced by sociocultural factors, such as the family unit, religion, geographical community, or virtual community. The *OTPF–4* defines ***values*** as "principles, standards, or qualities considered worthwhile by the client who holds them" (AOTA, 2020, p. 15) and uses the following definition for ***belief:*** "something that is accepted, considered to be true, or held as an opinion" (Merriam-Webster, n.d.).

A ***bias*** is a prejudgment or assumption that a person believes to be true. Everyone has biases, and those biases are often unconscious assumptions about others. Like all human beings, occupational therapy practitioners have biases that will influence the therapeutic relationship leading to harm, inefficient care, or missed opportunities. (*Note.* This is the first introduction to biases in this text, but because health care providers' biases significantly affect health disparities, we have included an entire chapter to the topic; see Chapter 4, "Sexuality, Bias, and Impact: Preventing Clinician Harm.") For now, consider how some of your beliefs might create bias about yourself or others. For example, if an occupational therapy practitioner received cultural messaging growing up that sex is inappropriate to talk about, it is likely they might find it difficult to discuss or be hesitant about discussing sex with their partners. This practitioner could also find it challenging to discuss sex with their clients, which in turn could make them think clients who bring up sex are acting inappropriately; in this way, the clinician ultimately causes harm to clients who needs intervention in this area.

As you engage in self-reflection in the next few sections, think of categorizing your thoughts as either values or beliefs, and think about how those values and beliefs were developed and then modified or solidified over time as the result of your life experiences. Development is fluid, but early life experiences are influential. The next section offers prompts to reflect on your early life development and the education and messages you received that have likely influenced your values, beliefs, and self-concept related to sexuality.

Early Concepts of Sex and Sexuality

Growing up, we all received direct and indirect messages regarding sex and sexuality. ***Direct messages*** are those that are explicitly communicated through information provided by family, siblings, friends, school, religious house of worship, books, community, and others. Examples include attendance at sexual health education classes at school or an elder sibling's teaching about periods and menstrual care. ***Indirect messages*** are those that are not taught directly to us but to which we are exposed through our family, communities, religious affiliations, media, and society—for example, how femininity is often portrayed in advertising or in television shows or the portrayal of sex and relationships in pornography.

Although we are asking you to reflect on direct and indirect messages you received growing up, those messages may not necessarily reflect what you currently think about sex and sexuality. Reflection Prompts 3.11–3.14 are intended to

REFLECTION PROMPT 3.11
Timeline of Sexual Health Information

Create a timeline, indicating different ages or stages, and reflect on your childhood and youth. Mark down at around what age you learned about sex, dating, relationships, puberty, menstruation, and other topics related to sexual health.

REFLECTION PROMPT 3.12
My Sexual Health Information Ecosystem

Think of your Sexual Health Information Ecosystem as all of the factors that influence your sexual health knowledge and understanding. Create a visual: Placing yourself at the center, and map out who (or perhaps also what) in your life growing up provided you with direct and indirect information about sexual health.

REFLECTION PROMPT 3.13
Messages I Received

1. What was my initial understanding of sex? Has this changed?
2. How did I understand why people had sex? What do I think about this currently?
3. Are there any sexual behaviors or practices that I engage in that I feel neutral or indifferent about? How or why did I start incorporating these practices?
4. Why do people have romantic relationships? How do I understand this now?
5. Who is desirable? Which bodies are desirable? Have my perspectives about this changed over time?
6. What did I learn about self-pleasure and masturbation? How do I feel about this now?
7. Do I carry any shame (i.e., a feeling of being inherently not worthy) around sex and sexuality? If so, why is that?
8. Do I have pride about myself as a sexual person? If so, why is that? What is the source of my pride, and is it internally driven or because I feel I am meeting what is expected of me by social standards?
9. What do I feel society tells me about how I should value myself as a sexual person? Where or from whom did I learn information about sexual health? How do I feel about this? What do I wish had been different?

REFLECTION PROMPT 3.14
Change Over Time

Think about your answers to Reflection Prompt 3.13. How have the answers changed over time? How have these messages influenced your current beliefs and values? Also consider the following questions:

1. Have I had experiences that made me question the validity of these messages? If so, what were they?
2. Are any of the messages I noted from childhood reinforced currently?
3. From these messages, what do I find potentially valuable? What do I find potentially harmful?
4. What messages informed some of my beliefs? As an adult, if those messages feel harmful and influence beliefs that are not supporting me as a sexual being, what can I do to begin to reframe them?

help you explore the sexual health information you received and how you feel about that information now.

Thought Experiments

Regardless of our identities and experiences, situations will arise in which we will be challenged to understand a client's perspectives and experiences, especially if we have not lived their same reality. ***Thought experiments*** allow us to imagine a world that is different from the one in which we currently live—a world in which all identities, genders, sexualities, and interests are given space to exist and be validated. This exercise is especially important for those privileged by their alignment with dominant paradigms, such as White, able bodied, monogamous, straight, and cisgender, because it might be the first time considering what a different world would be like. Reflection Prompt 3.15, a thought experiment, may support this perspective. In addition to noticing your responses to these questions, it may be worth noting what emotions come up for you as well.

Summary of Intrapersonal Reflection

Our sexual values, beliefs, and attitudes are shaped by our experiences. As we progress from childhood through adolescence and on to adulthood, we progressively

REFLECTION PROMPT 3.15
A Different World

1. What would it be like for you if we did not live in a heteronormative or cisnormative world?
2. How do you feel when sexual and gender minorities are centered either through experience or as characters in conversations about the general human experience of being a sexual being?
3. What would it be like if people from different racial, religious, and ethnic backgrounds had their sexualities uplifted and centered?
4. What biases or misunderstandings do you hold around the sexuality of those who are different from your own identity?

get more control over the information we consume and knowledge we acquire. In addition, we have progressively more acquired knowledge about ourselves because we have experiences that affect our understanding of ourselves as sexual beings. Our knowledge of sexual health and ourselves as sexual beings was always going to change throughout life and will continue to do so.

We encourage you to pause here and congratulate yourself for where you are right now in your self-knowledge. You have been integral in getting yourself to this point. Through strengthening self-reflection and by giving yourself permission to accept new versions of your sexual self, you will become well positioned to understand the complexities of sexuality for your clients and approach interventions without bias. The next section addresses knowing yourself with clients, which then segues into Chapter 4, "Bias and Clinician Harm," on understanding and reducing clinician bias and harm.

Interpersonal Self-Reflection: Knowing Yourself With Clients

The field of sexual health is complex and sensitive, and it brings with it many triggers. A ***trigger*** is a situation, stimulus, or experience that brings about distressing feelings, memories, or a combination of both, that pertain to sex, sexuality, and sexual health (see Reflection Prompt 3.16). These triggers can result in behaviors such as avoidance, hypervigilance, and emotional lability. As clinicians, it is important that we reflect on our triggers and their potential origin and then determine what we can do to ground ourselves when these triggers arise. Self-regulation strategies that are sensory based are important tools to use when triggered (see Chapter 9, "Trauma-Informed Care,"

REFLECTION PROMPT 3.16
My Triggers

1. What triggers (situations, stimuli, or experiences that result in distressing feelings) might you have in relation to sex, sexuality, and sexual health?
2. If you are unsure if you have triggers, are there aspects of sex, sexuality, and sexual health that bring you discomfort (e.g., emotionally, cognitively, physically, spiritually)?
3. Based on your responses to the previous question, can you anticipate what might trigger you in a professional setting?
4. Which of the following practices—in the moment of a trigger or discomfort—support your being present and feeling grounded:
   - diaphragmatic/deep breathing
   - progressive muscle relaxation
   - visualization strategies
   - use of calming scents
   - proprioceptive strategies, such as weighted blankets, walking, or exercising
   - auditory strategies, such as listening to calming music
   - cognitive strategies, such as journaling or repeating a meaningful phrase or mantra.
5. How can you begin to explore the origin of these triggers? How can you bring compassion and new understanding to them?

for more on the topic). Reflection Prompt 3.16 can guide you while you consider what your triggers might be and how you can navigate them in a professional setting.

Creating a Positive Client Experience

Sexual health, sex, and sexuality are perhaps the most challenging, personal, and nuanced areas that an occupational therapy practitioner will encounter in interacting with a client. As such, not only is intrapersonal reflection and processing space critical, as discussed earlier, but so, too, is setting a safe space for clients to share their challenges, concerns, and hopes about their sexual health. Given the complex nature of sexual health and the resulting feelings that may arise from such discussions, it may be helpful for you to explore community agreements with your client to create a brave space.

Community Agreements

Community agreements are typically used in group therapy or activities and educational settings to ensure, as much as possible, that the shared space is comfortable, equitable, and able to meet the needs of both the professional facilitator and the participants (Move to End Violence, n.d.). Common agreements that occupational therapy practitioners may set include those of confidentiality, equitable space and time for multiple people to engage in dialogue, or reflection on privilege and power dynamics within the group or on the client–professional dynamic. The following agreements may be helpful for the practitioner to not only hold internally with themselves but also share with their client when the therapeutic relationship is in its early stages (Move to End Violence, n.d.).

Simultaneity

The concept of ***simultaneity*** is that multiple truths and realities can exist at the same time. This is especially pertinent to sexuality, given its complicated and dynamic nature. It is important for the clinician–client relationship to hold simultaneity around sexuality rather than attempt to distill a particular situation. For example, a woman might experience pain with sex after childbirth, thus hindering participation in sexual intercourse. However, the client might continue to express and believe in herself as a sexual being as she explores nonpenetrative sex with her partner while undergoing treatment for the pain.

Depth without drowning

Sexuality can be complicated, as can addressing issues around it. To ensure that the client is progressing through their goals in a successful way, it is important that the clinician–client relationship find the "just-right challenge." Given the strong ties of sexuality to emotions, spirituality, trauma, memories, and so much more, the client must find depth within the work on sexuality without drowning and becoming overwhelmed.

Stay the whole time

Addressing sexuality is challenging and may require adaptations to the treatment plan, timing, and expectations. "Staying the whole time" acknowledges this and encourages both the client and the clinician to remain invested in the journey. This investment manifests as cognitive, emotional, and spiritual presence during the therapeutic relationship and the work and process outside of it. Staying the whole time is indicative of the need for investment by both parties in the therapeutic relationship and the work that lies ahead.

Struggle together

The relationship between clinician and client is essential during the natural peaks and valleys of the therapeutic process. It is furthermore important that the client not be made to feel that the therapeutic journey is theirs alone. The clinician's role is to act as ongoing support for the client, especially when problem solving and adaptations to the treatment plan may be needed to address issues that have arisen. Struggling together is both parties' understanding that although it is the client who is working toward their sexuality goals and outcomes, the clinician is beside them each step of the way.

Intersectional Lens

Intersectionality is a concept that was developed by Kimberlé Crenshaw, a legal scholar on civil rights, critical race theory, and Black feminist legal theory. Crenshaw (1989) used the term ***intersectionality*** to describe the experience of Black women's double bind of racial and gender prejudice in response to the feminist movement, which, too often, centered the White female experience by excluding discussions of racism. It is commonly defined as how race, class, gender, and other individual characteristics "intersect" and overlap with one another as well as connect with systems of oppression and discrimination. Given the intersectional nature of sexuality, it may be meaningful for the client to explore factors such as race, class, gender, and other social dynamics that may have affected their access to sexual health education or their sexual health overall. Intersectionality further lends credence to the important fact that sexuality cannot be distilled to a single experience or definition for everyone. It is up to each client to explore intersectionality, because it may have provided barriers that resulted in oppression of their sexuality or sexual identity (Coaston, 2019).

Therapeutic Use of Self

In addition to community agreements and the intersectional lens, therapeutic use of self is a powerful tool to use in discussions related to sexual health. A core concept in the field of occupational therapy, ***therapeutic use of self*** entails "working consciously with the interpersonal side of the therapeutic relationship to facilitate an optimal experience and outcome for the client" (Solman & Clouston, 2016, p. 1). Therapeutic use of self can be broken down into attunement, unconditional positive regard, self-disclosure, and balancing the power differential (Abson, 2019).

Attunement

Attunement is the ability to be completely present with your client, developing a feeling of connectedness with them. Attunement is even more critical when discussions of sexuality arise, given its sensitive, complex, and personal nature. With attunement, you should be considering what your body language is saying, how your tone of voice is delivering the message, whether your facial expressions and body language (including eye contact) match what you are saying, and whether you need to mirror the client for them to recognize that they have your full attention.

Unconditional positive regard

Unconditional positive regard is the ability to accept that the client is trying their best and accepting where they are at that time. Given the nature of sexuality, consider that a client's perspectives and needs around sexuality may be quite different from yours. Be aware of your triggers and how they might elicit biased thoughts and responses. The focus is always on providing client-centered care and treatment while allowing the client to make mistakes and encouraging their ability to make their own, self-determined choices.

Self-disclosure

Self-disclosure is a clinician's sharing of personal information (i.e., personal experiences) with clients and can occur intrasession (regarding what has happened within a session with a client) or extrasession (information from outside your client–clinician relationship; William & Mary School of Education, n.d.). Extrasession disclosure includes the sharing of information about yourself, whether that be previous experiences with other clients dealing with similar issues related to sexuality, your own experiences with sexuality, and other similar information. Both types of self-disclosure require a foundation of self-reflection.

Self-disclosure can be a positive experience for the client; it can help build rapport and develop a therapeutic alliance. In terms of considerations when self-disclosing, the clinician may want to reflect on the following before sharing personal information:

- Is this the right time and place to share your personal experiences?
- Is what you are about to share your own personal opinion or experiences (which should be stated), or is it factual?

- In terms of what you know about the client's values, is what you are about to share helpful?
- What possible effect(s) are you hoping that self-disclosure will have?

Balancing the power differential

Balancing the power differential between occupational therapy practitioners and clients is critical, because clients often believe that the practitioner has significant power over them. This belief can lead to passivity, whereas a practitioner should be promoting self-empowerment and self-help. Therefore, it is essential to understand the client in an intersectional way as it relates to sexuality as well as conduct an honest and vulnerable assessment of your own intersectionality as it relates to your own potential barriers to understanding and claiming your sexuality. The acknowledgment that you may know more about a possible solution to the client's problem based on your training and experience should be made while acknowledging that the client is the expert about themselves, their culture, their expectations, and their own lives. The client and the therapist should then be working together to problem solve how the "solution" that the therapist suggests can be integrated into the client's life based on the information the client has about themselves.

Summary

In this chapter, you have embarked on a journey from intrapersonal reflection to interpersonal reflection. Again, congratulate yourself on getting started doing the work so far to explore yourself as a sexual person—an activity many of us were never taught to do. As you continue this journey, we hope you feel better equipped to continue your self-reflection process with the questions and strategies we have provided. Knowing yourself as a sexual person is important to living a thriving life as an authentic sexual being in the way that you want to, but it is also imperative in order to address sexuality with clients.

Sameera Qureshi, MS, OTR, has worked at the intersections of Islam, mental health, and sexual health in school and community-based settings for the past 14 years. She is the founder of Sexual Health for Muslims, which is dedicated to providing online sexual health education and therapy services for Muslims and professionals who serve them. She is on the editorial board of the *American Journal of Sexuality Education;* serves as a contracted provider for Maven Clinic; and is a Wellness Advisor for the National Institutes of Health. Sameera is based in Virginia.

Kathryn Ellis, OTD, OTR/L, AASECT–SC, developed the Occupational Therapy Sexuality and Intimacy Clinic at Walter Reed National Military Medical Center in Bethesda, Maryland, and is the co-author of *Sex and Intimacy for Wounded Veterans: A Guide to Embracing Change.* She is the founder and CEO of a continuing education company, the Institute for Sex, Intimacy & Occupational Therapy. She is an American Association of Sexuality Educators, Counselors, and Therapists Certified Sexuality Counselor and a consultant on sexuality and intimacy projects and initiatives. Her private practice, Dr. Kathryn Ellis Sexual Wellness Counseling, is based in Delaware.

References

Abson, D. (2019, March 3). Therapeutic use of self. *The Occupational Therapy Hub.* https://www.theothub.com/post/therapeutic-use-of-self

American Occupational Therapy Association. (2020). Occupational therapy practice framework: Domain and process (4th ed.). *American Journal of Occupational Therapy, 74*(Suppl. 2), 7412410010. https://doi.org/10.5014/ajot.2020.74S2001

Betancourt, J., Green, A., & Carrillo, E. (2002). *Cultural competence in health care: Emerging frameworks and practical approaches.* The Commonwealth Fund.

Bordogna, A. L., Coyle, A. C., Nallamothu, R., Manko, A. L., & Yen, R. W. (2023). Comprehensive sexuality education to reduce pregnancy and STIs in adolescents in the United States: A systematic review and meta-analysis. *American Journal of Sexuality Education.* Advance online publication. https://doi.org/10.1080/15546128.2022.2080140

Bronfenbrenner, U. (1979). *The ecology of human development.* Harvard University Press.

Coaston, J. (2019, May 28). The intersectionality wars. *Vox.* https://www.vox.com/the-highlight/2019/5/20/18542843/intersectionality-conservatism-law-race-gender-discrimination

Crenshaw, K. (1989). Demarginalizing the intersection of race and sex: A Black feminist critique of antidiscrimination doctrine feminist theory, and antiracist politics. *University of Chicago Legal Forum,* Issue 1, 139–167. https://chicagounbound.uchicago.edu/cgi/viewcontent.cgi?article=1052&context=uclf

Cross, T. L. (1988). Services to minority populations: Cultural competence continuum. *Focal Point, 3*(1), 1–4. https://pathwaysrtc.pdx.edu/pdf/fpF88.pdf

Dahlberg, L. L., & Krug, E. G. (2002). Violence: A global public health problem. In E. Krug, L. L. Dahlberg, J. A. Mercy, A. B. Zwi, & R. Lozano (Eds.), *World report on violence and health* (pp. 3–21). World Health Organization.

Ellis, K. (2023). *This is how we do it: Sexuality and occupational therapy.* Lecture presented by The Institute for Sex, Intimacy and Occupational Therapy. www.sexintimacyot.com

Hammell, K. R. W. (2013). Occupation, well-being, and culture: Theory and cultural humility/Occupation, bien-être et culture: La théorie et l'humilité culturelle. *Canadian Journal of Occupational Therapy, 80,* 224–234. https://doi.org/10.1177/0008417413500465

Lorde, A. (2020). *Sister outsider: Essays and speeches.* Penguin Classics.

Merriam-Webster. (n.d.). Belief. In *Merriam-Webster.com dictionary.* https://www.merriam-webster.com/dictionary/belief

Move to End Violence. (n.d.). *Community agreements: Racial equity & liberation virtual learning series.* https://movetoendviolence.org/lp/relvirtuallearningcommunity-evergreen-registration

Nagoski, E. (2015). *Come as you are: The surprising new science that will transform your sex life.* Simon and Schuster.

Ott, K. (2017). Inviting perspective transformation: Sexual history awareness for professional formation. *Teaching Theology & Religion, 20,* 117–125. https://doi.org/10.1111/teth.12374

Planned Parenthood. (n.d.). *What is sex education?* https://www.plannedparenthood.org/learn/for-educators/what-sex-education

Planned Parenthood. (2016, November). *History of sex education in the United States.* https://www.plannedparenthood.org/uploads/filer_public/da/67/da67fd5d-631d-438a-85e8-a446d90fd1e3/20170209_sexed_d04_1.pdf

Sexuality Information and Education Council of the United States. (2022, July). *Sex ed state law and policy chart.* https://siecus.org/wp-content/uploads/2021/09/2022-Sex-Ed-State-Law-and-Policy-Chart.pdf

Solman, B., & Clouston, T. (2016). Occupational therapy and the therapeutic use of self. *British Journal of Occupational Therapy, 79,* 514–516. https://doi.org/10.1177/0308022616638675

Stayton, W. (1998). A curriculum for training professionals in human sexuality using the Sexual Attitude Restructuring (SAR) model. *Journal of Sex Education and Therapy, 23,* 26–32. https://doi.org/10.1080/01614576.1998.11074203

Tervalon, M., & Murray-García, J. (1998). Cultural humility versus cultural competence: A critical distinction in defining physician training outcomes in multicultural education. *Journal of Health Care for the Poor and Underserved, 9,* 117–125. https://doi.org/10.1353/hpu.2010.0233

West, L. M., Stepleman, L. M., Wilson, C. K., Campbell, J., Villarosa, M., Bodie, B., & Decker, M. (2012). It's *supposed* to be personal: Personal and educational factors associated with sexual health attitudes, knowledge, comfort and skill in health profession students. *American Journal of Sexuality Education, 7,* 329–354. https://doi.org/10.1080/15546128.2012.740945

Whitney, R. V., & Fox, W. W. (2017). Using reflective learning opportunities to reveal and transform knowledge, attitudes, beliefs, and skills related to the occupation of sexual engagement impaired by disability. *Open Journal of Occupational Therapy, 5.* https://doi.org/10.15453/2168-6408.1246

William & Mary School of Education. (n.d.). *The skill of self-disclosure.* https://counseling.education.wm.edu/blog/the-skill-of-self-disclosure

World Health Organization. (2006). *Defining sexual health—Report of a technical consultation on sexual health, 28–31 January 2002.* Sexual Health Document Series. Geneva.

World Health Organization. (n.d.). *Sexual health: Definitions.* https://www.who.int/health-topics/sexual-health#tab=tab_2

4

Sexuality, Bias, and Impact: Preventing Clinician Harm

Karrie L. Kingsley, *OTD, OTR/L;* **Joseph Christian Ungco,** *OTD, OTR/L; and* **Dominique H. Como,** *PhD, EdM, OTR/L*

CHAPTER HIGHLIGHTS

- Positionality
- Bias
- Clinician harm
- Historical context of occupational therapy and bias
- Bias in occupational therapy education
- Bias in research evidence
- How bias and clinician harm affect health care
- Addressing clinician bias and harm

KEY TERMS AND CONCEPTS

Advocates	Harm	Internalized bias
Allies	Homophobia	Nontargeted individuals
Bias	Implicit Association Test	Positionality
Context	Implicit bias	Targeted individuals
Critical self-reflection	Institutional bias	Transantagonism
Explicit bias		
Gender expansive		

Although sexual and intimate occupations are incredibly valuable and important to occupational therapy clients, many practitioners report barriers to addressing them in their routine occupational therapy practices (Conine et al., 1979; Lohman et al., 2017; McGrath & Sakellariou, 2016; McGrath et al., 2021). These occupations are often considered sensitive topics (i.e., requiring caution so as not to offend or be perceived as unprofessional or inappropriate).

But why are sexual and intimate occupations considered more sensitive than basic ADLs that frequently require client nudity, touch, and vulnerability, such as bathing or dressing? The answer relates to our society's sexual stigmas and taboos, which give rise to various biases. Therefore, enhancing occupational therapy practice to include sexual and intimate occupations requires practitioners to understand how bias influences their work and contexts as well as how it affects the clients and communities they serve. ***Bias,*** or prejudice in favor or against a person, group, or entity, influences our decision making and actions. Bias can be conscious or subconscious, and in both cases, it leads us to unfair actions and treatments toward others. When clinicians are influenced by bias, they practice in ways that can harm their clients.

Harm includes the many ways in which people can be negatively affected by action or inaction. Harm from bias results in physical, economic, psychological, and social detriment to individuals and groups. It can be internal, encompassing feeling excluded or unwelcome, having increased stress and mental distress, restricting oneself from accessing opportunities, and feeling less valuable. It can also be external, such as denial of treatment services, differential treatment, and doors closed to opportunity and participation.

In this chapter, readers will learn broadly about bias, clinician harm to clients resulting from bias, and strategies for reducing bias. This chapter also has several examples grounded in anti-LGBTQIA+[1] bias, because many LGBTQIA+ people's occupational experiences of bias overlap with aspects of the Occupational Therapy Sexual Assessment framework, including sexual activity as well as key constructs such as sexual self-view and sexual expression (Walker et al., 2020). Readers are reminded that many social identities are affected by bias in health care and bias surrounding sexual and intimate occupations. Readers are encouraged to seek additional resources on health care disparities for further understanding. Although occupational therapy practitioners may face a variety of biases based on their own personal identities (e.g., gender-based pay disparities), this chapter focuses on how practitioners can mitigate their own biases and risk of committing harm. In understanding bias and clinician harm, occupational therapy practitioners can improve their ability to address sexual and intimate occupations through a deeper understanding of contexts of practice and these occupational areas.

Positionality

Positionality is how someone is situated or positioned relative to systems of power and oppression in their society. This positioning is based on historical, cultural, and structural systems and how they either benefit or exploit one's social groups. Although everyone holds many social identities (e.g., race, gender, ability), the way

[1] The term *LGBTQIA+* communities refers to the diverse and unique communities formed by lesbian, gay, bisexual, transgender, queer, intersex, asexual, and other sexual and gender minoritized people. As greater awareness, social acceptance, and safety improve for these individuals and communities, new terms may emerge as language evolves to describe identities that exist outside of societal recognition and acceptance.

people experience their society and their environments is influenced by how these identities are positioned to be targeted or to act as agents within the system (i.e., society or environment).

Targeted individuals are those whose social identity groups are oppressed, marginalized, and exploited by an oppressor or dominant group's system of institutions (Nieto & Boyer, 2007). In the United States, these groups include Black, Indigenous, and other people of color; non-Christians; gender-expansive[2] people; women; LGBTQIA+ people; and people with disabilities. These groups are also sometimes labeled as "underprivileged," "disadvantaged," or "marginalized" communities. The use of the term *target* or *targeted* more accurately describes how the experiences of oppression and disadvantage in these groups are the result of systemic oppression and not of an inherent disadvantage or deficit within the groups.

Nontargeted individuals, also referred to as *agents,* are people who belong to dominant social groups who, through birth or acquisition, receive privileges, advantages, and benefits from the systems of power and oppression in their society (Nieto & Boyer, 2007). Agents can also be nontargeted groups. In the United States, agents include White people, Christians, cisgender men, heterosexual people, and people without disabilities. These groups are sometimes labeled as "privileged" or "advantaged." The use of *nontargeted* highlights that their lack of oppression is due to systems and institutions designed to not target their identities. The term *agent* captures the understanding that these groups (knowingly or unknowingly) have an active role in creating, sustaining, and perpetuating the inequities of our systems because their advantages are, in part, based on exploitation of targeted groups. This label is also a call to action because agents have the most power and influence to change systems and institutions so that they become more equitable for everyone.

It is important to understand positionality as we seek to raise awareness of our internalized biases because culture, history, and agency, or *targetedness,* influence these biases to a great degree. A person's positionality depends on context. For example, as an Asian American, chapter author Joseph Ungco's racial identity is targeted in the United States, but if they were to move to the Philippines, they would become a member of the dominant racial group and therefore acquire an agent, or nontargeted, positionality in terms of their race. Further, Tagalog, an official language of the Philippines, solely uses the gender-neutral third person pronoun *siya,*[3] so in this context, Dr. Ungco would not need to correct others on their pronouns and would likely experience less pronoun misuse than in the United States, where they are frequently misgendered with "he/him" pronouns or questioned about how to use the pronouns "they/them."

---

[2] ***Gender expansive*** is an umbrella term used to describe an ever-evolving range of individuals whose gender identity or expression differs from cultural norms prescribed by the dominant social group (e.g., transgender, gender nonconforming, nonbinary, genderqueer).

[3] *Siya* is the singular 3rd person pronoun in Tagalog used for people of any gender. This can be translated in English as "he/him," "she/her," and singular "they/them" simultaneously. In contrast, the pronoun *sila* is used for plural 3rd person (as in plural "they/them" in English).

An example of how racial targeting in the United States relates to sexuality can be seen in the history of anti-miscegenation laws. In the 1930s, cultural and political discourse stereotyped Filipino men as "assum[ing] the form of an American nativist-sculpted sexual beast, equipped with a penis impressive enough to penetrate all of white America, leaving a permanent stain of racial and social inferiority on its people (read: men)" (Tapia, 2006, p. 64). This anti-Filipino sentiment was used to rationalize proposed anti-miscegenation laws (Tapia, 2006), setting a unique context for Filipino men's racial experiences in the cultural context of the United States.

It is possible to understand how context and history shape perspectives by looking at LGBTQIA+ communities. A common perception in the United States is that transgender, nonbinary, and gender-expansive people are "new" or a sign of our contemporary and "progressive" world or that these identities are a sign of anti-religious ideology. These ideas are expressed by people saying, for example, "Back in the day, we just had men and women; all this new gender stuff is confusing." The idea that something is new because of the progressiveness of the time is an example of the influence that context and history have on shaping perspectives and bias. Gender-expansive people have existed throughout human history. Looking to other cultures and societies, however, can help lend perspective to assumptions within the U.S. context. For example, the Hindu American Foundation (HAF) asserts that Hinduism, the third largest religion in the world, holds LGBTQIA+ inclusion in its tenets and history (McDermott, 2021). Its religious texts (i.e., the *Vedas*) include *hijra*—or third-gender people—and treat same-sex relationships as normal parts of the spectrum of the human experience. The HAF stated, "In fact, it is bigotry towards LGBT people that is the Western and Abrahamic import into Indian society. This bigotry rose markedly during the time of British colonial rule, paralleling the Victorian-era view that homosexuality was one of the worst sins a person could commit" (McDermott, 2021, para. 5). Gender-expansive and same-gender-loving people are not new in our contemporary world; homophobia and transantagonism are the more recent changes in our society.

Authors' Note on Positionality

As authors it is important to take a moment to address our own positionality in relation to our identities, privilege, and experiences. Karrie Kingsley is White and middle class and was socialized as female. They are genderqueer and are partnered in a long-term monogamous queer relationship. Karrie experiences privilege in the areas of race, class, education level, ability, and size. Joseph Ungco is a queer person of color and first-generation American who has attained multiple levels of education, including their terminal degree. They were assigned male at birth and raised with masculine-attributed privileges in the northeast United States. Joe experiences privilege around perceived gender, education level, class, and ability. Pertinent to this chapter, as an Asian-American, they also experience privilege because of the "model minority" bias constructed and reinforced by U.S. society. Dominique Como is a cisgender, multiracial woman of color. Her intersecting identities have created both barriers to and facilitators of privilege. Dominique experiences privileges in the areas of sexuality, ability, and educational level.

Occupational Therapy's Positionality

To understand and address bias and the potential for doing harm, we must first understand our positionality in the context of U.S. society and the U.S. health care system. The *Occupational Therapy Practice Framework: Domain and Process* (4th ed.; *OTPF–4;* American Occupational Therapy Association [AOTA], 2020b) describes ***context*** as a "broad construct defined as the environmental and personal factors specific to each client (person, group, population)" (p. 9). The United States was founded on many principles that are now understood to be imperialist, capitalist, and White supremacist. Sociology professor Leland Saito (1998) summarized: "Throughout the history of the United States, race has been used by Whites for legitimizing and creating difference and social, economic and political exclusion" (p. 154). Occupational therapy practitioners born in the United States have been unavoidably raised, educated, and trained in an environmental context premised on these systems and ideologies. Practitioners born in colonized regions throughout the world may have been encultured with similar ideologies.

Although the *OTPF–4* describes the influence of the environmental component of context on clients, we occupational therapy practitioners are not immune to those factors, particularly the social attitudes, systems, and policies that have influenced the development of the profession and ourselves as practitioners. We draw from education, training, and policies that implicitly hold historic and institutional bias, and we replicate those perspectives in our cultural identification and attitudes toward others. These historic systems also affect our personal factors, including social background, status, upbringing, and life experiences, which formulate some of our psychological assets, habits, and behavioral patterns (see the *OTPF–4*, pp. 10–11).

The values of the occupational therapy profession are positively influenced by values from many cultural contexts that prepare occupational therapy practitioners to provide effective, inclusive, and client-centered care. For example, individualism, valued by U.S. culture and a hallmark of occupational therapy professional values, prepares practitioners for practicing client-centered care, upholding clients' autonomy and independence. This concept is a good fit for clients who come from individualistic cultures in the Global North, but it would be a poor fit for a client in the United States who values collectivism and interdependence with the people in their communities. In this example, culturally sensitive client-centered care would support the client and their community in mutual assistance rather than emphasize independence, as many occupational therapy measures do (e.g., the Executive Function Performance Test [Baum et al., 2008]; Katz Index of Independence in Activities of Daily Living [Katz et al., 1970]). However, this chapter is about bias and resulting clinician harm, so the content will focus on exploring the roots of bias, discussing ways to reconcile bias, and presenting antibias strategies.

The contexts in which we are raised hold social biases that later become internalized within our personal factors as we are educated and trained. Inevitably, we adopt these underlying biases into our personal attitudes and behaviors as practitioners. For example, if we are trained in biomedical models that identify sex as solely male or female, we may sustain and perpetuate historic and social biases of a binary view of sex that excludes people who are intersex. In addition, we may find it difficult to become accustomed to contemporary understandings of biological sex as a spectrum (Brusman, 2019; Montañez, 2017).

One way in which bias may manifest is by relying on gender norms in the occupational therapy assessment process without critically analyzing the extent to which a tool incorporates the biased idea of sex as aligning with gender as well as erroneously binary views on sex and gender. For example, an occupational therapy practitioner may wish to assess strength or fitness for a gender-expansive client by using a dynamometer to assess grip strength. Because the dynamometer is norm referenced according to binary gender (i.e., only men and women), the practitioner must decide how to interpret the results and how this interpretation will affect intervention decisions. If relying on assigned sex at birth, the practitioner risks misgendering and invalidating the client. They also risk delivering poor service from not having sufficient information and understanding of physiological changes through the client's transition (e.g., type and timing of hormone therapies). In addition, the client may be intersex and thus have a mixture of biological characteristics (e.g., hormones, chromosomes, anatomy) that are not captured by the limitations of a binary gender–based tool. By invalidating the client's gender, a practitioner can harm the client and introduce inaccuracies into the clinical decision-making process. Conversely, using tools that are nongendered or that include mixed-gender norms, such as the Bruininks–Oseretsky Test of Motor Proficiency (2nd ed.; Bruininks & Bruininks, 2005), may reduce the impact of gender bias in clinical decision making and validate the client's identity in the therapeutic process.

Many occupational therapy practitioners adopt the dominant social system's educational and systemic biases into their personal attitudes and behaviors. For these practitioners, relying solely on a gender-normed tool for their clients may be a manifestation of their own internalized bias influencing their behavior and clinical decision making. Other practitioners, however, may recognize that this approach will harm their client through invalidating their gender but feel unable to address this situation appropriately because of their biased education, training, and evidence-based practice. Being a more effective practitioner requires deep self-reflection to bring potential biases and their influence to light.

To understand how bias results in clinician harm, we must first critically reflect on our own positionality and our profession's position related to the society and systems in which we live. By understanding our societal and personal biases, we may begin the process of changing our behaviors to reduce the harm we may unknowingly commit in our practice.

Bias

Bias can play a detrimental role in clinical interactions and result in clinician harm. Bias includes explicit bias, implicit bias, and internalized bias. Typically, two forms of bias are discussed: implicit bias and explicit bias.

Implicit bias, sometimes referred to as *unconscious bias,* describes biased and stereotyped thinking that a person is not aware of (Kirwan Institute for the Study of Race and Ethnicity, 2012). We all carry implicit biases about many different things, but a person's implicit biases can affect their behavior toward others in negative ways without the person realizing it. Clinicians with implicit biases are at risk of perpetrating harm toward their clients. The following are examples of implicit bias and how it can harm patients or clients:

- A series of studies have demonstrated that medical professionals underestimate the level of pain experienced by Black patients. This implicit bias can lead to pain medications being recommended less frequently, not at all, or at smaller doses in Black patients compared with White patients with the same clinical presentation (Anderson et al., 2009; Hoffman et al., 2016).
- People often assume that someone who is overweight is not healthy and, conversely, that someone who is thin is healthy. In a medical setting, this bias may mean that bloodwork for health indicators is either deemed unnecessary or overrecommended, depending on the weight of the patient. Patients may not receive the care they need, resulting in harm.
- An occupational therapist assumes that an 85-year-old client does not engage in sexual activity and therefore does not address hip precautions for sexual activities, placing the client at risk for hip dislocation.
- An occupational therapy practitioner who is a specialist in pelvic floor issues does not include pain management techniques for a Black woman reporting pain with penis–vagina penetrative sex because of implicit bias underestimating the level of pain experienced by Black patients.
- When working with autistic youth, an occupational therapy practitioner assumes that the clients are cisgender and heterosexual. This implicit bias toward autistic clients is harmful because 69% of autistic people are LGBTQIA+ (George & Stokes, 2018) and are up to almost 7 times more likely to be transgender or gender expansive (Strang et al., 2014). The actions and behaviors of the practitioner, whether through commission or omission, may result in the client disengaging from occupational therapy treatment, experiencing negative mental health consequences, and not getting access to sexual health information that matches their sexual activity. The harm related to these biases places autistic youth at risk for victimization, sexually transmitted infections (STIs), suicide, and pregnancy. See Case Example 4.1, "Jenny," later in this chapter for an analysis of this type of biased scenario.

When confronted with implicit bias, a person's inclination may be to say that because it is unintentional, it is not harmful. This attitude is precisely what makes this bias *implicit* and why it often leads to harm, even when clinicians think they are being well-meaning.

Explicit bias is overt, intentional bias. Examples of explicit bias include expressions of racism, transantagonism,[4] homophobia,[5] sexualization or asexualization, and antireligious attacks. A person expressing explicit bias is doing so intentionally but may not view the actions as expressions of personal bias—rather, they might attribute the bias to "policy," "my religion," or "budget issues." Explicit bias is often cached in White supremacy and supports the oppression of another group based on negative beliefs toward that group. The following are examples of explicit bias and how occupational therapy practitioners and others use explicit bias to exclude specific people from treatment or reject particular topics in therapy or education:

- In health care, a doctor cites religious beliefs to justify denying care for a transgender patient. An emergency department turns away homeless or low-income patients because of their inability to pay for services.
- In occupational therapy regarding sexual and intimate occupations, an occupational therapy practitioner intentionally avoids discussing sexual activity with an LGBTQIA+ client because they "disapprove of the lifestyle" and consider queer sex to be "abhorrent." A practitioner who is personally against premarital sex provides sexual and intimate occupation interventions only for married couples.
- In academia, a professor approves a student's sex and intimacy doctoral project only if it involves sex regarding straight, married clients because of their hatred toward LGBTQIA+ people. A faculty member states that "sex and intimacy isn't important to focus on. Disabled people have much more important things to think about, like toileting."

Internalized bias is bias toward one's own in-group that occurs through socialization. This kind of bias values the dominant group over their own identity. An example of internalized bias would be an LGBTQIA+ person who has been socialized that their identity as an LGBTQIA+ person is "bad"; they therefore develop biases about their own identity as inferior to heterosexual people. This internalized bias leads to harm, such as a closeted politician who promotes anti-gay legislation, or a transgender person believing they deserve poor treatment from providers because they have internalized messages that being transgender is "abhorrent."

---

[4] ***Transantagonism*** refers to hostility toward transgender people and those who are perceived as transgender.

[5] Although phobias are generally thought of as an extreme fear, ***homophobia*** refers to hostility, hatred, or prejudice against same-gender-loving people or those perceived to not be heterosexual.

Clinician Harm

Clinician harm occurs when a clinician's biases affect their interactions with clients or patients and their clinical care decisions. To prevent harmful client interactions, occupational therapy practitioners first need to become aware of implicit, unconscious biases and then use active strategies to prevent expressing them. All forms of clinician harm reinforce health care disparities for minoritized communities.

Two mechanisms are hypothesized to link implicit bias to health disparities. The first is that health care providers make different decisions regarding care based on their implicit bias, which in turn can negatively affect recovery and overall health and cause harm (Zestcott et al., 2016). The second is that provider behaviors convey their bias, which, in turn, erodes trust on the part of the patient; as a result, they do not follow the provider's recommendations, leading to harm (Zestcott et al., 2016).

An occupational therapy practitioner's assumption that older adults do not engage in sexual activity and resulting avoidance of the topic places the client at risk for increased STIs and engaging in contraindicated sexual activities. (See Chapter 5, "Sexual and Intimate Occupations Across the Lifespan," for further discussion on ageism and sexuality, and Case Example 4.2, "Theo," later in this chapter, which describes how ageism may influence a provider's approach to sex and intimacy treatment.) Assuming a client is heterosexual, cisgender, and monogamous influences the practitioner's interactions and therapeutic use of self in a way that prompts the client to protect themself by not disclosing specific occupations, including ADLs and sexual and intimate occupations, leading to increased risk for a variety of negative outcomes. For example,

- A gay client recovering from hip or back surgery might not feel safe disclosing sexual positioning, leading to increased risk of contraindicated movements.
- A straight, polyamorous client with posttraumatic stress disorder might not mention all of their romantic partners, who are key parts of their social support system.
- A nonbinary client with impaired sensation in their hands might engage in chest compression wrapping as an ADL, but because of fear of the practitioner's judgment, they are at increased risk of pneumonia or cracked ribs without an appropriate compensatory strategy for their hand function.

Studies have also shown that when adolescents experience a negative health care encounter, they are less likely to return for follow-up care (Tobin et al., 2018). This bad experience can affect a client's long-term engagement in the health care system and health management occupations. It is critical that occupational therapy practitioners actively reduce the risk of bias and harm in their practices because these problems can have lifelong implications for their clients.

Historical Context of Occupational Therapy and Bias

The occupational therapy profession was birthed from several social and philosophical paradigms around the turn of the 20th century (Andersen & Reed, 2017). Those paradigms included mental hygiene, moral treatment, arts and crafts, pragmatism, and the settlement house movement. Each contributing influence contained biased and problematic perspectives. The founders of the profession all were White middle- to upper-class men and women. The mental hygiene movement was informed and led by eugenicists. The settlement movement was strongly informed by religious beliefs related to helping the less fortunate without much consideration given for the systemic reasons that kept some people disadvantaged while privileging others. In addition, occupational therapy was designed to be a "women's profession," and early recruitment efforts for students and faculty focused on White upper-class women (Mahoney, 2020). It is important to point out that the men who helped to found the occupational therapy profession had no intention of participating as practitioners because they believed that occupational therapy was women's work, not worthy of their participation (Frank, 1992). The profession did not graduate its first Black students until 1946 and advised against admitting people with disabilities into the profession until the passing of Section 504 of the Rehabilitation Act in 1973 (P. L. 93-112), which made it illegal to exclude such people (Mahoney, 2020).

It should not be surprising that as a profession today, occupational therapy remains disproportionately composed of White women and does not reflect the diversity of the U.S. population (AOTA, 2020c). The huge disparity between the profession's demographics in the United States and the diversity of the U.S. population historically and today has implications for the breadth and depth of perspectives on occupation and health. Further research is needed to understand how our historical context influences other demographic disparities such as sexual orientation, gender identity, socioeconomic status, ability, and religion compared with client and population diversity (AOTA, 2020c).

Occupational therapy theorists insist that all occupations fall into three basic categories: self-care, work, and play. Insisting on universal experience of purpose has been called into question as perpetuating ableist, individualistic, and patriarchal ideologies. In addition, in the face of evidence that occupations may live outside these categories, the profession has been accused of being dogmatic (Hammell, 2009). Many rich and meaningful activities, including sexual activity, are grouped under the umbrella of self-care. As a profession, we situate sexuality as perfunctory, which does not capture the richness and nuance of the experience or of the breadth of expressions of sexual activity. It is probable that many people experience sexual activity as an occupation in and of itself and would object to categorizing it alongside brushing one's teeth.

Bias in Occupational Therapy Education

Based on data collected during 2020 academic year, occupational therapy programs graduated 73% White and 91% female students at the doctoral level, 73% White and 89% female students at the master's degree level, and 70% White and 85% female students at the occupational therapy assistant level (Harvison, 2021). Note that data captured only the sex categories of male, female, and other. Faculty in occupational therapy education doctoral-level programs is 79% White and 91% female (Harvison, 2021). The current accreditation requirement for faculty to have a doctoral degree to teach in a professional occupational therapy program perpetuates a faculty pool that is overwhelmingly White and female. This disproportionate representation has a cascading effect across education, practice, and research in the occupational therapy profession. If prospective students, research subjects, and clients do not see themselves reflected in the profession, it will adversely affect student recruitment and retention, research validity, and client care.

Educational standards are one way to hold professional occupational therapy educational programs and their faculty accountable to teaching and preparing future occupational therapists to be effective clinicians and researchers across points of difference. The Accreditation Council for Occupational Therapy Education (ACOTE®; 2018) recently updated the required educational standards for implementation in 2020. Not a single standard requires that programs explicitly address race, racism, or discrimination in health care; furthermore, no standard explicitly includes sexuality. Occupational therapy educators are disproportionately White and are under no specific guidelines to teach beyond that perspective or to even consider that they might be teaching only from their own perspective. In addition, current ACOTE standards, in the context of requirements for "diversity factors" (Standard B.1.2), include the problematic phrase "lifestyle choices," which for decades has been used to oppress LGBTQIA+ communities. Using this phrase implies that LGBTQIA+ people can equally choose to be cisgender and heteronormative, likening one's inner concept of self to choosing a lifestyle practice such as becoming a vegan.

One example of how an aspect of White culture can dictate the occupational therapy profession is to consider the impact of purity culture on the professional attitudes and tendencies for sexuality and intimacy. *Purity culture* is a teaching in some White evangelical Christian churches and youth groups that dictates absolute sexual abstinence before heterosexual marriage. The teachings are directed mostly toward women and teach "the oppression of their bodies, restricting sexual agency, and teaching a shame response to pleasure" (Natarajan et al., 2022, p. 316). Purity culture views men as unable to control themselves sexually and women as the gatekeepers of men's sexual desire (Owens et al., 2020).

Considering the lack of occupational therapy educational content related to sexuality and intimacy, occupational therapy practitioners raised in the context of purity culture could easily carry such biases with them into the clinic. For example, a female practitioner might worry that she is responsible if her male clients flirt with her. If her occupational therapy curriculum did not center pleasure, and if she feels a general hesitancy to speak about sex because she was taught that women should not talk about sex, then this practitioner could overlook addressing clients' sexual occupations and cause clinical harm (Case Example 4.3, "Kara," illustrates how purity culture can influence a provider approaching sexual and intimate occupational therapy). To help divest from the influences of purity culture in occupational therapy education, occupational therapy professors can look toward feminist and queer literature that position pleasure as worthy of discussion and also tend not to pathologize common sexual issues such as low desire and pain (Jones, 2019). Using this lens, the occupational therapy profession can begin to see occupational therapy's role in discussing the factors that influence desire, pain management strategies, and techniques for pleasure.

In *Queering the Color Line: Race and the Invention of Homosexuality in American Culture,* Somerville (2006) described how negative attitudes toward LGBTQIA+ people in the United States developed in alignment with negative attitudes toward racial minorities. According to Somerville, White ideologies around racial inferiority were applied to LGBTQIA+ people as a way to justify discrimination based on "sexual deviance" beginning in the late 19th century. Given the historical role of White racial ideologies in defining racial and sexual deviance, it is worth critically reflecting on how these historical narratives persist in a majority White profession founded in the early 20th century. How might these histories and ideologies influence views on sexual and intimate practice? The persistence of negative historical narratives causes harm and sets the tone for the profession to perpetrate harm toward LGBTQIA+ communities.

Bias in Research Evidence

Much of the worldwide research evidence in health care is focused on Western, educated, industrialized, rich, and democratic (WEIRD) societies (Masuda et al., 2020). There has been rising criticism in fields such as medicine and psychology regarding bias in the research data based on an overrepresentation of White men and lack of representation of many groups, including

- people from racial and ethnic groups minoritized in WEIRD societies;
- LGBTQIA+ people;
- women;
- children;
- older adults;

- people with disabilities, barriers to accessing health care, lower incomes, or limited educational attainment; and
- residents of rural areas (National Institutes of Health, 2019).

A recent study used qualitative methods to explore barriers perceived by researchers when recruiting diverse people into clinical trials for cancer treatment and found many iterations of explicit bias influencing patient selection (Niranjan et al., 2020). Among these biased perspectives were the views that patients who are non-English speaking or are Black are not protocol compliant and therefore are excluded from clinical trials (Niranjan et al., 2020). Another study found that surgical research is likely to reflect the sex bias of the surgical profession, with evidence suggesting that male authors in surgical research include more male than female patients in their studies (Xiao et al., 2018).

In 2018, the *American Journal of Occupational Therapy* reported 74% of articles represented U.S. authors despite submissions from 24 countries (Richards, 2019). Of the international submissions that were published, a majority were from European countries or Canada, which also fall within the WEIRD umbrella. Other leading occupational therapy journals (e.g., the *British Journal of Occupational Therapy,* the *Canadian Journal of Occupational Therapy,* the *Australian Occupational Therapy Journal*) also tend to represent WEIRD societies. Like other sciences, occupational therapy and its practitioners are at risk for informing clinical decisions with research data that are gleaned from a limited population. These data reflect only the "minority world," meaning only 7% of the global population falls into the WEIRD category (Hammell, 2009). As the U.S. population becomes increasingly diverse, we are at a point where the majority of our clinical populations fall outside of the existing body of evidence.

It is critical for us, as evidence-based occupational therapy practitioners, to understand that bias and limitations in theory and evidence both perpetuate historic harm and exclusion and reduce our capacity to provide high-quality care. Although bias can often be thought of as a lack of education, in reality, it can be learned or reinforced by our education and training. A study in the *Proceedings of the National Academies of Science* found that half of a sample of White medical students and residents endorsed false beliefs about biological differences between Black and White people, such as "Black people's skin is thicker than White people's skin," "Black people's nerve endings are less sensitive than White people's," and "Black people's blood coagulates more quickly than White people's" (Hoffman et al., 2016, p. 4298). This example illustrates how historical eugenicist beliefs in biological race differences, dominance of limited perspectives in education and training (i.e., White, cisgender, upper-middle class, Western educated), and exclusion of the full representation of our country and world demographics in research saturate health care and become normalized in the work we do within it.

How Bias and Clinician Harm Affect Health Care

Over the past decade there has been greater attention to the role of institutional and interpersonal mechanisms of oppression in the health care field (Egede et al.,

2021; Sabin, 2022; Williams & Rucker, 2000; Yearby et al., 2022). Looking at bias at the institutional level can elucidate the mechanisms contributing to social determinants of health and how medical institutions cause further harm through practices that create additional barriers for targeted, minoritized, and historically oppressed communities. People who experience disparities also often experience negative care interactions, which make them more likely to avoid seeking care and therefore further exacerbate the disparity, trapping them in a negative feedback loop.

Institutional bias includes policies and practices within institutions (e.g., health care, education, criminal justice system) that, regardless of intent, result in different outcomes for different racial or ethnic groups (Serchen et al., 2021). Institutional bias in the medical industrial complex is well established (Serchen et al., 2021). Additionally, there is a long history of medical atrocities perpetrated against members of minoritized and oppressed communities, including Black, Indigenous, immigrant, and Latine/Latinx[6] people. The Tuskegee experiments, forced sterilizations, and other callous acts have had lasting effects on trust of the medical community. Health care environments are full of biases and barriers, including ableism, fat phobia and shaming, devaluation of interdependent family units,[7] and noninclusive forms and records. Access issues, including health insurance access and coverage, privatization and price gouging of medications, and lack of translation services are also problems. Specifically regarding sexuality, LGBTQIA+ people in many places are still unprotected, criminalized, and considered to have mental health and identity disorders by the medical community (Neumann et al., 2021). Historically, LGBTQIA+ people have been subjected to corrective methods, including electroshock, aversion therapy, lobotomies, castration, and sedatives (Hipp et al., 2019). Conversion therapy is still practiced across the United States despite condemnation by the American Psychological Association and the American Medical Association.

A study by Zestcott et al. (2016) measured bias in health care providers and found biases toward African Americans, Latinos, gay and lesbian people, Native Americans, people who are obese, people with low socioeconomic statues, drug users, and wheelchair users.[8] Beyond identifying the existence of these biases, multiple studies have suggested that these biases affect client care. For example, when given the exact same clinical scenarios and patient presentation information, health care providers made different treatment recommendations for patients who were identified as Black on the documentation (Zestcott et al., 2016). Several studies have found that compared with White patients, Black patients, including children,

---

[6] *Latinx* is used here as a gender-neutral term in standard American English to refer to people of Latin American origin or descent. We would like to draw attention to the associated term *Latine*, which is a more common gender-neutral term within Latinx communities because it draws from Spanish linguistic structure versus the Anglicized "Latinx."

[7] Interdependent family units include a variety of familial constellations beyond the White cisnormative nuclear family structure, such as intergenerational cohabitating families, "chosen family" structures, single parents coraising children with other single parents, blended families, and polyamorous families.

[8] The social identity terms listed are the ones named and measured by Zestcott et al. (2016).

are underprescribed pain medications (Hoffman et al., 2016). In addition, medical students who had greater racial bias in assessing the pain of Black patients also had greater racial bias in treatment recommendations for Black patients (Hoffman et al., 2016).

Societal biases also apply to sexual and intimate occupations in a variety of ways along lines of race, ability, age, and additional identities. WEIRD society oversexualizes or fetishizes some people and considers others nonsexual beings. Specific racial and ethnic groups are subject to a range of sexual biases. Examples include bias toward Black people as having larger than average genitalia, Latinx people as being more passionate, and Asian people as having smaller than average genitalia. In addition, trends in either devaluing the sexuality of people with disabilities or fetishizing such people have been reported (Mona et al., 2017). Older adults are not considered as sexual as younger people. If clinicians have implicit biases around race, ethnicities, sexual minority communities, ages, and disabled individuals, these biases can be expressed through the clinical decisions made about addressing clients as sexual beings.

Addressing Clinician Bias and Harm

Bias exhibited by clinicians, whether explicit (conscious) or implicit (unconscious), can drastically affect clinical care decisions, treatment, and client–provider interactions. To reduce the expression of bias, it is first essential to acknowledge that bias exists and identify where it may show up (i.e., within oneself, encounters, and contexts). Second, it is crucial to increase knowledge of specific communities to yield positive change and take action. Done in conjunction, these steps can lead to dismantling oppression, improving health disparity outcomes, and providing accessible and equitable care. This section details some of the resources available to identify biases and take action.

Identifying Bias

One of the first steps to identifying bias is to prime oneself to look for it. Camara Jones is a family physician, epidemiologist, and the past president of the American Public Health Association. Her work focuses on the effects of racism on health and well-being. As a teacher, her allegories on race and racism illuminate topics that are otherwise difficult for many to understand and discuss.

One of Jones's more prominent allegories, sometimes referred to as the dual reality of racism, or the restaurant saga, showcases how what is evident to some may be simultaneously invisible to others (Jones, 2016). In this story, Jones shares that when she was a medical student, after a night of studying, she headed out to find somewhere to eat. While sitting in a late-night eatery, the restaurant had closed, but she saw a sign on the door that read "open." She recognized that the sign on the door was double-sided, and although it read "open" to her and everyone inside the restaurant, it read "closed" to everyone outside the restaurant. So, what is the big deal?

The duality of the sign meant that some, such as Jones and her friends, could continue to eat and remain comfortably inside the restaurant while those outside would likely remain hungry and unserved. Unlike Jones, others may not recognize that the sign is double-sided. In fact, for many already seated in the restaurant, there may be no impetus to look at the sign at all. They may not believe that those outside want to get in, because if they did want to come in, why would they not just walk in like those seated had? They may choose to consciously block out those on the outside because their discomfort is of no concern to them. This example highlights the dual reality of many experiences, showing how those in a position of privilege may not even recognize systems of inequity. Therefore, one must be primed to look for biases—to see both sides of the sign.

Critical self-reflection (e.g., being open to admitting shortcomings) is a crucial next step to identifying potential bias. One way to do this is to complete the ***Implicit Association Test*** (IAT; Greenwald et al., 1998). The IAT measures associations between concepts and stereotypes or evaluations. The IAT is an online assessment that asks people to associate evaluative words with concepts (e.g., fat people/good). An implicit preference is identified when categorization occurs quickly (e.g., associating positive words such as *happy, delight*, and *magnificent* with straight people and associating negative words such as *awful, humiliate*, and *horrible* with gay people).

Upon completion of the IAT, the user is provided with a summary of groups that they have an automatic preference for compared with other groups. This report could be used to aid further self-reflection. Asking and honestly answering the following questions may be an excellent first step in recognizing an area requiring additional self-work: What was surprising? What was in alignment with what I believe to be true about myself? How do I feel about the results? (For more information about the IAT, see Project Implicit, https://implicit.harvard.edu/implicit.)

It is essential to consider how biases may reveal themselves. As previously mentioned, bias is ever present and can be found in many contexts. For example, there is a tendency to surround oneself with similar people. In and of itself, this inclination is not negative, but it has been cited as a rationale for why disparities persist in areas such as employment and real estate. Research has shown that people with typical Anglo-sounding names get more interviews than those with international- and "Black"-sounding names and frequently are offered a higher salary when hired (Boyd-Swan & Herbst, 2019; Lippens et al., 2022; Mobasseri, 2019). Additionally, research has shown that bias exists in housing practices (Asplund et al., 2020; Faber, 2018). In majority Black or Hispanic communities, homeowners typically experience lower property evaluations, which can contribute to less economic mobility, keeping these homeowners in the same community.

These critical experiences shape how members of these targeted groups are positioned in our society (e.g., their sense of belonging) and affect their occupational opportunities. Home ownership affects a family's educational opportunities and, thus, their education-related occupations, and employment discrimination directly affects the occupations of work. Both areas, particularly health literacy and access to health care, influence health status and health management. Occupational therapy practitioners need to understand these interrelated structures and how bias manifests in them to better understand the complex context of our clients. Reflection Prompt 4.1 includes questions to consider.

Aging is an inevitable outcome for everyone, if they are lucky. In the United States, however, age bias is prevalent but often overlooked. It is especially common in the media. For example, it is well documented that women in Hollywood are often shamed for growing older, and the number of starring roles available for older women remains limited compared with those available for men. Reflection Prompt 4.2 provides questions for consideration regarding aging and sexuality.

Taking Action

Bias in ourselves is unavoidable, but critical self-reflection provides a solid foundation upon which to begin the antibias journey. This section describes ways to take action.

REFLECTION PROMPT 4.1
Encountering Diversity

- How diverse are your social groups and workplace?
- How diverse was your community growing up?
- How diverse is your current neighborhood?
- How might differences in neighborhoods, workplace, and upbringing affect perspectives on sexual and intimate occupations?
- If you received sexual health education, how diverse was it?
- Did you mostly learn about people who belonged to different racial identities through being friends, romantic partners, classmates, teammates, roommates, or coworkers or mostly through media outlets, for example, rap music or watching telenovelas?

REFLECTION PROMPT 4.2
Aging and Sexuality

- What do you think about aging adults?
- Do you consider older adults to be less valuable?
- How do you feel when you think about older adults as sexual beings?
- How has your view of yourself shifted as you age? How might it continue to shift in the future?
- How do you see yourself as an older adult? What about as a sexual older adult?
- How do you see the sexual desirability of older adults portrayed in the media? In your community?
- What kind of role models do you have for aging as a sexual and intimate being?

Educate yourself

Take the time to learn about others. Seek first-person accounts about other races, religions, and genders to understand better. This education can be accomplished through various methods, including reading books and listening to podcasts. You can also seek connections with those who are unlike you. Look at your community; is it diverse? If not, find ways to expand your circles. Maybe that means attending a different church, enrolling your child in a different Little League, or joining a support group in the next town. The goal of expanding these communities is to learn from others, have more diverse experiences, engage in difficult conversations, actively listen, and constantly reevaluate your biases. Remember, however, that the onus is not on people in targeted groups to educate agents. More formal ways to educate yourself include taking culturally responsive training courses or reading journal articles written by scholars from targeted groups.

Encourage inclusivity

Some strategies to encourage an antibias environment range from advocating for organizational change to displaying inclusive materials. For example, universal design, which creates an environment that is usable and beneficial to all, can ensure that everyone can access services and spaces regardless of common barriers. Another tool is to create accessible materials, pamphlets, and resources. In addition to making materials accessible, they can also be inclusive. For example, having images in a waiting room representative of our diverse society may make people feel more comfortable. Another approach is to develop policies that support inclusivity, such as creating intake forms that allow the client to write in their demographic information without being forced into checking traditional boxes. This strategy could include an open textbox for "gender identity" instead of providing only "male, female, and other"[9] as options.

Be an ally or, better yet, an advocate

Allies are people with power and privilege who recognize that some members of society are targeted. They empathize with people of targeted groups when they are mistreated and take action to minimize the impact through support and assistance. ***Advocates*** are similar to allies in their position of power and privilege; however, their approach to supporting targeted groups extends beyond individual protections. They instead proactively attempt to advocate for systemic change and dismantle systems of oppression.

[9] There are some problems with this example. The option of "other" implies that the respondent is abnormal and undesirable. It asserts the provider's expectations of who is included in their community (i.e., male and female only) and who by definition is atypical or unwelcome. Additionally, *male* and *female* are sex terms, not gender identities (e.g., *hijra, kathoey*, man, nonbinary person, two-spirit person, woman).

Allyship is often interpersonal and addresses an immediate concern (e.g., when an occupational therapist corrects a colleague who misgenders a client). One way to be an ally is to speak out against bias. For example, interrupt when you hear a biased comment, question why someone has made a hateful statement, educate others about the offensive language used, or echo someone who has spoken up about an injustice (Delacroix, 2018).

Although being an ally is terrific, some literature suggests that advocates are necessary to effect change. Advocacy can be thought of as acting for a cause; it includes systemic and proactive action to address the underlying issues of bias and inequity. An example of an occupational therapy practitioner advocate is one who takes initiative on organization-wide changes such as updating health record forms to include space for pronouns, bringing in trainers on gender-affirming care, and working with the team on a process for triaging when biased incidents occur in their practice. (Note that these strategies all address the original issue and client while benefiting future clients and others in the organization.) Advocates participate in talks, rallies, and protests; they promote the equitable distribution of power and opportunities; and they support those in positions of power who want to increase equity (Pulsely, n.d.).

Allies and advocates can come from all backgrounds and social groups, but it is important to emphasize that those from nontargeted or agent groups have even more ability (and therefore, more responsibility) to influence structural change. When people first learn they are agents in systems of power, they might feel guilt or shame for benefiting from exploitation of targeted groups. Remember that although agents perpetuate the system (unintentionally or not), they also have greater influence within the system to make change. The following are a few key points to keep in mind as you work to support targeted groups:

- Be open to listening.
- Do the inner work to figure out how you participate in oppressive systems.
- Amplify the voices of others.
- Do not act as an expert when you are not.
- Do not assume that every member of a group feels oppressed and needs to be "saved" (Guide to Allyship, n.d.).

Be prepared to make mistakes

Mistakes will happen, no matter how much introspection you do, how much you educate yourself, and how much of an ally or an advocate you have been. What is important is how you handle the mistake. It can be tough to be confronted with a shortcoming or to think that your actions have caused harm, especially if that was not your intention. Your instinct might be to protect yourself by becoming defensive, your mistake is an opportunity for growth. Most people easily respond to everyday offenses (e.g., bumping into someone on the sidewalk). In that instance, your instinct is to apologize and keep walking. It rarely feels like it should be that simple when you make a mistake involving bias, but it should. When an offense is identified, it is vital to recognize that regardless of intent, impact matters, so focus on the affected person, listen, and apologize. After the incident, you can determine the extent to which this area needs further reflection (i.e., a previously unseen bias or a misstep on your journey).

Exhibit 4.1 summarizes foundational, reactive, and proactive strategies for mitigating bias. Exhibit 4.2 is an example of a patient handout designed to minimize bias.

EXHIBIT 4.1
Strategies for Mitigating Bias

Learning About Bias: Foundational Strategies

- Take the Implicit Association Test (Greenwald et al., 1998) or other implicit bias test and reflect on the results:
  - Engage in practices of critical self-reflection and cultural humility practices (see Chapter 3, "Guided Self-Reflection of Self as a Sexual Being," for additional Reflection Prompts to guide this practice).
  - Reflect on what contextual factors influenced your results, and actively seek out opportunities to learn about and engage with your "less preferred" groups.
  - Consider ways to compensate for your implicit preferences, and be intentional about how you approach interactions with these groups (e.g., be kinder, be more thorough, pause to reflect before responding).
- Learn more about systems of oppression and how bias manifests in health care:
  - Read journal articles, books, and other media on systems of oppression and bias in health care.
  - Seek out continuing education sessions on health disparities and social determinants of health.
  - Work with your institution to understand where gaps in care are occurring, and look for patterns consistent with health disparity or targeted identity group research.
- Build your capacity for identifying and mitigating bias:
  - Start a journal club, community of practice, or mentoring circle focused on addressing bias and equity.
  - Work with colleagues to practice how you would respond to biased incidents: Avoid role-playing where one of you pretends to be a targeted identity, and focus on addressing the biased incident from your own positionality.
  - Engage in activities to build resilience and accountability: Work with trusted colleagues on apologizing for missteps when implicit bias arises, avoid centering yourself, and create solutions that focus on the person affected or harmed.

(Continued)

EXHIBIT 4.1
Strategies for Mitigating Bias *(Cont.)*

Responding to Bias (in the Moment): Reactive Strategies

- *Interrupt.* Speak up against biased remarks, even when they are labeled as jokes. For example, say "That joke isn't funny" or "I know we're talking about your sexual and intimate occupations, but saying that women are only good for sex is demeaning and unacceptable."
- *Ask simple, direct questions.* Question why the speaker made the comment, or lead them to assess their own bias. For example, ask "What do you mean by that?" or "Are you saying that all people with disabilities aren't interested in sex?"
- *Recognize that ignorance or lack of exposure to diverse people may be at the root of the issue, and provide an opportunity to educate.* Use facts and knowledge to bring better understanding to the speaker. For example, say
  - "That term is antiquated because it's harmful. Do you know the history of that word? I can tell you more about it."
  - "I used to call older adults 'cute' too, but I learned that infantilizing older adults is one of the reasons I feel so uncomfortable using a sexuality and intimacy assessment with them."
  - "Actually, only 15–25% of females orgasm from penis–vagina penetration, but 75–85% of females orgasm from clitoral stimulation. That said, what we really need to do is ask her how she orgasms because we really have no way of knowing otherwise."
- *Amplify the messages of others who intervene.* If someone else interjects, uplift and echo what they did. This action helps create momentum for change. For example, say "Thank you for saying that, Johnny. I agree that term is derogatory and offends me as someone who cares about our community here." (Note that the speaker is including themself as someone offended by the bad behavior instead of saying that it is offensive to the target group. This response is one way to show solidarity and model collective action).
- *Redirect colleagues to their professional ethics and responsibility.* If a colleague violates the profession's or workplace's code of ethics, remind them of their professional responsibilities. For example, say, "I am not suggesting you need to revoke your religion, but as providers we have a responsibility to provide ethical care for all people, including LGBTQIA+ people, to our best ability. What you did was against our code of ethics, so let's talk about how we can correct this and improve the health of the clients you harmed."
- *Call for a time out and hold a quick meeting to intervene.* Some teams select a code word, such as "purple flag," when bias may be showing up. This term is used to signal concerns that warrant assessment, conversation, and reflection specifically about situations of bias (as opposed to concerns regarded as "red flags"). A purple flag signals a pause in the action to assess whether bias is at play. For example, as practitioners set up in a pediatric clinic, Kaia calls out "Purple flag," which gets everyone's attention. She then states, "I noticed that everyone's grabbing toys for only one gender with their clients: GI Joes for the ones assigned male at birth, Barbies for the ones assigned female at birth. We may be reinforcing gender norms that don't actually apply to some of these kids. Maybe we can all take a moment to make sure we have both GI Joes and Barbies at-hand. And we can also grab an extra toy or two that's gender neutral, like Legos. That way, we're not limiting the clients, and they can have a range to choose from as they like."

(Continued)

EXHIBIT 4.1
Strategies for Mitigating Bias *(Cont.)*

- *Reflect as a group after an initial bias intervention and analyze the response for additional opportunities.* Bias intervention often comes up "in the moment," such as when someone says something problematic or a client voices a complaint. After applying the above strategies, occupational therapy practitioners and teams can hold a debrief meeting to reflect on what went well and other concerns that the team can address related to bias. For example, after Kaia calls "purple flag" in the previous example, the team could meet at their next break or at the end of the day to talk about how applying Kaia's recommendation went with their clients. This can reinforce for the team when positive encounters happen: "My new client surprised me by only picking the new toys I grabbed this session instead of the ones I had tried last time." Reflection also opens opportunities for new thinking: "Thanks, Kaia, for the suggestion! I also noticed that all of the dolls here are White. Can we find some more appropriate toys, either race neutral or reflective of our clients' demographics?"

Reducing Risk of Bias (In the Future): Proactive Strategies

- Seek to prevent opportunities for bias to manifest:
  - Remove names from résumés when hiring.
  - Use open-ended questions or forms when assessing clients.
  - Provide multiple ways of interacting (e.g., written, visual, verbal).
- Diversify the automatic messages you receive from society or culture:
  - Follow diverse perspectives on social media.
  - Intentionally seek media, books, and resources from people in targeted groups (e.g., searching online for "sex and disability" or "race, gender, sexuality, and disability" or for specific targeted identities such as "Black, disabled, and sexuality" will yield a variety of resources, collections, and authors with perspectives beyond those of nontargeted identity groups).
  - Engage in continuing education provided by people in targeted groups (e.g., Multicultural, Diversity and Inclusion Network, Occupational Therapy and Disability Studies Network).
- Review intake forms and materials in your setting with a critical eye:
  - Ensure that forms use gender-neutral or gender-inclusive language (e.g., "Are you dating?" vs. "Do you have a boyfriend/girlfriend?").
  - Rewrite handouts to have a wide representation of identities and to reflect the community you are serving (e.g., use multiple languages in handouts; include images with a mix of races, genders, and abilities).
  - Make sure materials are accessible across a variety of disabilities (e.g., physical, cognitive, emotional), languages, cultures of the people you serve (e.g., are meal-planning activities for dates centered on White American foods despite serving a primarily Latin American community?), and socioeconomic conditions (e.g., provide options for low- or no-cost positioning equipment for sexual activities).
- Engage all staff in training and problem solving:
  - Determine how your team will recognize, address, and prevent biased incidents in clinical care (e.g., use a "purple flag" system, follow up with a patient questionnaire, use the reflective Extended PLISSIT [*p*ermission, *l*imited *i*nformation, *s*pecific *s*uggestions, and *i*ntensive *t*herapy; Taylor & Davis, 2007] model).
  - Choose journal articles or in-services that will help your team have a shared language and foundational knowledge to be effective in reducing bias.
  - Agree on how your team will work together to increase comfort and competence with incorporating sex and intimacy into the practice setting.
  - Determine what resources and mutual support will help the team start providing sex and intimacy services for the first time.
  - Establish how clinicians will document and bill for sexual and intimate occupations. Make sure administrators are aware and understand how these occupations fit into the scope of occupational therapy.

EXHIBIT 4.2
Example of Inclusive Handout

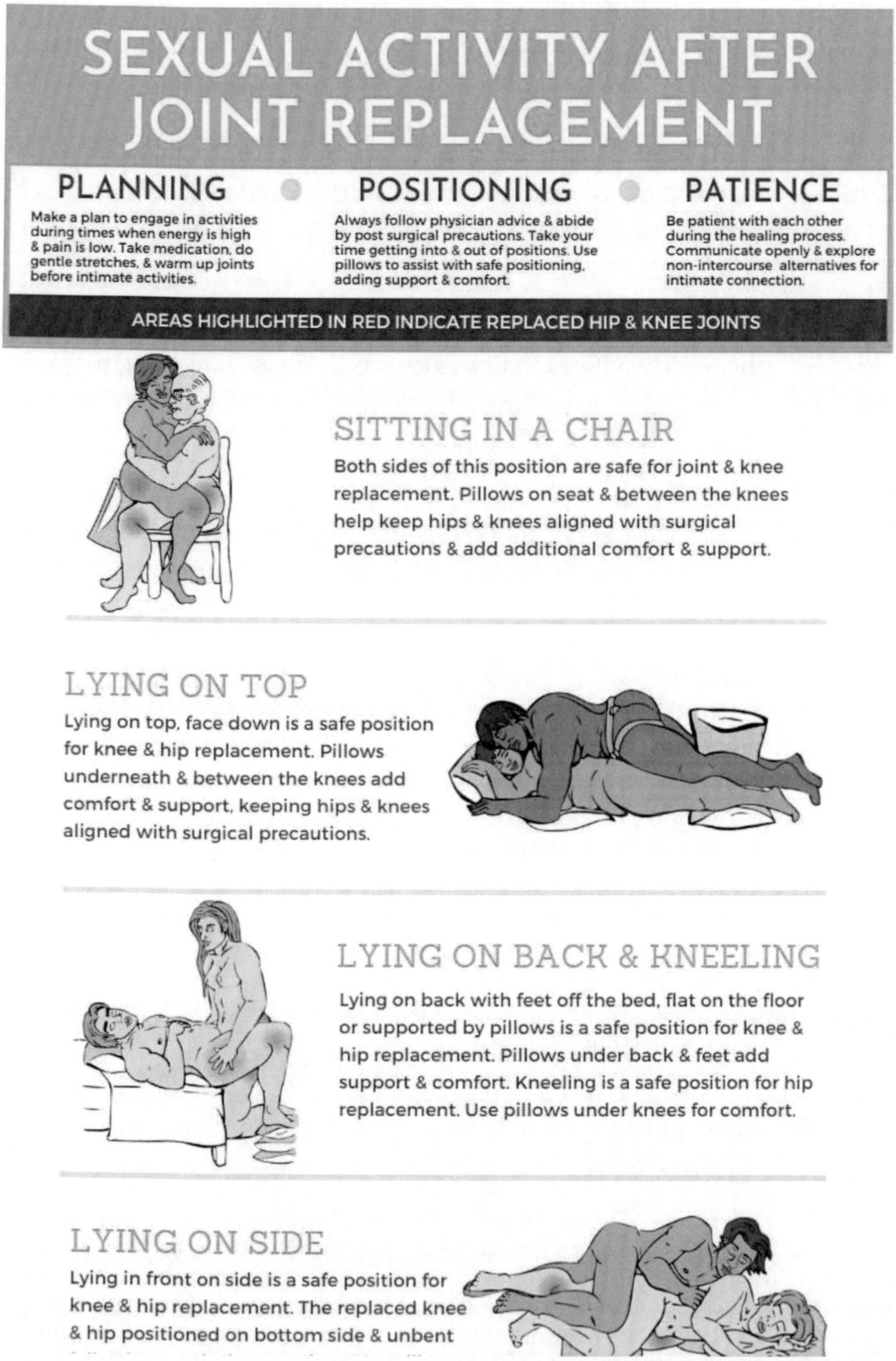

Source. From "Inclusive Infographic and Handout on Safe Sexual Positioning After Joint Replacement Surgery," by J. Hutchinson. EnbyOT. https://www.enbyot.com/sex-after-joint-replacement/. Copyright © 2020 by J. Hutchinson. Used with permission.

CASE EXAMPLE 4.1. JENNY: TRANSANTAGONISM HARMING CLIENT SELF-VIEW

An occupational therapist has a client who is a 3-year-old transgender girl, **Jenny.** The therapist writes a goal for Jenny to increase their engagement in "play appropriate for boys." The clinical director reviewing the therapist's documentation caught the goal before the parents received it. During a follow-up observation of a clinical session, the director observed the therapist gender policing[10] the child during a session by stating, "Those toys are for girls; you can't play with them."

How bias shows up

The occupational therapist has strong values and beliefs that "there are only two genders." The therapist wanted Jenny to behave in ways that reflected her sex assigned at birth. This aim was in direct conflict with the family's goals and desires.

Impact of bias

This example is a case of explicit bias. Lack of acceptance and misgendering are highly associated with suicide risk for transgender children and youth (Haas et al., 2014; Lefevor et al., 2019; The Trevor Project, 2019). In addition, the occupational therapist's bias is detrimental to the client's identity development, which can shape how their sexual self-view develops as they age. For example, if the child experienced gender policing from the therapist and continued to experience gender-policing messages and aggressions throughout their development, they may, as an adult, experience anxiety and shame around their gender identity. In the short term, they may be distressed because the occupational therapist denied them the toys they wanted to play with. If they continue to experience gender-policing and biased encounters, they could internalize them over time. These feelings may lead them to engage in sexual and intimate occupations in negative and unhealthy ways, for example, posturing a masculine versus a feminine expression during sex. They may also learn to distrust the health care system and avoid routine care such as STI screenings.

Bias intervention

The parents were distressed when Jenny reported the occupational therapist told her she couldn't play with girl toys but appreciated the clinical director for intervening before the therapist could further harm Jenny. The clinical director reprimanded the

[10] *Gender policing* consists of acts that impose or enforce "normative gender expressions on an individual who is perceived as not adequately performing these via their appearance or behavior" (British Columbia's Office of the Human Rights Commissioner, 2020, para. 1). Often, gender-expansive individuals experience gender policing in how providers and other people impose or enforce gender conformity (e.g., telling a gender-fluid person "only girls wear dresses; that's not for you.").

(Continued)

CASE EXAMPLE 4.1. JENNY: TRANSANTAGONISM HARMING CLIENT SELF-VIEW *(Cont.)*

therapist because their actions were a direct violation of the *AOTA Occupational Therapy Code of Ethics* (AOTA, 2020a); reassigned the client; and made sure more inclusive, client-centered goals were written. To prevent this issue from recurring, the clinical director brought in consultants to review intake forms as well as provide in-service training on gender-affirming care. In addition, the team advocated for a more robust nondiscrimination policy at their institution and instituted a diversity statement as part of their application process when hiring new therapists.

Risks without bias intervention

The following risks to the client could occur if bias intervention is not initiated:

- Health care encounters that traumatize clients set the stage for ineffective health management and increased risk of a variety and severity of conditions as a result of clients avoiding routine and necessary care.
- The biases of Jenny's occupational therapist introduced and reinforced patterns of transphobia, affecting the child's safety and social participation. Transphobia is known to increase risk for a variety of health conditions, including anxiety, self-harm, and suicidal ideation. In addition, it sets an example that the child's gender identity will not be accepted and may negatively affect the child's sexual self-view in later life. It also deprives them of meaningful occupations related to their roles as a young girl.
- If the child adopts negative attitudes toward their gender identity and sexual self-view, they will be placed at increased risk of victimization for sexual assault and intimate partner violence because they may engage in risky behaviors to keep their identity secret. This maladaptive coping strategy is the result of internalizing the belief that they deserve poor treatment.

CASE EXAMPLE 4.2. THEO: AGEISM TOWARD SEXUAL OCCUPATIONS

An occupational therapist is working with **Theo,** a 63-year-old man with a new diagnosis of Parkinson's disease. When the therapist asks questions about his occupational profile, he states that he has recently started dating again after the death of his wife. The therapist adds goals for going to restaurants and theaters for date-night activities. Theo asks if they could also talk about occupations for "late night date-night activities." The therapist interprets this correctly as being about sexual activities, becomes uncomfortable, and says, "That sort of thing isn't part of therapy."

(Continued)

CASE EXAMPLE 4.2. THEO: AGEISM TOWARD SEXUAL OCCUPATIONS *(Cont.)*

How bias shows up

The occupational therapist has adopted implicit messages from society infantilizing older adults, with the assumption that they are not sexually active. She adds dating activities to the occupational profile because she thinks it's "cute" for Theo to date, but she stops short of affirming his full sexuality as a human being. She also states her explicit belief that sex and intimacy are not a part of occupational therapy, despite their inclusion in the *OTPF–4*.

Impact of bias

A combination of explicit and implicit bias is present in this case. A common stereotype of older adults is that they are nonsexual, and they are often infantilized (i.e., considered "cute"), which in this case affects the occupational therapist's ability to view Theo as an autonomous adult who deserves access to the full range of occupations that he finds meaningful. People with new diagnoses often have questions about how their most meaningful occupations might be affected, making it critical for occupational therapy practitioners to provide clients with compassionate and accurate information. The result of this therapist's biases may prompt the client to develop erroneous beliefs about his ability to engage in sexual activity. In addition, because the therapist denied that these occupations are a part of the scope of occupational therapy practice, the client may not follow up on the subject with future providers.

Bias intervention

Theo, who believed he asked for assistance from the incorrect health care professional, asked one of the nursing staff from the same care agency for support. The nurse referred him to a support group for people with Parkinson's disease and brought his question to a team meeting. When the occupational therapist expressed her awkwardness, the team encouraged her to reflect on the biases causing her discomfort and suggested she increase her knowledge and skills regarding sexuality. They advised her about participating in continuing education opportunities and mentorship and learning how to use the Occupational Performance Inventory of Sexuality and Intimacy (Walker et al., 2020) and the Extended PLISSIT [*p*ermission, *l*imited *i*nformation, *s*pecific *s*uggestions, and *i*ntensive *t*herapy; Taylor & Davis, 2007] Model to support her in future client care situations.

Risks without bias intervention

The following risks to the client could occur if bias intervention is not initiated:

- This experience reinforces ageism that the client may have experienced.

(Continued)

CASE EXAMPLE 4.2. THEO: AGEISM TOWARD SEXUAL OCCUPATIONS *(Cont.)*

- The client may be at increased risk of STIs (see Chapter 5, "Sexual and Intimate Occupations Across the Lifespan").
- The client may not receive the care needed to engage in sexual activity safely, placing him at increased risk for falls and injuries during sexual activity.
- The client will have a limited understanding of the impact of his health condition on sexual and intimate occupations.
- The occupational therapist will continue to avoid providing guidance to clients about sexual activity, placing all future clients at risk.
- The occupational therapist's response perpetuates erroneous understanding of occupational therapy services.

CASE EXAMPLE 4.3. KARA: BIAS IMPEDING CARE

Kara is a certified occupational therapy assistant in her mid-20s. She works in acute rehabilitation on a cancer unit. She never addresses sexuality with her clients, and neither do her fellow occupational therapy practitioners. A 25-year-old male client, with whom Kara has worked for about 5 weeks and maintained a strong therapeutic rapport, flirts with her during treatment in the therapy gym one day. Kara immediately feels ashamed, unprofessional, and worried about whether other clients and practitioners heard the flirtation. She abruptly ends the treatment session and tells the client, "That's inappropriate."

How bias shows up

Kara's reactions are likely based on implicit biases, such as the idea that advances from men are ultimately the responsibility of women to manage, possibly developed from cultural messages around purity culture (see the "Bias in Occupational Therapy Education" section). She is worried that her coworkers may have heard the flirtation and that she will get in trouble for it. She feels ashamed for "bringing it on" and wonders whether she did something to provoke or invite the flirtation. Kara also believes that a playful flirtation is always unprofessional. She acknowledges that her place of work is not likely to be a place she should be initiating flirtations; however, she fails to acknowledge that her client is not at his place of work. In addition, the client may not be familiar with the social norms

(Continued)

CASE EXAMPLE 4.3. KARA: BIAS IMPEDING CARE *(Cont.)*

of a hospital setting and may view it as an appropriate place to meet a potential romantic partner. Although the occupational therapy practitioner is in her place of work, the client is living his real life.

An additional personal factor for Kara that could create a bias within the therapeutic relationship is that the flirtation from the client reminds her of the continual unwanted advances she receives from men outside of work and within work from other hospital staff. She used to correct such advances with tact and kindness, but she realized this approach was not effective. She found a direct and firm approach was more effective with stopping flirtation when it was unwanted, so she felt this would be the best approach to use with the client.

Impact of bias

The impact of these biases leads Kara to message shame to the client by saying his flirtations are inappropriate without explanation about why and terminating the treatment session. Given the context of life-altering experiences from the cancer diagnosis and treatment, it is possible that the client was practicing the social skill of flirting again with someone with whom he felt safe, given their strong therapeutic rapport. The resulting negative outcome could be the client thinking that his behavior was inappropriate because he is disabled, not desirable, or both. Moreover, the flirtation may have been the client's only way to communicate that he is a sexual being, because sexuality was never addressed with him.

Bias intervention

In this case, bias intervention can include several strategies, such as

- *Self-reflection.* Occupational therapy practitioners should ask, "Am I taking too much accountability for this client's behavior?" "Is this harassment, degrading communication, or playful flirtation?" "Will I get in trouble for this?" They should also recognize the difference in context (workplace for the practitioner vs. not for the client).
- *Proactively addressing sexuality.* Addressing sexuality with clients up front will avoid clients' having to communicate indirectly, through jokes or flirtation.
- *Discussion on problem solving.* Clinic leadership can facilitate a dialogue on problem solving that includes
  - Explicitly stating that client flirtations are not the responsibility of the clinician
  - Differentiating among playful flirtation, degrading communication, and harassment and acknowledging it is sometimes hard to distinguish among them

(Continued)

CASE EXAMPLE 4.3. KARA: BIAS IMPEDING CARE *(Cont.)*

- o Clarifying strategies for responding to playful flirtation, degrading communication, and harassment, such as setting verbal boundaries in response to flirting and reporting harassment to the charge nurse and occupational therapy supervisor
- o Scripting responses that practitioners can use when a client flirts with them, such as, "Oh, I think you're either asking me out or flirting with me. I can't accept or flirt back, and I'd appreciate it if you didn't flirt with me again. That said, it sounds like you might have a goal for meeting a romantic partner, which is definitely something we can talk about in our treatment sessions. Is that the case?"

Risks without bias intervention

Without bias intervention, this client may begin to internalize that he is not a desirable partner or asexualize himself. Especially if the client lacks affirmation in other realms of his life, this encounter could tip the balance toward internalizing the negativity of Kara's reaction as reflective of his desirability and sexuality. This internalization may be reinforced in subsequent encounters with Kara and other health care providers and contribute to the following risks:

- The client might seek sexual experiences that are secretive and risky because he may feel he no longer has access to romantic and sexual partners. He may want to ask women on dates but defer to friend relationships because he does not see himself as worthy of a romantic relationship.
- Due to a sexual self-view that he is deficient, the client may overcompensate by giving, either emotionally, sexually, or materially, in romantic relationships without consideration of his own sexual wants because he is "just glad to have someone and is afraid they'll leave him." This self-view also puts him at risk for exploitation or abuse from intimate partners.
- The occupational therapy practitioner may have contributed to mental health difficulties the client already has as a result of the stigma from his cancer diagnosis. Therefore, the client may become less motivated to engage in therapy, diminishing his progress in all aspects of the process, including in occupations not involving sexuality and intimacy.

Summary

Acknowledging that bias exists within ourselves and in our encounters and contexts is the first step in dismantling oppression, improving disparities in health outcomes, and providing accessible and equitable care for all occupational therapy clients. This acknowledgment includes understanding that although environmental and cultural contexts have positively influenced occupational therapy professional values, bias is embedded within the profession's history, education, research, and practices. In addition, sexual and intimate occupations are often ignored, avoided, or inadequately addressed in occupational therapy practice as a result of these biases and historical influences.

Biases (whether conscious or unconscious) exhibited by clinicians can drastically affect clinical care decisions, treatment, and client–provider interactions. These institutional and interpersonal mechanisms of oppression contribute to disparities experienced by targeted, minoritized, and historically oppressed communities. Therefore, occupational therapy practitioners must diminish their expression of bias by learning about bias, actively responding to it, and reducing the risk of future bias.

Karrie Kingsley, OTD, OTR/L (they/them/theirs), is the associate chief inclusion and diversity officer and an associate professor of clinical occupational therapy in the Chan Division of Occupational Science and Occupational Therapy at the University of Southern California in Los Angeles. Their scholarly activities are largely focused on increasing the knowledge and skills of health professionals to become more inclusive practitioners.

Joseph Christian Ungco, OTD, OTR/L (they/them), is the associate director for diversity, equity, and inclusion (DEI) education, client services, and data analytics for the Fred Hutchinson Cancer Center in Seattle. They lead several organization-wide diversity, equity, and inclusion initiatives, including the bias mitigation education program and gender-inclusive and accessible spaces initiative. They also continue to serve in DEI roles in occupational therapy, including serving as cochair of the national Network for LGBTQIA+ Concerns in Occupational Therapy and sitting on the executive council for the Occupational Therapy Multicultural, Diversity and Inclusion National Network. Dr. Ungco's work is centered on amplifying the voices of those most affected by systems of oppression and actualizing structural change.

Dominique H. Como, PhD, EdM, OTR/L (she/her/hers), is a postdoctoral associate in the Department of Occupational Therapy, School of Health and Rehabilitation Sciences, at the University of Pittsburgh. Dr. Como's research interests include reducing disparities by improving the overall health care experiences of underserved populations who are affected by social injustices based on policies implemented at the systemic level and manifested on the societal, interpersonal, and individual levels.

References

Accreditation Council for Occupational Therapy Education. (2018). Accreditation Council for Occupational Therapy Education (ACOTE®) Standards. *American Journal of Occupational Therapy, 72*(Suppl. 2), 7212410005. https://doi.org/10.5014/ajot.2018.72S217

American Occupational Therapy Association. (2020a). AOTA 2020 occupational therapy code of ethics. *American Journal of Occupational Therapy, 74,* 7413410005. https://doi.org/10.5014/ajot.2020.74S3006

American Occupational Therapy Association. (2020b). Occupational therapy practice framework: Domain and process (4th ed.). *American Journal of Occupational Therapy, 74*(Suppl. 2), 7412410010. https://doi.org/10.5014/ajot.2020.74S2001

American Occupational Therapy Association. (2020c). Occupational therapy's commitment to diversity, equity, and inclusion. *American Journal of Occupational Therapy, 74*(Suppl. 3), 7413410030. https://doi.org/10. 5014/ajot.2020.74S3002

Andersen, L. T., & Reed, K. L. (2017). *The history of occupational therapy: The first century.* Slack.

Anderson, K. O., Green, C. R., & Payne, R. (2009). Racial and ethnic disparities in pain: Causes and consequences of unequal care. *Journal of Pain, 10,* 1187–1204. https://doi.org/10.1016/j.jpain.2009.10.002

Asplund, J., Eslami, M., Sundaram, H., Sandvig, C., & Karahalios, K. (2020). Auditing race and gender discrimination in online housing markets. *Proceedings of the International AAAI Conference on Web and Social Media, 14,* 24–35. https://doi.org/10.1609/icwsm.v14i1.7276

Baum, C. M., Connor, L. T., Morrison, T., Hahn, M., Dromerick, A. W., & Edwards, D. F. (2008). Reliability, validity, and clinical utility of the Executive Function Performance Test: A measure of executive function in a sample of people with stroke. *American Journal of Occupational Therapy, 62*(4), 446–455. https://doi.org/10.5014/ajot.62.4.446

Boyd-Swan, C., & Herbst, C. M. (2019). Racial and ethnic discrimination in the labor market for child care teachers. *Educational Researcher, 48,* 394–406. https://doi.org/10.3102/0013189X19867941

British Columbia's Office of the Human Rights Commissioner. (2020). *Gender policing.* https://bchumanrights.ca/glossary/gender-policing/

Bruininks, R. H., & Bruininks, B. D. (2005). *Bruininks–Oseretsky Test of Motor Proficiency* (2nd ed.). Pearson.

Brusman, L. (2019, June 14). *Sex isn't binary, and we should stop acting like it is.* Massive Science. https://massivesci.com/articles/sex-gender-intersex-transgender-identity-discrimination-title-ix/

Conine, T. A., Christie, G. M., Hammond, G. K., & Smith, M. F. (1979). An assessment of occupational therapists' roles and attitudes toward sexual rehabilitation of the disabled. *American Journal of Occupational Therapy, 33*(8), 515–519.

Delacroix, J. (2018, November 14). *Speak up against hateful rhetoric.* Learning for Justice. https://www.learningforjustice.org/magazine/speak-up-against-hateful-rhetoric

Egede, L. E., Walker, R. J., & Williams, J. S. (2021). Intersection of structural racism, social determinants of health, and implicit bias with emergency physician admission tendencies. *JAMA Network Open, 4*(9). https://doi.org/10.1001/jamanetworkopen.2021.26375

Faber, J. W. (2018). Segregation and the geography of creditworthiness: Racial inequality in a recovered mortgage market. *Housing Policy Debate, 28,* 215–247. https://doi.org/10.1080/10511482.2017.1341944

Frank, G. (1992). Opening feminist histories of occupational therapy. *American Journal of Occupational Therapy, 46,* 990–999. https://doi.org/10.5014/ajot.46.11.989

George, R., & Stokes, M. A. (2018). Gender identity and sexual orientation in autism spectrum disorder. *Autism, 22,* 970–982. https://doi.org/10.1177/1362361317714587

Greenwald, A. G., McGhee, D. E., & Schwartz, J. L. (1998). Measuring individual differences in implicit cognition: The Implicit Association Test. *Journal of Personality and Social Psychology, 74,* 1464–1480. https://doi.org/10.1037//0022-3514.74.6.1464

Guide to Allyship. (n.d.). *The work of allyship.* https://guidetoallyship.com/#the-work-of-allyship

Haas, A. P., Rodgers, P. L., & Herman, J. L. (2014, January). *Suicide attempts among transgender and gender non-conforming adults: Findings of the National Transgender Discrimination Survey.* American Foundation for Suicide Prevention and The Williams Institute. https://queeramnesty.ch/docs/AFSP-Williams-Suicide-Report-Final.pdf

Hammell, K. W. (2009). Sacred texts: A sceptical exploration of the assumptions underpinning theories of occupation. *Canadian Journal of Occupational Therapy, 76,* 6–22. https://doi.org/10.1177/000841740907600105

Harvison, N. (2021). *Academic programs annual data report: Academic year 2019–2020.* American Occupational Therapy Association.

Hipp, T. N., Gore, K. R., Toumayan, A. C., Anderson, M. B., & Thurston, I. B. (2019). From conversion toward affirmation: Psychology, civil rights, and experiences of gender-diverse communities in Memphis. *American Psychologist, 74,* 882–897. https://doi.org/10.1037/amp0000558

Hoffman, K. M., Trawalter, S., Axt, J. R., & Oliver, M. N. (2016). Racial bias in pain assessment and treatment recommendations, and false beliefs about biological differences between Blacks and Whites. *PNAS: Proceedings of the National Academy of Sciences, 113,* 4296–4301. https://doi.org/10.1073/pnas.1516047113

Jones, A. (2019). Sex is not a problem: The erasure of pleasure in sexual science research. *Sexualities, 22,* 643–668. https://doi.org/10.1177/1363460718760210

Jones, C. (2016). How understanding of racism can move public health to action: Allegory highlights dual reality of privilege. *The Nation's Health, 46*(1), 3.

Katz, S., Downs, T. D., Cash, H. R., & Grotz, R. C. (1970). Progress in the development of the index of ADL. *The Gerontologist, 10*(1), 20–30. https://doi.org/10.1093/geront/10.1_Part_1.20

Kirwan Institute for the Study of Race and Ethnicity. (2012, May 29). *Understanding implicit bias.* https://kirwaninstitute.osu.edu/article/understanding-implicit-bias

Lefevor, G. T., Boyd-Rogers, C. C., Sprague, B. M., & Janis, R. A. (2019). Health disparities between genderqueer, transgender, and cisgender individuals: An extension of minority stress theory. *Journal of Counseling Psychology, 66,* 385–395. https://doi.org/10.1037/cou0000339

Lippens, L., Baert, S., Ghekiere, A., Verhaeghe, P. P., & Derous, E. (2022). Is labour market discrimination against ethnic minorities better explained by taste or statistics? A systematic review of the empirical evidence. *Journal of Ethnic and Migration Studies, 48,* 4243–4276. https://doi.org/10.1080/1369183X.2022.2050191

Lohman, H., Kobrin, A., & Chang, W. (2017). Exploring the activity of daily living of sexual activity: A survey in occupational therapy education. *Open Journal of Occupational Therapy, 5,* 1–11. https://doi.org/10.15453/2168-6408.1289

Mahoney, W. J. (2020). A historical overview of occupational therapy education. In S. D. Taff, L. C. Grajo, and B. R. Hooper (Eds.), *Perspectives on occupational therapy education: Past, present, future* (pp. 13–30). Slack.

Masuda, T., Batdorj, B., & Senzaki, S. (2020). Culture and attention: Future directions to expand research beyond the geographical regions of WEIRD cultures. *Frontiers in Psychology, 11,* 1394. https://doi.org/10.3389/fpsyg.2020.01394

McDermott, M. (2021, June 11). *Homosexuality isn't a Western import to India, but bigotry against LGBT people is.* Hindu American Foundation. https://www.hinduamerican.org/blog/homosexuality-not-western-import-india-bigotry-is

McGrath, M., Low, M. A., Power, E., McCluskey, A., & Lever, S. (2021). Addressing sexuality among people living with chronic disease and disability: A systematic mixed methods review of knowledge, attitudes, and practices of health care professionals. *Archives of Physical Medicine and Rehabilitation, 102,* 999–1010. https://doi.org/10.1016/j.apmr.2020.09.379

McGrath, M., & Sakellariou, D. (2016). The Issue Is—Why has so little progress been made in the practice of occupational therapy in relation to sexuality? *American Journal of Occupational Therapy, 70,* 7001360010. https://doi.org/10.5014/ajot.2016.017707

Mobasseri, S. (2019). Race, place, and crime: How violent crime events affect employment discrimination. *American Journal of Sociology, 125,* 63–104. https://doi.org/10.1086/703883

Mona, L. R., Cameron, R. P., & Clemency Cordes, C. (2017). Disability culturally competent sexual health care. *American Psychologist, 72,* 1000–1010. https://doi.org/10.1037/amp0000283

Montañez, A. (2017, September 1). Beyond XX and XY: The extraordinary complexity of sex determination. *Scientific American, 317,* 50–51. https://doi.org/10.1038/scientificamerican0917-50

Natarajan, M., Wilkins-Yel, K. G., Sista, A., Anantharaman, A., & Seils, N. (2022). Decolonizing purity culture: Gendered racism and White idealization in evangelical Christianity. *Psychology of Women Quarterly, 46,* 316–336. https://doi.org/10.1177/03616843221091116

National Institutes of Health. (2019, November 22). *Notice of NIH's interest in diversity* (Notice No. NOT-OD-20-031). https://grants.nih.gov/grants/guide/notice-files/NOT-OD-20-031.html

Neumann, N., Neu, D., & Ungco, J. C. (2021). Addressing LGBTQIA+ trauma: Your role and your responsibility. In A. Lynch, R. Ashcraft, & L. Tekell (Eds.), *Trauma, occupation, and participation: Foundations and population considerations in occupational therapy* (pp. 195–221). AOTA Press.

Nieto, L., & Boyer, M. F. (2007, March). Understanding oppression: Strategies in addressing power and privilege, Part 3: Skill sets for agents. *ColorsNW Magazine, 6,* 34–38.

Niranjan, S. J., Martin, M. Y., Fouad, M. N., Vickers, S. M., Wenzel, J. A., Cook, E. D., . . . Durant, R. W. (2020). Bias and stereotyping among research and clinical professionals: Perspectives on minority recruitment for oncology clinical trials. *Cancer, 126,* 1958–1968. https://doi.org/10.1002/cncr.32755

Owens, B. C., Hall, M. E., & Anderson, T. L. (2020). The relationship between purity culture and rape myth acceptance. *Journal of Psychology and Theology, 49,* 405–418. https://doi.org/10.1177/0091647120974992

Pulsely. (n.d.). *Advocacy vs allyship: Understanding the differences.* Pulsely. https://pulsely.io/blog/advocacy-vs-allyship-understanding-the-differences

Rehabilitation Act of 1973, Pub. L. 93-112, 29 U.S.C. §§ 701–796l.

Richards, L. G. (2019). Editorial—State of the journal, 2019. *American Journal of Occupational Therapy, 73,* 7306070010. https://doi.org/10.5014/ajot.2019.736003

Sabin, J. A. (2022). Tackling implicit bias in health care. *New England Journal of Medicine, 387,* 105–107. https://doi.org/10.1056/nejmp2201180

Saito, L. (1998). *Race and politics: Asian Americans, Latinos, and Whites in a Los Angeles suburb.* University of Illinois Press.

Serchen, J., Doherty, R., Atiq, O., & Hilden, D. (2021). A comprehensive policy framework to understand and address disparities and discrimination in health and health care: A policy paper from the American College of Physicians. *Annals of Internal Medicine, 174,* 529–532. https://doi.org/10.7326/m20-7219

Somerville, S. B. (2006). *Queering the color line: Race and the invention of homosexuality in American culture.* Duke University Press.

Strang, J. F., Kenworthy, L., Dominska, A., Sokoloff, J., Kenealy, L. E., Berl, M., . . . Wallace, G. L. (2014). Increased gender variance in autism spectrum disorders and attention deficit hyperactivity disorder. *Archives of Sexual Behavior, 43,* 1525–1533. https://doi.org/10.1007/s10508-014-0285-3

Tapia, R. (2006). Just ten years removed from a bolo and a breech-cloth: The sexualization of the Filipino "menace." In A. T. Tiongson, Jr., E. V. Gutierrez, & R. V. Gutierrez (Eds.), *Positively no Filipinos allowed: Building communities and discourse* (pp. 43–60). Temple University Press.

Taylor, B., & Davis, S. (2007). The Extended PLISSIT model for addressing the sexual well-being of individuals with an acquired disability or chronic illness. *Sexuality and Disability, 25,* 135–139. https://doi.org/10.1007/s11195-007-9044-x

The Trevor Project. (2019). *National survey on LGBTQ youth mental health 2019.* https://www.thetrevorproject.org/survey-2019/

Tobin, V., Bockting, W. O., & Hughes, T. L. (2018). Mental health promotion for gender minority adolescents. *Journal of Psychosocial Nursing and Mental Health Services, 56,* 22–30. https://doi.org/10.3928/02793695-20180601-02

Walker, B., Otte, K., LeMond, K., Hess, P., Kaizer, K., Faulkner, T., & Christy, D. (2020). Development of the Occupational Performance Inventory of Sexuality and Intimacy (OPISI): Phase one. *Open Journal of Occupational Therapy, 8*(2), 1–18. https://doi.org/10.15453/2168-6408.1694

Williams, D. R., & Rucker, T. D. (2000). Understanding and addressing racial disparities in health care. *Health Care Financing Review, 21,* 75–90.

Xiao, N., Mansukhani, N. A., Mendes de Oliveira, D. F., & Kibbe, M. R. (2018). Association of author gender with sex bias in surgical research. *JAMA Surgery, 153,* 663–670. https://doi.org/10.1001/jamasurg.2018.0040

Yearby, R., Clark, B., & Figueroa, J. F. (2022). Structural racism in historical and modern US health care policy. *Health Affairs, 41,* 187–194. https://doi.org/10.1377/hlthaff.2021.01466

Zestcott, C. A., Blair, I. V., & Stone, J. (2016). Examining the presence, consequences, and reduction of implicit bias in health care: A narrative review. *Group Processes and Intergroup Relations, 19,* 528–542. https://doi.org/10.1177/1368430216642029

5

Sexual and Intimate Occupations Across the Lifespan

Temor "Tay" Amin-Arsala, *MS, OTR/L;* **Elizabeth K. Schmidt,** *PhD, OTR/L;* *and* **Joseph Christian Ungco,** *OTD, OTR/L*

CHAPTER HIGHLIGHTS

- Historical context of sexuality in the United States
- Current trends in sex and intimacy occupations across the lifespan
- A lifespan look at sex and intimacy occupations

KEY TERMS AND CONCEPTS

Adverse childhood experiences
Cissexism
Cumulative life stage effects
Enthusiastic consent
Eugenics
Generational cohort effects
Heterosexism
LGBTQIA+
Patriarchal
Queering
Social mores
Sociosexuality
Toxic masculinity

Sexual and intimate occupations are a key area for people at any stage of life. Although it may seem that sexual and intimate occupations are restricted to adults, in actuality this set of occupations follows a developmental sequence that begins at birth and influences people as sexual and intimate beings throughout their life. This chapter explores the context, occupation, performance, and person domains of sexual and intimate occupations pertaining to life stages from birth to death.

In interpreting and producing the content of this chapter, we, the authors, acknowledge our own positionality as it shapes the text. Two of us bring experiences of Whiteness or attributed-Whiteness in our work, whereas the third brings experiences of being a person of color in the United States. Additionally, we possess a mixture of heterosexual, cisgender, and queer identities among the three of us. Although we bring different backgrounds and relationships to race, gender identity, sexual orientation, socioeconomic status, and more, we want to highlight the importance of understanding the White-dominant, cisnormative, heteronormative, ableist, ageist, and capitalist societal backdrop in which occupational therapy practice takes place.

An example of how this backdrop produces implicit bias is the common cultural conception of "sex" or "sexual activity" as being synonymous with penis-in-vagina penetrative intercourse with "man on top of woman" positioning. We see this particular configuration frequently in media and in both formal and informal early education on sexual activity, revealing a bias toward a cisgender, heterosexual, male pleasure–focused, female pleasure–erased view of sexual occupations. These same biases affect the sources used in this chapter as well as the cissexist,[1] heterosexist,[2] patriarchal,[3] and White-centric sources of information that have long come from academia and other research institutions. Against this backdrop of systemic privileges and oppressions, we approached this chapter with the intention of beginning to dismantle those structures that affect occupational therapy's understanding of sexual and intimate occupations.

Throughout this text, *sexual activity* refers to the broadest range of acts, including masturbation, foreplay, anal sex, fingering, sexual fantasies, cunnilingus, kink/bondage dominance sadomasochism (BDSM), sexual training, and reproductive sex, among many others. Although the occupational therapy profession is dominated by White, cisgender, female perspectives, in this chapter, we intentionally emphasize a ***queering***[4] of the literature in an attempt to liberate understandings of occupation from historically White, cisgender, patriarchal, and heterosexual-centered influences.

This chapter is organized by developmental life stages beginning with infancy and ending with older adulthood. Each life stage includes key concepts and milestones organized by the domains (context, occupation, performance and person) described in the *Occupational Therapy Practice Framework: Domain and Process* (4th ed.; *OTPF–4;* American Occupational Therapy Association, 2020). This chapter will guide readers in recognizing broad and diverse facets of human sexuality, integrating previous knowledge of human development with specific analysis of sexual and intimate occupations across the life course and analyzing context, occupations, performance, and person factors associated with human sexuality.

---

[1] ***Cissexism*** is explicit or implicit discrimination or prejudice against transgender people. This discrimination is rooted in considering cisgender as "normal" or superior to transgender.

[2] ***Heterosexism*** is attitudes and biases presuming that heterosexual or opposite-sex relationships are "normal" and therefore superior to same-sex attractions or relationships, which are seen as deviating from that "norm."

[3] ***Patriarchal*** refers to a society that is primarily controlled by men and is male-centric in its norms and privileges.

[4] ***Queering*** refers to applying queer theory to critically analyze areas that presume heterosexuality and identity binaries as dominant and "normal." In "queering the literature," we seek to understand ways in which these assumptions are replicated and institutionalized in our professional knowledge and thus continue to oppress sexual and gender diverse individuals.

Historical Context of Sexuality in the United States

Because of the importance of context in understanding individual experiences around sex and intimacy throughout their life, it is critical for occupational therapy practitioners to understand the historical context contributing to the experiences of many people today as well as the body of literature and evidence currently informing health care. This history includes a variety of key topics such as medical trauma (e.g., experiments on Black women without anesthesia carried out by J. Marion Sims, the "father of gynecology"; see Ojanuga, 1993), pathologization of LGBTQIA+[5] people (e.g., "homosexuality" and "gender identity disorder" categorized as mental illnesses in previous editions of the *Diagnostic and Statistical Manual of Mental Disorders* [e.g., American Psychiatric Association, 1968; see Neumann et al., 2021]), medicalization of women's sexuality (e.g., use of clitoral stimulation and the invention of vibrators to relieve "hysteria"; see Castleman, 2013), hypersexualization of children (e.g., young Black girls; see Epstein et al., 2017), and eugenics, among others. Although it is beyond the scope of this chapter to go into these areas in depth, it is crucial for readers to continue learning about these topics and broaden their understanding of the historical context influencing people's sexual and intimate occupations today.

Eugenics, in particular, warrants critical analysis as a malpractice that is directly connected to occupations of sexual activity and intimacy. ***Eugenics*** is a set of beliefs and practices aimed to improve the genetic quality of the human population (Galton, 1904). The belief and perspective that certain people are unfit to procreate or may damage society by passing their genes onto a child permeated policies, recommendations, and practices of forced sterilization. People with mental health conditions or disabilities, prisoners, people with low socioeconomic status, and people of color were forcibly sterilized or coerced into using birth control as a form of eugenics (Lawrence, 2014; Pegoraro, 2014; Stern, 2005; Tilley et al., 2012; Torpy, 2000). Although forced sterilization is no longer legal, sterilization and eugenic beliefs continue to this day. Specifically, people with disabilities are more likely to be sterilized (Brown et al., 2018; Li et al., 2018; Wu et al., 2017) or prescribed contraception (Brown et al., 2018; Greenwood & Wilkinson, 2013; McCarthy, 2009; Tilley et al., 2012; Wu et al., 2018).

Some evidence also suggests that many people with intellectual and developmental disabilities who may be sterilized or prescribed contraception may not have the information necessary to make empowered decisions regarding their own sterilization or contraception (Horner-Johnson et al., 2018; McCarthy, 2009). In fact, health care providers are less likely to initiate contraceptive counseling with their

[5] The term ***LGBTQIA+*** refers to the diverse and unique communities formed by lesbian, gay, bisexual, transgender, queer, intersex, asexual, and additional sexual and gender-diverse people. As greater awareness, social acceptance, and safety improve for these individuals and communities, new terms may emerge as language evolves to describe identities that exist outside of societal recognition and acceptance.

patients with intellectual and developmental disabilities than with those without disabilities or with other disabilities (Taouk et al., 2018). Providers are also more likely to provide contraceptive counseling to the parents or caregivers of people with intellectual and developmental disabilities instead of the patients themselves (Taouk et al., 2018). Thus, health care providers and families heavily influence these decisions based on their own eugenic beliefs, including misconceptions about the ability of people with disabilities to serve in parenting roles, manage menstrual hygiene, and comply with contraceptives (Agaronnik et al., 2020; McCarthy, 2009; Tilley et al., 2012).

With this historical perspective in mind, we turn to the Occupational Therapy Sexual Assessment Framework (OTSAF), which provides a conceptual outline for understanding various constructs of occupational performance for sexuality and intimacy (Walker et al., 2020). These constructs can be embedded into occupational therapy as depicted in Figure 5.1. The purpose of this chapter is to provide an occupation-centered analysis of sexuality and intimacy for each life stage from birth to death at the level of the context, occupation, performance, and person. Because human development is a part of foundational occupational therapy education and training, this chapter assumes that the reader is generally familiar with life stages and development over the lifespan. This chapter is not a comprehensive and exhaustive source for human development but highlights aspects specifically related to sexual and intimate occupations and models a way for readers to deepen their understanding of human development in the context of sexuality and intimacy.

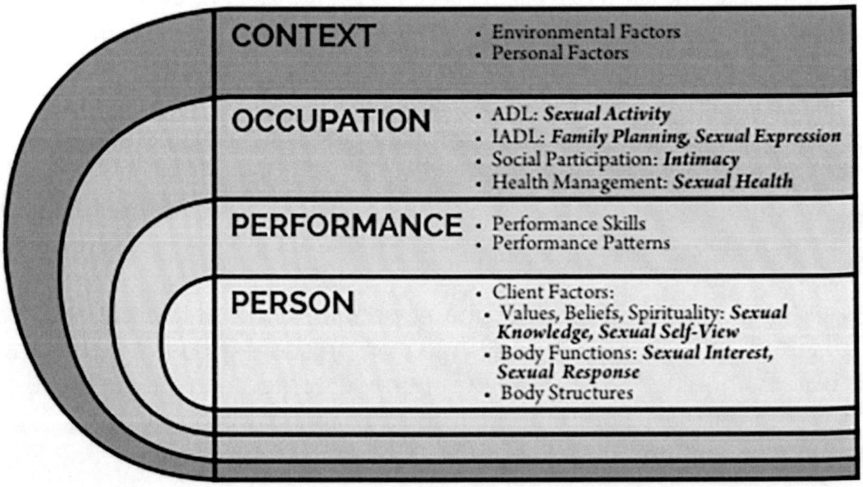

FIGURE 5.1
Occupational Therapy Sexual Assessment Framework for sex and intimacy evaluation.

Source. From "The Occupational Performance Inventory of Sexuality and Intimacy (OPISI)," by B. A. Walker, 2020. Copyright © 2020 by Beth Ann Walker and the University of Indianapolis. https://opisi.uindy.edu. Used with permission.

Sexual and Intimate Occupations Across the Lifespan

This section is organized by developmental life stages beginning with infancy and ending with older adulthood. Each subsection follows the *OTPF–4* and OTSAF by presenting sexual and intimate occupations through context, occupation, performance, and person.

Infancy and Toddlerhood (Prebirth to Age 3 Years)

Context

Sexual well-being of infants and toddlers is rarely considered outside of the context of healthy physiological development. However, a variety of ***adverse childhood experiences*** (ACEs) that occur during this period can affect sexual well-being during this period and later in life. An *ACE* is a "traumatic event or situation that a person identifies as having directly experienced or observed from birth through the age of 18 years" (Atchison & Suarez, 2021, p. 4). ACEs include experiencing or witnessing violence, abuse, neglect, a death in the family, or mental health problems (Felitti et al., 1998). ACEs can influence various aspects of health and function later in life, including sexual and intimate occupations.

In addition to ACEs, social norms imparted on children early in life can affect sexual well-being throughout a person's lifetime. Western culture emphasizes alignment between one's gender and their assigned sex (based on sex chromosomes, physical traits, and hormones) and begins to push gender stereotypes and norms as early as gestation. *Gender-reveal parties* are gatherings of family, friends, and communities to share or "reveal" a fetus's assigned sex, often using stereotypic symbols of gender (i.e., pink for female and blue for male). These parties have been critiqued for assigning a gender to a person who has not yet been able to consider their identity and for emphasizing binary concepts of sex and gender (Gieseler, 2017; Guignard, 2015).

The harm of loudly and boisterously assigning gender to the unborn can have immediate and even harmful effects (e.g., explosive pyrotechnics inadvertently starting forest fires; Peñaloza, 2020). More often, however, the harm of these events is not immediate, but they perpetuate and contribute to gender stereotypes that follow infants throughout the rest of their lives (Gieseler, 2017; Guignard, 2015; Perry, 2020). People typically emphasize clothing, toys, and activities traditionally viewed as feminine for children with an assigned sex of female and those viewed as masculine for children with an assigned sex of male. Gender stereotypes centering on a binary view of gender can have short- and long-term health effects for everyone (e.g., increased eating disorders and depression, limited ideas of "permissible" sex positions based on gender roles), but they are particularly detrimental for people who are gender nonconforming or transgender (Fiani & Han, 2019; Newcomb et al., 2020; Weber et al., 2019).

Occupation

From prebirth to age 3 years, children rely on their parents for sexual health management and sexual expression and engage in few sexual and intimate occupations. Occupations they do engage in include social participation (i.e., intimacy and bonding with parents or caregivers) and sexual activity (i.e., self-exploration). Immediately after birth, infants can begin bonding with their parents or caregivers. Strong attachment to caregivers is vital in infancy for healthy social and emotional development and for healthy relationship attachment styles later in life (Masten, 2018).

Infants between 6 and 11 months begin to discover their genitals during diaper changes. They may respond to exploration and touch of their genitals by experiencing penile erections or vaginal lubrication (Martinson, 1976; Mesman et al., 2019). Although research is limited in this area, theorists primarily attribute these reactions to reflexive responses. However, theorists also hypothesize that young children experience pleasure but may be less likely to engage in pleasure-seeking behaviors because of limited experiences, attention, and other factors associated with their age (Martinson, 1976). Children in preschool also engage in exploratory behaviors with their bodies and can experience penile erections or vaginal lubrication; they begin to show more interest in others who are nude, may walk around without clothes, or may touch their mother's breasts (Larsson & Svedin, 2002; Mesman et al., 2019).

Performance

From prebirth to age 3 years, children develop a variety of performance skills, including motor, social interaction, and process skills. According to Smet and Lucas (2020), motor skills develop from reflexes to coordinated movements to engage in self-exploration. Additionally, social interaction skills develop from neurophysiological modulation (from birth to 2 or 3 months), where infants are reliant on their parents or caregivers for soothing and then can independently self-soothe. Infants begin to demonstrate an awareness of social demands between ages 12 and 18 months, which leads to their ability to exhibit self-control in accordance with social expectations between 24 and 48 months (Smet & Lucas, 2020). This ability is an important component of sexual development because children may now identify gender norms and stereotypes, which contribute to their developing sense of identity.

Infants and toddlers also engage in a variety of play that may contribute to their overall sexual development, including social play (i.e., parallel play, imitation of parents and peers, playing in groups of children, observing other children; Smet & Lucas, 2020) as a mechanism to learn social behaviors. Again, these social behaviors are often situated in the context of children's upbringing and the gender norms or stereotypes that are impressed upon them. Process skills, such as temperament, activity level, approach or withdrawal, distractibility, intensity of reactions, attention span, quality of mood, threshold of response, and adaptability, begin to develop during this time. Temperament may contribute to the development of adaptive, successful relationships later in life and is heavily influenced by children's caregivers, environment, and social experiences (Smet & Lucas, 2020). This association suggests the importance of social development and opportunities for a variety of play with diverse people and in diverse settings.

Person

Cultural and familial values and beliefs can strongly influence the gender norms and stereotypes that are impressed upon youth from prebirth to age 3 years, which can have significant effects on children's identity development and health (Weber et al., 2019). Body functions and structures—specifically chromosomes, gonads, and hormones—also contribute to assigned sex in Western culture, which again can influence the norms and stereotypes imposed upon people. Additionally, some people are born with variations in sex characteristics that differ from those associated with the medical definitions for *male* and *female.* Some parents, physicians, and surgeons choose to assign a sex to intersex infants and children using various medical interventions, including surgery, despite no available evidence supporting the necessity of this approach (Minto et al., 2003). Some intersex children who receive medical intervention then go on to experience gender dysphoria or sexual dysfunction later in life (Kreukels et al., 2018; Minto et al., 2003).

Childhood and Youth (Age 3 Years to Puberty)

Context

Childhood is strikingly marked by an increase in social network size and diversity. Social interaction during the infant and toddler years is usually limited to family members and family friends. Enrollment in elementary school increases social scope to other, novel, children and adults who may be of differing races, gender identities, abilities, and backgrounds (Rucinski et al., 2021).

This sudden increase in social relationships leads to several important circumstances for a child. First, the development of friendships with peers in school or in the community during childhood is often the first instance of extrafamilial intimacy a child may experience. For the only child, childhood friendships may be the first opportunity for intimacy with someone of a similar age (Dunn, 2004). Additionally, at this stage, social influences become more pronounced, including the internalization of ***social mores:*** the socially constructed, culture-specific customs, values, and concepts that serve as determinants of what is and is not moral for a culture or group. Because social norms and mores regarding other children and adults in the community may be different from in a child's household, children must learn to effectively navigate different social environments (Berns, 2016).

Social boundaries and culture-specific morals affect perception of sex and intimacy for all children. Compiling research on sex and intimacy occupations during childhood reveals stark differences among the results of different studies, depending on the study's perspective. For example, in Friedrich et al. (1998), in which sexual activity in children is considered via parent report, sexual activity in children (e.g., exploration of their own bodies in public, genital touching of themselves and peers, purposeful observation of others who are nude) decreases across childhood until the start of puberty. Conversely, when adults were asked retroactively about their childhood sexual behaviors, many reported that these behaviors continued throughout childhood, though they may have moved from the view of others (Haugaard, 1996; Larsson & Svedin, 2002).

The contrast between the results of these two studies serves to highlight two interconnected phenomena that affect views on sex and intimacy occupations during childhood. First, a gradual embedding of cultural mores around sexual behaviors may change how children interact with their own bodies and sexuality—for most, the outcome is to move these practices into more private settings as a result of either positive or negative experiences altering their conceptions. Those who do not shift to more private settings of exploration often find themselves, and their caregivers, shamed for their actions. Second, in contrast to puberty, which is often portrayed as an oversexualized period of development, childhood is seen as a period of time in which adults may ignore, intentionally or unintentionally, any signs of developing sexuality in children (LeVay et al., 2021; Robinson, 2012). This willful ignorance and exclusion of sexuality from childhood often stems from the idea that sexuality is for "adults only." Moreover, the exclusion of children from discussions of sexuality, no matter the topic, is framed as "preserving the innocence" of a child as a way of protecting them from the perceived dangers of sexuality (Robinson, 2012).

Robinson (2012) argued that this cultural regulation of childhood sexuality and insistence that children must be protected from the topics of sex and intimacy serve to further the replication of heteronormative societal norms as children age and their access to education on sexuality is controlled. Additionally, children who more openly display sexual behaviors during this time may find themselves the targets of shaming by adults or pathologization by health care professionals. This shame can have further consequences as children age, because children experiencing more shame in childhood have an increased likelihood of unprotected sexual encounters and substance use as they reach young adulthood (Stuewig et al., 2015).

Socially constructed gender norms become further reinforced during childhood. Children often experience pressure from various sources to conform to certain gender norms related to sex assigned at birth. Although many laugh off gender stereotyping during childhood as something to be expected (e.g., "boys will be boys," girls receiving messages to "be nice"), this push for gender conformity often creates a lifelong impact on sex and intimacy occupations at both the individual and societal levels.

Toxic masculinity, whereby masculinity and the pressure for men to present as masculine become dangerous to both men and others around them, is one of the most often referred to results of excessive pressure to conform to gender norms. For preadolescent boys, toxic masculinity insidiously decreases the likelihood of self-reporting of childhood sexual trauma while simultaneously increasing the likelihood of bullying other children, especially those assigned male at birth not conforming to typical gender norms (Ford, 2019; Morrison, 2020). These toxic ideologies around masculinity continue past childhood, influence adolescence, and affect adulthood. Adult men who align themselves with more traditional models of masculinity (often associated with toxic masculinity) demonstrate increased levels of dysfunctional and sometimes dangerous sexual beliefs as well as lower levels of sexual inhibition linked to fears of performance failure than do adult men who embrace less prescriptive and more modern concepts of masculinity (Clarke et al., 2015).

Occupation

Children's curiosity about and exploration of themselves and others are hallmarks of sex and intimacy occupations in childhood. Although most preadolescent children do not engage in sexual intercourse with others, a minority of 3% have participated in the act before age 13 years (Szucs et al., 2020). More common expressions of sexuality come in the form of touching one's own genitals, trying to look at others who are nude, beginning to develop infatuations or "crushes" on other children, and beginning to talk about sex with their peers (Friedrich et al., 1998; Kellogg, 2010; Mesman et al., 2019).

Play and sexual and intimate occupations are interconnected in childhood. Although many children may not truly understand sexual intercourse, they may recognize ideas around sex and intimacy and replicate them through play. At the younger end of childhood, these ideas may resemble mimicking the social relationships they see in adolescents and adults, from playing house and pretending to be married to holding hands and kissing. Play may also serve as the first steps of sexual exploration with other children. For example, children may play games involving purposeful sexual behavior with other children, such as "doctor," "truth or dare," or others that include both visual and physical interaction with the bodies of other children, regardless of gender identity or sexual orientation (Okami et al., 1997).

Performance

Performance patterns and performance skills for sex and intimacy occupations during childhood are more fluid and amorphous than at many other ages, given the vast differences in participation. Many childhood performance skills set up future participation in more direct sex- and intimacy-related occupations. Increases in gross motor and fine motor coordination across childhood (Belsky, 2013) improve the capacity of children to engage in more complex physical tasks as they age. Additionally, cognitive and socioemotional developments across childhood begin to cultivate the analytical and social skills people need to effectively navigate both interpersonal relationships and relationships with their own body (Belsky, 2013).

Person

Although childhood is not marked by the same rapid growth and development as is often associated with adolescence and puberty, physical changes are associated with body structures and functions during this phase of life. Most notable is the change in height of children across childhood. From the end of toddlerhood to the beginning of adolescence, physical height can more than double. At least three distinct growth spurts are measurable in childhood (preschool, mid-childhood, and late childhood), with a fourth prepubertal growth spurt for children who begin puberty late (Bock, 2004; Butler et al., 1990).

Physically, children are able to engage in sexual behaviors despite being prepubescent and lacking the secondary sex characteristics that develop during puberty. Children with penises will likely continue to experience erections, both through manual stimulation and involuntarily. Although not common for many reasons, penetrative insertion of the penis is possible for these children, whether inserting vaginally, orally, or anally. With sexual stimulation of their genitals, some children may find orgasm possible (Martinson, 1976). Manual stimulation of sensitive structures (e.g., penis, clitoris) can result in a pleasurable sensation for children. For children with a penis or testes, ejaculation is unlikely, and if any ejaculate is expelled, the fluid will not contain sperm (Campbell et al., 2013). For children with vaginas, manual stimulation of the clitoris does not produce the same quantity or type of lubrication within the vagina that pubescent and postpubescent females often produce (Campbell et al., 2013).

Outside of larger cultural mores on sexual behaviors in children, individual reactions from peers and adults in a child's life regarding the child's sexual exploration may cause the child to view current and future sexual experiences as either positive or negative. Throughout childhood, sexual knowledge varies greatly by individual. By age 10 years, many children have a basic understanding of puberty, reproductive processes, and childbirth (National Center on the Sexual Behavior of Youth, 2020), but their understanding may vary depending on culture, family dynamics, and biases associated with disability status.

Adolescence (Puberty Through Age 18 Years)

Context

Adolescence is a pivotal time for increased independence and autonomy in occupations associated with sexuality and intimacy. However, independence and autonomy are strongly influenced by family upbringing and morals; cultural values and beliefs; and even policy at the school, state, and federal levels.

Adolescents often have little control over their sexual health education. For example, they require inclusive, comprehensive sexuality education to access and apply information to engage in safe sexual practices, manage sexual health and family planning, and feel supported in their intimate relationships and sexual expression (Kirby & National Campaign to Prevent Teen and Unplanned Pregnancy, 2007). Yet, sexuality education is not federally mandated, and therefore access to this information differs by state, school and, sometimes, family. Moreover, not all youth have rights to make decisions for themselves in all aspects of their sexual health care, depending on state and federal legislation (Guttmacher Institute, 2021). Thus, some youth must rely on their parents or caregivers for final decisions regarding family planning and sexual health management. This lack of autonomy may contribute to adverse outcomes for youth, including unplanned pregnancies and sexually transmitted infections (STIs). In fact, the birth rate among 15- to 19-year-olds, although decreased in recent years, is 26 per 1,000 women (Kost et al., 2017); adolescents ages 15 to 19 years and young adults ages 20 to 24 years experience the highest rates of STIs (Centers for Disease Control and Prevention [CDC], 2019).

Issues concerning enthusiastic consent are certainly relevant during this life stage, but given states' variance in age-of-consent laws, we address these issues in more detail in the young adult section. Adolescents are considered minors until age 18 years, but states and districts vary in their regulation of age of consent for sexual activities (Age of Consent, 2021). Depending on the state, adolescents may be able to consent to sexual activities with someone 2 to 5 years within their age, on average, when they are between ages 16 and 18 years (Age of Consent, 2021; World Population Review, 2021). These laws are in place to protect adolescents from coercion and sexual assault and abuse, given that their prefrontal cortex is still developing until young adulthood (Arain et al., 2013).

The prefrontal cortex affects executive functioning and people's ability to make decisions regarding their sexual or reproductive health. For adolescents, underdeveloped executive functioning skills may make them more likely to make impulsive decisions regarding sexual activities without thinking through the related consequences (Arain et al., 2013). Rates of sexual activity, however, are low among those in early adolescence (age 15 years or younger) but increase as the adolescent ages (Martinez & Abma, 2015). Specifically, 44% of 17- to 18-year-olds and 69% of 19-year-olds in the United States report that they are sexually active (Martinez & Abma, 2015). Inclusive, detailed, and timely sexual health education in childhood and adolescence has been shown to decrease many of the potentially negative outcomes of teenage sexual encounters such as STIs, unwanted pregnancies, and sex while under the influence of drugs and alcohol (Reis et al., 2011).

Occupation

Adolescents experience a shift in their social relationship priorities, changing focus from their families to their friends and, for some, intimate partners. They may explore variations in their sexual expression to learn their preferences; it is often through such intimate experiences that they begin exploring the occupation of sexual activity. As adolescents experience many new intimate life experiences, they may begin refining their sexual identity. Adolescents who engage in partnered sexual activities may also be considering family planning (i.e., contraception) and health management (i.e., initiation of routine gynecological or prostate exams, increasing autonomy of annual medical visits).

Performance

Although adolescents may explore the occupation of sexual activity, few identify their preferences or fully develop habits, routines, and rituals at this stage, which means they may be malleable. The malleability of youth's engagement in sexual activity emphasizes the importance of sexuality education for safe sexual practices, positive exploration experiences, and health management and maintenance.

Person

Adolescents experience a variety of body function and structure changes associated with their sexual and intimate occupations. Puberty is the initial indicator of adolescence. Puberty is characterized by a complex interaction of hormones, in which the hypothalamus and pituitary gland stimulate the release of sex-related hormones, causing physical growth and the development of secondary sex characteristics. Puberty typically starts between ages 8 and 14 years and lasts approximately 4 years. This time frame is similar for most people, including those with disabilities (Autism Society, n.d.; Rosenfield et al., 2000). Adolescents with cerebral palsy and autism spectrum disorder may start puberty slightly earlier or later than their peers, according to some research, but this finding has not been consistently demonstrated (Corbett et al., 2020; Knickmeyer et al., 2006; Sheridan, 2020; Worley et al., 2002).

Hormonal changes affect not only physical development but also emotion and behavior. Specifically, youth further develop their understanding, expression, and regulation of their emotions consistent with emotional maturity. This process of development is vital for social participation and intimate relationships. Cognitive processes also develop significantly during adolescence. Youth may initially engage in more risk-taking behaviors as their social demands and interests change. As the adolescent ages, the amygdala and prefrontal cortex of the brain are also rapidly developing, leading to improved judgment control, planning abilities, and understanding of consequences (Crone & Dahl, 2012; Peper & Dahl, 2013). The brain continues to develop and refine these abilities well beyond the pubertal physical changes and into adulthood (Luna et al., 2001).

The experience of puberty can be a challenging time for all youth. They may experience contrasting emotions during puberty, such as anxiety, fear, confusion, and pride, particularly youth who menstruate early (Short & Rosenthal, 2008). Feelings of anxiety, fear, and confusion may be exacerbated in youth with disabilities. However, it is suggested that sexuality education to prepare for the upcoming changes may ease such feelings (Fouquier & Camune, 2015). In addition, many youth experience challenges with body image acceptance and self-esteem during puberty. These challenges may also be exacerbated in youth who are perceived as disabled or different by their peers without disabilities (Hassouneh-Phillips & McNeff, 2005; Kościński, 2007; Okkerse et al., 2001; Workman et al., 2020).

All occupations associated with sexuality and intimacy are also influenced by values, beliefs, and spirituality. Sexual expression is an important occupation associated with identity development, and a positive self-identity is vital for all youth because it is associated with positive self-esteem and improved mental health outcomes (Chen, 2019). Thus, supporting sexual expression is critical to affirm self-esteem and improve mental health.

Young Adulthood (Ages 18 to 39 Years)

Context

Culture dictates which sexual and intimate occupations are socially acceptable and which are not. Premarital sex, hook-up culture, and same-sex sexual relations are three areas in which culture may heavily influence those participating. Sex before marriage has become more socially acceptable over the past half century, from almost 40% of the U.S. population believing premarital sex was wrong in 1972 to just under 20% believing it was wrong in 2018. There is a much greater acceptance of sex outside of marriage (Smith et al., 2019). Hook-up culture, otherwise known as ***sociosexuality,*** or the willingness to engage in casual sex (LeVay et al., 2021), occurs across all sexual orientations and gender identities. As opposed to monogamy (discussed more in Chapter 7, "Intimate Partnerships"), sociosexuality involves engagement in sexual occupations without prior or subsequent commitment. Many young adults actively participate in this practice while single, and some continue to participate in hook-up culture while partnered or married (Monto & Carey, 2014). Others may choose not to engage in sociosexuality, preferring to have relationships with their potential sex partners before engaging in sexual occupations.

Despite relaxation of attitudes toward sex in the United States, ableism, heterosexism, racism, and cissexism continue to affect minoritized[6] young adults as they engage in sexual and intimate occupations. For these minoritized groups, prevailing cultural attitudes affect not only engagement in sexual partnerships (see Chapter 7 for more details) but also personal safety. For example, sexual and gender minorities or young adults with disabilities face increased sexual and intimate partner violence (Codina et al., 2020; Dammeyer & Chapman, 2018; Flores et al., 2020). Many religious institutions, political parties, and sociocultural groups continue to denounce nonheterosexual or gender-diverse identities as deviant, which in turn creates discriminatory practices in employment, education, housing, and more. These systemic and cultural prejudices then trickle down to the individual level, for example, increasing the danger of seeking out sex partners for LGBTQIA+ individuals. Trans women of color in particular find themselves targeted by culturally perpetrated violence and hate crimes (Gamarel et al., 2020).

The United States has a history of controlling who is legally allowed to have sex and how they have sex. *Sodomy laws,* or laws prohibiting certain sexual acts (often anal sex, oral sex, or "homosexual sex"), were federally legal until 2003, when *Lawrence v. Texas* deemed such laws unconstitutional. Although these laws appeared to target sexual acts that any couple might engage in, they were often designed specifically for and largely only enforced against same-sex sexual activity. Of note, several of the laws specifically outlined sodomy restrictions for "homosexual couples," whereas married heterosexual couples were exempt from the law. Despite the Supreme Court's decision, in 2020, 15 states continue to have sodomy

[6] *Minoritized* refers to the process of marginalization and creation of "minority" groups through dominant social processes of power, privilege, and exclusion.

laws on the books, and 3 states specifically target same-sex relations (American Civil Liberties Union, n.d.).

Occupation

Upon reaching young adulthood, options for sexual activity occupations become both more numerous and more possible than at previous stages of life. Although most of these occupations are physically possible during adolescence, cultural and personal factors often limit access to them. Self-pleasure and masturbation continue throughout adulthood, with people of all genders participating. With greater economic independence, young adults may choose to purchase sex toys to augment and enrich their own experiences with self-pleasure. For many, this period of life may be the first time certain sexual acts are conducted with other people. Kissing, fondling, mutual masturbation, oral sex, and vaginal or anal intercourse may all be performed with peers their own age or older or younger individuals. Sexual relations may involve two or more people of any combination of gender identities and body structures, regardless of sexual orientation. In addition to being an ADL, sexual activity may be a part of other ADLs (e.g., dressing), IADLs, health management, social participation, leisure, play, education, or work areas of occupation for young adults (LeVay et al., 2021).

Sexual health and family planning are key occupations in young adulthood (see Chapter 7 for more information on family planning). With the increase in sexual activities that often occurs during this period of life comes the need to appropriately manage potential outcomes of these activities. Sexual health covers a wide range of topics but may include birth control to avoid pregnancy (e.g., condoms, hormones, intrauterine devices; Frost et al., 2012), STI prophylaxis (e.g., condoms, pre- and post-exposure prophylactics, dental dams), and screening or testing for sexual activity–related diseases. Sexual health may also include medication management and the management of other conditions or diseases that may affect sexual performance and function. Family planning may include birth control, fertility treatments, and health condition management.

Of note, outside of condoms and *vasectomy* (a procedure in which the vas deferens is cut, preventing sperm from leaving the testes), there have, historically, not been many commercially available contraception options for individuals with penises and testes. Market limitations, failure rates, side effects, and social conceptions of masculinity all result in excessive responsibility for contraception falling on individuals with uteri (Kanakis & Goulis, 2015; Thirumalai & Page, 2019). In a global study, only 14% of contraception use was by cisgender men, indicating the failure of patriarchal society to hold cisgender men as accountable as their partners for their own and their partners' sexual health (Kanakis & Goulis, 2015).

Intimacy is another important occupation in young adulthood (see Chapter 7 for performance skills related to building intimacy). Intimacy for young adults may involve giving and receiving affection from others, whether they be friends, casual sex partners, romantic partners, or strangers on the Internet. There is no one right way for intimacy to look. For some, intimacy involves in-person discussion of important topics or the physical intimacy of sleeping together. For others, intimacy might involve long-distance phone or video calls or require text messaging while lying in bed at night. Intimacy for young adults may or may not involve sexual activity, and it may have differing meanings to those involved.

Sexual expression in young adults is extremely person dependent because it is the lived manifestation of an individual as a sexual being through the interaction of sexual orientation and gender identity. Sexual expression in young adults may span all areas of occupation. They may choose to manifest their sexual being through clothing choice, career choice, educational opportunities, choice of play and leisure activities, and even sleeping and living arrangements. Social participation may be affected by sexual expression. For example, a trans woman may choose to join a women's roller derby group to affirm her identity as a woman. Conversely, a young, heterosexual man might avoid joining a cheer team despite an interest in the sport to prevent questioning of his heterosexuality.

Performance

The performance skills needed for young adults to engage in occupations of sex and intimacy vary from person to person (see Chapter 8, "Sexual Activity as an ADL"). However, the most important performance skills for young adults participating in sexual and intimate occupations revolve around ***enthusiastic consent*** and its recognition. Rather than the historical "No means no" theory governing consent, whereby consent is revoked only if one party says no or is unable to answer, enthusiastic consent highlights the need for all sexual partners involved to be able to give an enthusiastic yes to engage in sexual acts (Agbasiere, 2022). Enthusiastic consent can be verbal (spoken, signed, or given through augmentative messages) or gestural (e.g., thumbs up). Sexually active people must be able to recognize enthusiastic consent when it is given and be able to disengage or terminate from the encounter if enthusiastic consent is not given or is withdrawn. Similarly, participants must also be able to give their own enthusiastic consent to participate.

Performance patterns (roles, habits, and routines) in young adults are heavily influenced by both their environment and their personal experiences. During young adulthood, people may find that many of their performance patterns change and shift as a result of a combination of life events (e.g., moving out of their childhood home, leaving grade school, moving in with roommates or partners, being exposed to more diverse groups, exploring their sexual orientation or gender identity).

Young adulthood is a period during which many new routines involving sexual and intimate occupations may develop. Preparation for these occupations may involve cleaning one's body before engaging in sexual acts. Cleaning can range from a full shower and brushing teeth to simply wiping oneself down with a wet wipe or washing one's face. Individuals engaging in anal sex may develop routines such as douching their rectum with water to remove fecal matter or using antidiuretics to decrease the chance of feces moving into the rectum during anal play (e.g., anal training, fingering, penetrative sex). Routines involving potential sex partners may also start to take shape. For some, Friday night may always be date night with their significant other(s), with a high likelihood of intercourse occurring at the end of the evening. For others, routines might involve spending part of the day searching for potential sexual partners on hook-up apps, chatting, exchanging photos, and reaching an agreement for time and location to meet.

Person

Physical, cognitive, and physiological changes continue to occur across adulthood despite the cessation of puberty in the late teens and early 20s. With increasing skills and development comes the ability for young adults to navigate increasingly complex sexual and interpersonal relationships with others. The slow process of cognitive maturation in the young adult is particularly visible in the actions of young college-aged individuals. Although they physically resemble adults, they are still developing cognitively and emotionally and may not have the capacity to approach sexuality and intimacy in the same way as someone in their late twenties or thirties.

In the late 30s, testosterone and estrogen begin to decrease, a change that may influence sexual response and interest (LeVay et al., 2021). This decrease is only one of many factors influencing sexual desire. As previously stated, people at this age may also have increased capacity for sexual and intimate occupations as a result of further cognitive and emotional maturation. In a study of cisgender, heterosexual men, the following core ideas were also correlated with increases or decreases of sexual desire and interest: one's idea of feeling desired, the ability to experience novel and unexpected sexual encounters, intimate communication, rejection, physical ailments and disability, and level of emotional connection with one's partner (Murray et al., 2017). Across multiple settings, partner responsiveness, intimacy, and personal histories with attachment are all correlated with increased or decreased sexual desire over time (van Lankveld et al., 2021).

Values, beliefs, and spirituality regarding occupations of sex and intimacy continue to develop over the course of young adulthood. Although context plays a large role in the development of these client factors, personal experience and autonomy influence changes in these factors as well. Values and beliefs regarding sexual and intimate partnerships continue to be refined and explored, including views on monogamy and polyamory, sociosexuality, marriage and relationships, and more. Values and beliefs around sexual health practices may change over time as well, incorporating new information or discarding old beliefs as change occurs (e.g., feelings about abortion, the meaning of safe sex).

Young adults find themselves continuing to build upon the sexual knowledge they gained during previous life stages. Although formal curricula on sexual health and wellness inform some aspects of sexual knowledge, much knowledge about sexual practices and health is gained through social networks and trial and error. Gay, lesbian, trans, and queer young adults, having received next to no formal education about LGBTQIA+ sexual health and wellness, often have to seek out most of this information on their own in a process described as "reading up" (Devine & Nolan, 2011). Similarly, people with disabilities may be limited in their understanding and knowledge of sexual health because they have limited access to sexuality education and to the "hidden curriculum," or learning through social networks (Barnard-Brak et al., 2014; Gougeon, 2009).

Middle Adulthood (Ages 40 to 64 Years)

Context

People in middle adulthood often face misperceptions from younger individuals that they are no longer sexually active. It is important for occupational therapy practitioners to understand that people in middle adulthood continue to engage in occupations associated with sexuality and intimacy and that their sexual health still needs to be addressed (Gewirtz-Meydan et al., 2019).

In Western culture, current slang (e.g., sugar daddies, zaddies, DILFs, MILFs, cougars) has become increasingly more common, with the misunderstanding that these are the only adults in middle or older adulthood who are sexually active. All these terms refer to people in middle or older adulthood who date or engage in sexual activities with younger individuals. *Sugar daddies* and *sugar mamas* are people in middle or older adulthood who provide allowances, monetary gifts, gifts, or travel for their *sugar babies,* younger people who consensually enter a relationship with the older person for these specific perks. Websites and organizations help sugar daddies and sugar mamas meet sugar babies and come to an agreement on what they are looking for in the relationship (Padawer, 2009). A *zaddy*[7] is an attractive older man; a *DILF* refers to an attractive older man or a father who may elicit interest from younger partners without the financial benefits associated with the "sugar" relationship. A *cougar* is a woman who uses similar "predatory sexual advances" as men to gain the attention of younger men (Harris & Asthana, 2009), and a *MILF* is an attractive mother (or someone who is perceived to be a mother) who may elicit interest from younger partners.

Based on these terms, it is clear that age, gender, socioeconomic status, and appearance influence others' perceptions of whom people choose as sexual partners. For example, although middle adults around the world continue to engage in sexual activity at high rates (Nicolosi et al., 2004), often only those who are perceived as conventionally attractive are given these labels. Oversexualizing a particular set of adults in this way may feed into cultural narratives that middle adults, particularly older ones, are less sexual than people in younger life stages.

Other personal factors that influence occupations associated with intimate partnerships and sexual activities in middle adulthood include an individual's physical appearance and physique. In recent years, cosmetic surgery has increased,

[7] The term *zaddy* refers to middle-aged men who are seen as mature, stylish, and attractive.

specifically among women in middle adulthood, although cosmetic surgery has increased among young adults as well (American Society of Plastic Surgeons, 2019). As cosmetic surgery is becoming increasingly common in Western culture for women, men are experiencing different norms. Specifically, *dad bods,* defined as the body of "a man between the ages of 20 and 54, with a [body mass index] between 24 and 29.9" (Ingraham, 2015), and belly size somewhere between a six-pack and beer gut (Ingraham, 2015) are being seen as desirable. These changing norms suggest that women must maintain good physical fitness and stay healthy and active to look young and be considered attractive, whereas men have more flexibility because a wider range of body types are considered acceptable for them.

Occupation

Sexual activity occupations during middle adulthood often echo the occupations of young adulthood, though they may change in frequency, duration, or other ways. Both masturbation and partnered sexual acts continue throughout this period, partnered sex continuing to involve one or more additional adults. For some, additional exploration of sexual acts may occur during this time, bringing in kink and play into their occupations (e.g., BDSM, swinging, bondage, pup play; LeVay et al., 2021). Dating, marriage, divorce, separation, and cohabitating may all occur at different times during middle adulthood. Monogamy, polyamory, and remaining single all are viable relationship options during this period (Anapol, 2010).

Family planning and sexual health occupations may shift over middle adulthood. Pregnancy, with or without medical assistance, is possible for many across middle adulthood (LeVay et al., 2021), so birth control and contraception continue to be used. Changes in fertility, relationship status, intimacy patterns, or other personal decisions may alter the use of these methods at any time. For some middle adults, adoption results in parenting occupations. For those who began parenting in young adulthood, middle adulthood may bring continual adjustments to their lives as their children age. Parents and caregivers may begin to educate their children on topics of sex and intimacy.

Sex and intimacy occupations more common to young people (e.g., first-time sexual encounters, new forms of intimacy, self-education, sexual expression) may reoccur or occur for the first time as life circumstances change. For example, some middle adults may come out as LGBTQIA+, and others may be negotiating their relationship or gender identity. This expansive new growth or change in occupational engagement may be like a second puberty to some experiencing it (Johnston & Jenkins, 2008; Moore-Ramirez et al., 2017; Witten, 2008).

Performance

A variety of performance skills, patterns, and roles are associated with intimate partner relationships and maintenance of sexual health throughout adulthood. Whether these skills, patterns, and roles change in middle adulthood is largely dependent on the person and their unique life circumstances, preferences, and relationships. For some people, these elements of performance are finally refined, whereas for others, age-related changes require modification of these elements.

Similarly, some people may be in stable, long-term, committed relationships and may not experience significant changes in habits, routines, roles, and rituals within their intimate partnerships. These structures can either support their sexual and intimate engagements or stifle engagement if the habits, routines, roles, or rituals contribute to a monotonous sexual or intimate routine. Others may experience a rapid shift in these structures through separation, divorce, or dating. In addition, some individuals in middle adulthood may create new habits, routines, roles, and rituals in response to the co-occupations of parenting or grandparenting because they are experiencing these co-occupations for the first time or are experiencing novel stages of parenthood (i.e., raising teenagers).

Person

As previously mentioned, people in middle adulthood may experience age-related changes that influence their sexual health. These changes may include postpartum, menopausal, hormonal, physical, and physiological issues. These changes may affect arousal patterns and lead to erectile dysfunction and decreased vaginal lubrication (Fisher et al., 2020; Mert, 2018). In addition to physical and physiological changes, people may experience novel life stressors associated with this stage of life (e.g., parenting challenges, changes in long-term relationships, losing or caring for parents or older family members, new pressures at work) that can affect their sex and intimacy (Yazdanpanahi et al., 2016).

Although the sexual health changes that may occur during this stage of life must be taken into consideration, note that other personal factors continue to be important for participation in intimate partnerships in middle adulthood. For example, the types of relationships (e.g., monogamy, polyamory) that people are interested in still vary.

Older Adulthood (Ages 65 Years or Older)

Older adulthood may include many of the same phenomena and experiences as in middle adulthood, because there is significant variability in life circumstances, aging experiences, and occupational engagement. This stage is defined for the purpose of this chapter as beginning at age 65 years for consistency with U.S. policies around Social Security benefits, Medicare eligibility, and population health measures.

Context

People older than age 65 years "consistently identify sexual well-being as integral to overall quality of life" (Syme et al., 2012, p. 232). However, prevailing societal attitudes often depict older adulthood as marked by asexuality, with those who express sexual interest as abnormal or lecherous (e.g., "dirty old men"). Ageist attitudes held by society at large as well as internalized by many older adults themselves also contribute to challenges experienced by older adults in engaging in sexual activity and intimate partnerships.

Occupation

Older adults may engage in a wide variety of sexual and intimate occupations. These occupations may involve a longtime partner, themselves, or a new relationship. Family planning may take new forms, including taking care of grandchildren and helping their own children as they enter parenthood. Sexual health is an area of occupation that may be complicated by the presence of age-related health risks and conditions. For those in institutional or care settings, sexual expression may become restricted because of limited access to clothing of choice, limited range of role fulfillment opportunities, not feeling safe authentically expressing themselves, or policies restricting their ability to fully express themselves as a sexual being.

Performance

For older adults, many of the performance patterns (habits, routines, roles) of sexual and intimate occupations stem from cumulative life stage and generational cohort effects. ***Cumulative life stage effects*** are the impact and influence of individual experiences from all previous life stages on the current stage of development. For example, a bisexual woman who came out later in life and became partnered in middle adulthood may have social relationships and roles at this age that are different from a heterosexual woman who married during young adulthood. ***Generational cohort effects*** are differences between age cohorts (e.g., baby boomers vs. Gen X) that may be attributed to the unique historical circumstances experienced by cohort members, particularly when these circumstances occurred at critical developmental stages for the cohort (e.g., being a young adult during the Vietnam War vs. being in early childhood). In older adulthood, many people may have profound changes in their social lives and intimate partners that affect their occupations, such as the need to care for grandchildren or loss of a spouse. The loss of a longtime spouse or companion may decrease opportunities for sexual activity but may also present new opportunities for dating and other intimacy-building occupations.

Generational cohort effects may influence occupational choices and habits, including those involving sexual health. Sexually active older adults are at significant risk for HIV or AIDS and other STIs. According to data from athenahealth (Watertown, MA), the biggest increase of in-office STI treatments was in adults older than 60 years, in part because this group has the lowest condom use of any population (Pereto, 2018).

Some of this increased risk may be attributed to generational cohort effects or life stage effects. For example, baby boomers grew to sexual maturity when oral contraceptive pills first became widely available, and as such, they may have experienced sexual freedom with limited concern for unwanted pregnancy. By the time widespread awareness and concern about STIs occurred during the HIV/AIDS crisis of the 1980s, many boomers were already in long-term monogamous relationships and largely inoculated from this risk. As they enter older adulthood, many may be dating again for the first time in decades after a divorce or loss of a partner and engaging in less safe sexual practices because of a lack of contemporary sex education and information. Further complicating this issue, many STIs may resemble other issues attributed to aging (e.g., syphilis presents with muscle aches and fatigue and, in late stages, dementia-like symptoms; HIV or AIDS may first present as normal flu-like symptoms coinciding with decreased immune function associated with aging). This example is just one way in which life stage and generational cohort effects influence performance patterns involving sexual and intimate occupations for older adults.

Person

Typical aging includes many changes that may alter a person's sexual expression, including changes to body structures and functions that affect performance skills. Sexual activity in older adulthood may be affected by decreased physical energy and increased physical discomfort (Karraker et al., 2011). Additional age-related changes include decreased sex hormones (e.g., estrogen, testosterone), increased time and techniques for sexual response (i.e., vaginal lubrication, erection), decreased intensity of orgasm (e.g., fewer contractions, shorter ejaculation time), and longer or more pronounced refraction periods (i.e., rapid loss of erection).

In addition to these typical age-related changes, many common conditions and illnesses among older adults also affect physical factors regarding sexual activity. For example, cerebrovascular disease may lead to impaired motor skills needed for sexual activity, and anxiety can affect intimate communication. Chronic conditions, such as arthritis, hypertension, and obesity, may reduce arousal, decrease desire to continue with sexual activity, and require restricting activity to certain positions.

Prescription medications for a wide variety of conditions, including depression and hypertension, may also affect an older adult's sexual expression. Possible side effects of these medications include changes in desire and arousal, erectile dysfunction, and delayed orgasm. Medications to address issues related to sexual expression may require medication reconciliation or be contraindicated by certain conditions associated with older adults. For example, sildenafil may be used to treat erectile dysfunction but is contraindicated for people with certain cardiac conditions. Additionally, physical changes associated with a medical condition or illness may alter older adults' sexual self-view. For example, arthritis-related hand deformity may be considered "ugly" by some and diminish their self-esteem, or a woman who has had a mastectomy may feel less feminine.

Summary

This chapter highlighted some current trends in sexual and intimate occupations across the lifespan as well as the interplay of personal and contextual factors on these occupations. An important contextual factor is a person's generational cohort (e.g., millennial, boomer). Generational cohort effects are present throughout life and affect how each life stage may be experienced. For example, the experiences of sexual freedom for boomers in young adulthood may be a factor in their increased risk for STIs in older adulthood. Although we may not yet know how Gen Z will experience older age, it is useful to consider how generational trends may affect their later sexual and intimate occupations.

Although we discussed various contextual factors at different points throughout the lifespan, it is critical to acknowledge that these concepts are not static and may occur during other life stages as well. The key point is that there is no universal average human being but rather innumerable permutations of experiences and occupational engagement based on personal histories, life changes, collective identities, traumas, environmental changes, and more. Blackness, indigeneity, queerness, disability, education, geographic location, and countless other factors all interplay to create the brilliant and multitudinous expressions of sexuality and intimacy that humanity creates and experiences.

It is also crucial that we, as occupational therapy practitioners, recognize that these factors may affect people differently depending on when in the life course they experience them. Some people have experiences in childhood that influence their occupations of sexuality and intimacy as adolescents, young adults, middle adults, and older adults, whereas others may experience a similar sexual or intimate occupation for the first time in middle adulthood, thereby creating a different developmental experience. We are likely to experience some factors in the future, as will our clients. For example, at the very least, age-related changes may influence how we participate in these occupations. Therefore, it is critical that occupational therapy practitioners recognize the impact of people's lived experiences and consider the lifespan perspective when addressing sexual and intimate occupations with their clients, regardless of the age range or population they primarily work with.

We, the authors, acknowledge the impact of our own biases and perspectives on the content and structure of this chapter. Although our own mix of experiences tied to our identities helps to give us a certain amount of perspective, we cannot help but highlight the White-dominant, heterosexist, cissexist world in which we exist. Attempting to work through the structural and ideological biases inherent in culture, education, and health care to dismantle oppressive systems requires continual reflective practice and positioning and repositioning ourselves in our own context (see Chapter 3, "Guided Self-Reflection of Self as a Sexual Being," and Chapter 4, "Sexuality, Bias, and Impact: Preventing Clinician Harm," for guidance on engaging in reflective practice and mitigating bias in occupational therapy practice).

As society changes and adapts, content such as this also will change and adapt. The way people age and experience sexuality and intimacy is likely to look different in forthcoming generations because of the influence of societal changes on people's lived experiences. Thus, we challenge occupational therapy practitioners to continue learning and growing with the ever-evolving concepts and experiences of sexuality and intimacy. This knowledge is vital in supporting clients in their sexual and intimate occupations at every point in their lives.

Temor "Tay" Amin-Arsala, MS, OTR/L (he/him/they/them), is a queer, half-Afghan occupational therapy practitioner who completed his master's degree at Tufts University in Medford, Massachusetts. He also has a graduate certificate in LGBT Health Policy and Practice from George Washington University in Washington, DC. Amin-Arsala's personal and professional interests include occupational justice, inclusive and equitable health care education, and a general queering of the occupational therapy profession. He currently serves as the treasurer for the Network for LGBTQIA+ Concerns in Occupational Therapy and is the state delegate from Massachusetts to the American Occupational Therapy Association's Representative Assembly. During the workday, he is a school-based practitioner who resides in Boston.

Elizabeth K. Schmidt, PhD, OTR/L (she/her/hers), is a straight, White cisfemale who completed both her master's degree in occupational therapy and PhD in health and rehabilitation sciences at The Ohio State University in Columbus. She completed her postdoctoral training at Boston University and is currently an assistant professor of occupational therapy at the DeBusk College of Osteopathic Medicine at Lincoln Memorial University–Knoxville. She has grant funding from the National Institute of Disability, Independent Living, and Rehabilitation Research in Washington, DC, to conduct a participatory approach research study alongside queer autistic researchers to better understand supports and barriers to community participation for queer autistic adults. Schmidt's research is primarily focused on accessibility of sexuality education for adolescents and adults with neurodevelopmental disabilities. She is passionate about occupational justice and sexual and reproductive health autonomy for people with neurodevelopmental disabilities.

Joseph Christian Ungco, OTD, OTR/L (they/them/he/him), is the associate director for diversity, equity, and inclusion (DEI) education, client services, and data analytics for the Fred Hutchinson Cancer Center in Seattle. They lead several organization-wide DEI initiatives, including the bias mitigation education program and gender-inclusive and accessible spaces initiative. They also continue to serve in DEI roles in occupational therapy, including serving as co-chair of the national Network for LGBTQIA+ Concerns in Occupational Therapy and sitting on the executive council for the Occupational Therapy Multicultural, Diversity and Inclusion National Network. Dr. Ungco's work is centered on amplifying the voices of those most affected by systems of oppression and actualizing structural change.

References

Agaronnik, N., Pendo, E., Lagu, T., Dejong, C., Perez-Caraballo, A., & Iezzoni, L. I. (2020). Ensuring the reproductive rights of women with intellectual disability. *Journal of Intellectual and Developmental Disability, 45,* 365–376. https://doi.org/10.3109/13668250.2020.1762383

Agbasiere, C. L. (2022, January). *What is affirmative, enthusiastic consent?* Leda Health. https://www.leda.co/blog/what-is-affirmative-enthusiastic-consent

Age of Consent. (2021). *United States age of consent map.* https://www.ageofconsent.net/states

American Civil Liberties Union. (n.d.). *Why sodomy laws matter.* https://www.aclu.org/other/why-sodomy-laws-matter

American Occupational Therapy Association. (2020). Occupational therapy practice framework: Domain and process (4th ed.). *American Journal of Occupational Therapy, 74*(Suppl. 2), 7412410010. https://doi.org/10.5014/ajot.2020.74S2001

American Psychiatric Association. (1968). *Diagnostic and statistical manual of mental disorders* (2nd ed.).

American Society of Plastic Surgeons. (2019). *Plastic surgery statistics report.* https://www.plasticsurgery.org/documents/News/Statistics/2020/plastic-surgery-statistics-full-report-2020.pdf

Anapol, D. (2010). *Polyamory in the 21st century: Love and intimacy with multiple partners.* Rowman and Littlefield.

Arain, M., Haque, M., Johal, L., Mathur, P., Nel, W., Rais, A., . . . Sharma, S. (2013). Maturation of the adolescent brain. *Neuropsychiatric Disease and Treatment, 9,* 449–461. https://doi.org/10.2147/NDT.S39776

Atchison, B. J., & Suarez, M. (2021). Introduction to trauma and the role of occupational therapy. In A. Lynch, R. Aschcraft, & L. Tekell (Eds.), *Trauma, occupation, and participation: Foundations and population considerations in occupational therapy* (pp. 1–18). AOTA Press.

Autism Society. (n.d.). *Living with autism: Puberty and children on the autism spectrum.* https://www.autism-society.org/wp-content/uploads/2014/04/LWA_Puberty.pdf

Barnard-Brak, L., Schmidt, M., Chesnut, S., Wei, T., & Richman, D. (2014). Predictors of access to sex education for children with intellectual disabilities in public schools. *Intellectual and Developmental Disabilities, 52,* 85–97. https://doi.org/10.1352/1934-9556-52.2.85

Belsky, J. (2013). *Experiencing the lifespan* (3rd ed.). Worth Publishers.

Berns, R. M. (Ed.). (2016). *Child, family, school, community: Socialization and support.* Cengage Learning.

Bock, R. D. (2004). Multiple prepubertal growth spurts in children of the Fels Longitudinal Study: Comparison with results from the Edinburgh Growth Study. *Annals of Human Biology, 31,* 59–74. https://doi.org/10.1080/03014460310001636570

Brown, H. K., Kirkham, Y. A., Lunsky, Y., Codigo, V., & Vigod, S. N. (2018). Contraceptive provision to postpartum women with intellectual and developmental disabilities: A population-based cohort study. *Perspectives on Sexual and Reproductive Health, 50,* 93–99. https://doi.org/10.1363/psrh.12060

Butler, G. E., McKie, M., & Ratcliffe, S. G. (1990). The cyclical nature of prepubertal growth. *Annals of Human Biology, 17,* 177–198. https://doi.org/10.1080/03014469000000952

Campbell, C., Mallappa, A., Wisiniewski, A. B., & Silvosky, J. F. (2013). Sexual behavior of prepubertal children. In D. S. Bromberg & W. T. O'Donohue (Eds.), *Handbook of child and adolescent sexuality* (pp. 145–170). Academic Press. https://doi.org/10.1016/B978-0-12-387759-8.00006-4

Castleman, M. (2013). *"Hysteria" and the strange history of vibrators.* https://www.psychologytoday.com/us/blog/all-about-sex/201303/hysteria-and-the-strange-history-vibrators

Centers for Disease Control and Prevention. (2019). *Sexually transmitted disease surveillance 2018: STDs in adolescents and young adults.* https://www.cdc.gov/std/stats18/STDSurveillance2018-full-report.pdf

Chen, K.-H. (2019). Self-identity and self-esteem during different stages of adolescence: The function of identity importance and identity firmness. *Chinese Journal of Guidance and Counseling, 55,* 27–56. https://doi.org/10.3966/172851862019050055002

Clarke, M. J., Marks, A. D. G., & Lykins, A. D. (2015). Effect of normative masculinity on males' dysfunctional sexual beliefs, sexual attitudes, and perceptions of sexual functioning. *Journal of Sex Research, 52,* 327–337. https://doi.org/10.1080/00224499.2013.860072

Codina, M., Pereda, N., & Guilera, G. (2020). Lifetime victimization and poly-victimization in a sample of adults with intellectual disabilities. *Journal of Interpersonal Violence, 37,* 2062–2082. https://doi.org/10.1177/0886260520936372

Corbett, B. A., Vandekar, S., Muscatello, R. A., & Tanguturi, Y. (2020). Pubertal timing during early adolescence: Advanced pubertal onset in females with autism spectrum disorder. *Autism Research, 13,* 2202–2215. https://doi.org/10.1002/aur.2406

Crone, E. A., & Dahl, R. E. (2012). Understanding adolescence as a period of social-affective engagement and goal flexibility. *Nature Reviews Neuroscience, 13,* 636–650. https://doi.org/10.1038/nrn3313

Dammeyer, J., & Chapman, M. (2018). A national survey on violence and discrimination among people with disabilities. *BMC Public Health, 18*(355), 1–9. https://doi.org/10.1186/s12889-018-5277-0

Devine, R., & Nolan, C. (2011). Sexual identity and human occupation: A qualitative exploration. *Journal of Occupational Science, 3,* 154–161. https://doi.org/10.1080/14427591.2007.9686596

Dunn, J. (2004). *Understanding children's worlds. Children's friendships: The beginnings of intimacy.* Blackwell.

Epstein, R., Blake, J. J., & González, T. (2017). *Girlhood interrupted: The erasure of Black girls' childhood.* Georgetown Center on Poverty and Inequality. https://www.law.georgetown.edu/poverty-inequality-center/wp-content/uploads/sites/14/2017/08/girlhood-interrupted.pdf

Felitti, V. J., Anda, R. F., Nordenberg, D., Williamson, D. F., Spitz, A. M., Edwards, V., . . . Marks, J. S. (1998). Relationship of childhood abuse and household dysfunction to many of the leading causes of death in adults: The Adverse Childhood Experiences (ACE) Study. *American Journal of Preventive Medicine, 14,* 245–258. https://doi.org/10.1016/s0749-3797(98)00017-8

Fiani, C. N., & Han, H. J. (2019). Navigating identity: Experiences of binary and non-binary transgender and gender non-conforming (TGNC) adults. *International Journal of Transgenderism, 20,* 181–194. https://doi.org/10.1080/15532739.2018.1426074

Fisher, J. S., Rezk, A., Nwefo, E., Masterson, J., & Ramasamy, R. (2020). Sexual health in the elderly population. *Current Sexual Health Reports, 12,* 381–388. https://doi.org/10.1007/s11930-020-00278-0

Flores, A. R., Langton, L., Meyer, I. H., & Romero, A. P. (2020). Victimization rates and traits of sexual and gender minorities in the United States: Results from the National Crime Victimization Survey, 2017. *Science Advances, 6,* 1–10. https://doi.org/10.1126/sciadv.aba6910

Ford, C. (2019). *Boys will be boys: Power, patriarchy, and toxic masculinity.* Oneworld.

Fouquier, K. F., & Camune, B. D. (2015). Meeting the reproductive needs of female adolescents with neurodevelopmental disabilities. *Journal of Obstetric, Gynecologic and Neonatal Nursing, 44,* 553–563. https://doi.org/10.1111/1552-6909.12657

Friedrich, W. N., Fisher, J., Broughton, D., Houston, M., & Shafran, C. R. (1998). Normative sexual behavior in children: A contemporary sample. *Pediatrics, 101,* 1–8. https://doi.org/10.1542/peds.101.4.e9

Frost, J. J., Duberstein Lindberg, L., & Finer, L. B. (2012). Young adults' contraceptive knowledge, norms and attitudes: Associations with risk of unintended pregnancy. *Perspectives on Sexual and Reproductive Health, 44,* 107–116. https://doi.org/10.1363/4410712

Galton, F. (1904). Eugenics: Its definitions, aims and scope. *The Sociological Review, sp1(1),* 43–51. https://doi.org/10.1177/0038026104SP100104

Gamarel, K. E., Jadwin-Cakmak, L., King, W. M., Lacombe-Duncan, A., Trammell, R., Reyes, L. A., . . . Harper, G. W. (2020). Stigma experienced by transgender women of color in their dating and romantic relationships: Implications for gender-based violence prevention programs. *Journal of Interpersonal Violence, 37,* NP8161–NP8189. https://doi.org/10.1177/0886260520976186

Gewirtz-Meydan, A., Levkovich, I., Mock, M., Gur, U., & Ayalon, L. (2019). Promoting a discussion on later life sexuality: Lessons from sexologist physicians. *Sexual and Relationship Therapy, 34,* 193–210. https://doi.org/10.1080/14681994.2018.1437258

Gieseler, E. (2017). Gender-reveal parties: Performing community identity in pink and blue. *Journal of Gender Studies, 27,* 661–671. https://doi.org/10.1080/09589236.2017.1287066

Gougeon, N. A. (2009). Sexuality education for students with intellectual disabilities, a critical pedagogical approach: Outing the ignored curriculum. *Sex Education, 9,* 277–291. https://doi.org/10.1080/14681810903059094

Greenwood, N. W., & Wilkinson, J. (2013). Sexual and reproductive health care for women with intellectual disabilities: A primary care perspective. *International Journal of Family Medicine, 2013,* 642472. https://doi.org/10.1155/2013/642472

Guignard, F. P. (2015). A gendered bun in the oven. The gender-reveal party as a new ritualization during pregnancy. *Studies in Religion/Sciences Religieuses, 44,* 479–500. https://doi.org/10.1177/0008429815599802

Guttmacher Institute. (2021). *An overview of consent to reproductive health services by young people.* https://www.guttmacher.org/state-policy/explore/overview-minors-consent-law#

Harris, P., & Asthana, A. (2009). *Female 'cougars' are on the prowl. Or are they just a male fantasy?* https://www.theguardian.com/lifeandstyle/2009/sep/27/cougar-courtney-cox-older-women

Hassouneh-Phillips, D., & McNeff, E. (2005). "I thought I was less worthy": Low sexual and body esteem and increased vulnerability to intimate partner abuse in women with physical disabilities. *Sexuality and Disability, 23,* 227–240. https://doi.org/10.1007/s11195-005-8930-3

Haugaard, J. J. (1996). Sexual behaviors between children: Professionals' opinions and undergraduates' recollections. *Families in Society: The Journal of Contemporary Social Sciences, 77,* 81–89. https://doi.org/10.1606/1044-3894.850

Horner-Johnson, W., Moe, E. L., Stoner, R. C., Klein, K. A., Edelman, A. B., Eden, K. B., . . . Guise, J. (2018). Contraceptive knowledge and use among women with intellectual, physical, or sensory disabilities: A systematic review. *Disability and Health Journal, 12,* 139–154. https://doi.org/10.1016/j.dhjo.2018.11.006

Ingraham, C. (2015). *Do you have a dad bod? This flow chart will tell you.* https://www.washingtonpost.com/news/wonk/wp/2015/05/11/do-you-have-a-dad-bod-this-flow-chart-will-tell-you/

Johnston, L. B., & Jenkins, D. (2008). Coming out in mid-adulthood: Building a new identity. *Journal of Gay and Lesbian Social Services, 16*(2), 19–42. https://doi.org/10.1300/J041v16n02_02

Kanakis, G. A., & Goulis, D. D. (2015). Male contraception: A clinically-oriented review. *Hormones, 14,* 598–614. https://doi.org/10.14310/horm.2002.1623

Karraker, A., DeLamater, J., & Schwartz, C. R. (2011). Sexual frequency decline from midlife to later life. *Journals of Gerontology, Series B: Psychological Sciences and Social Sciences, 66B*, 502–512. https://doi.org/10.1093/geronb/gbr058

Kellogg, N. D. (2010). Sexual behaviors in children: Evaluation and management. *American Family Physician, 82*, 1233–1238.

Kirby, D., & National Campaign to Prevent Teen and Unplanned Pregnancy (U.S.). (2007). *Emerging answers, 2007: Research findings on programs to reduce teen pregnancy and sexually transmitted diseases.* National Campaign to Prevent Teen and Unplanned Pregnancy.

Knickmeyer, R. C., Wheelwright, S., Hoekstra, R., & Baron-Cohen, S. (2006). Age of menarche in females with autism spectrum conditions. *Developmental Medicine and Child Neurology, 48*, 1007–1008.

Kościński, K. (2007). Facial attractiveness: General patterns of facial preferences. *Anthropological Review, 70*, 45–79. https://doi.org/10.2478/v10044-008-0001-9

Kost, K., Maddow-Zimet, I., & Arpaia, A. (2017). *Pregnancies, births and abortions among adolescents and young women in the United States, 2013: National and state trends by age, race and ethnicity.* https://www.guttmacher.org/report/us-adolescent-pregnancy-trends-2013

Kreukels, B. P. C., Köhler, B., Nordenström, A., Roehle, R., Thyen, U., Bouvattier, C., . . . Cohen-Kettinis, P. T. (2018). Gender dysphoria and gender change in disorders of sex development/intersex conditions: Results from the dsd-LIFE Study. *Journal of Sexual Medicine, 15*, 777–785. https://doi.org/10.1016/j.jsxm.2018.02.021

Larsson, I., & Svedin, C. (2002). Sexual experiences in childhood: Young adults' recollections. *Archives of Sexual Behavior, 31*, 263–273. https://doi.org/10.1023/A:1015252903931

Lawrence, M. (2014). *Reproductive rights and state institutions: The forced sterilization of minority women in the United States.* Senior Theses, Trinity College, Hartford, CT. https://digitalrepository.trincoll.edu/theses/390

LeVay, S., Baldwin, J., & Baldwin, J. (2021). *Discovering human sexuality* (5th ed.). Oxford University Press.

Li, H., Mitra, M., Wu, J. P., Parish, S. L., Valentine, A., & Dembo, R. S. (2018). Female sterilization and cognitive disability in the United States, 2011–2015. *Obstetrics and Gynecology, 132*, 559–564. https://doi.org/10.1097/aog.0000000000002778

Luna, B., Thulborn, K. R., Munoz, D. P., Merriam, E. P., Garver, K. E., Minshew, N. J., . . . Sweeney, J. A. (2001). Maturation of widely disrupted brain function subserves cognitive development. *NeuroImage, 13*, 786–793. https://doi.org/10.1006/nimg.2000.0743

Martinez, G. M., & Abma, J. C. (2015). *Sexual activity, contraceptive use, and childbearing of teenagers aged 15–19 years in the United States.* NCHS Data Brief, 209. https://www.cdc.gov/nchs/data/databriefs/db209.pdf

Martinson, F. M. (1976). Eroticism in infancy and childhood. *Journal of Sex Research, 12*, 251–262. https://doi.org/10.1080/00224497609550945

Masten, A. S. (2018). Resilience theory and research on children and families: Past, present, and promise. *Journal of Family Theory and Review, 10*, 12–31. https://doi.org/10.1111/jftr.12255

McCarthy, M. (2009). Contraception and women with intellectual disabilities. *Journal of Applied Research in Intellectual Disabilities, 22*, 363–369. https://doi.org/10.1111/j.1468-3148.2008.00464.x

Mert, M. (2018). Can programmed aging theory adequately explain sexual dysfunction among the elderly? *Studies by Undergraduate Researchers at Guelph.* https://doi.org/10.21083/surg.v10i1.3199

Mesman, G. R., Harper, S. L., Edge, N. A., Brandt, T. W., & Pemberton, J. L. (2019). Problematic sexual behavior in children. *Journal of Pediatric Health Care, 33*, 323–331. https://doi.org/10.1016/j.pedhc.2018.11.002

Minto, C. L., Liao, L., Woodhouse, C. R. J., Ransley, P. G., & Creighton, S. M. (2003). The effect of clitoral surgery on sexual outcome in individuals who have intersex conditions with ambiguous genitalia: A cross-sectional study. *Lancet, 361*, 1252–1257. https://doi.org/10.1016/S0140-6736(03)12980-7

Monto, M. A., & Carey, A. G. (2014). A new standard for sexual behavior? Are claims associated with the "hookup culture" supported by general social survey data? *Journal of Sex Research, 51*, 605–615. https://doi.org/10.1080/00224499.2014.906031

Moore-Ramirez, A., Kautzman-East, M., & Ginicola, M. M. (2017). LGBTQI+ persons in adulthood. In M. M. Ginicola, C. Smith, & J. M. Filmore (Eds.), *Affirmative counseling with LGBTQI+ people* (pp. 49–60). American Counseling Association. https://doi.org/10.1002/9781119375517.ch5

Morrison, C. J. (2020). *Toxic masculinity: Male childhood sexual trauma, and the challenges to how young men heal* (Pub. No. 79604) [Masters thesis, Dalhousie University]. Faculty of Graduate Studies Online Theses.

Murray, S. H., Milhausen, R. R., Graham, C. A., & Kuczynski, L. (2017). A qualitative exploration of factors that affect sexual desire among men aged 30–65 in long-term relationships. *Journal of Sex Research, 54*, 319–330. https://doi.org/10.1080/00224499.2016.1168352

National Center on the Sexual Behavior of Youth. (2020). *Normative sexual behavior.* http://www.ncsby.org/content/normative-sexual-behavior

Neumann, N., Neu, D., & Ungco, J. C. (2021). Addressing LGBTQIA+ trauma: Your role and your responsibility. In A. Lynch (Ed.), *Trauma, occupation, and participation* (pp. 195–221). AOTA Press.

Newcomb, M. E., Hill, R., Buehler, K., Ryan, D. T., Whitton, S. W., & Mustanski, B. (2020). High burden of mental health problems, substance use, violence, and related psychosocial factors in transgender, non-binary, and gender diverse youth and young adults. *Archives of Sexual Behavior, 49*, 645–649. https://doi.org/10.1007/s10508-019-01533-9

Nicolosi, A., Laumann, E. O., Glasser, D. B., Moreira, E. D., Paik, A., & Gingell, C. (2004). Sexual behavior and sexual dysfunctions after age 40: The global study of sexual attitudes and behaviors. *Urology, 64*, 991–997. https://doi.org/10.1016/j.urology.2004.06.055

Ojanuga, D. (1993). The medical ethics of the 'father of gynaecology', Dr J Marion Sims. *Journal of Medical Ethics, 19*, 28–31. https://doi.org/10.1136/jme.19.1.28

Okami, P., Olmstead, R., & Abramson, P. R. (1997). Sexual experiences in early childhood: 18-year longitudinal data from the UCLA Family Lifestyles Project. *Journal of Sex Research, 34*, 339–347. https://doi.org/10.1080/00224499709551902

Okkerse, J. M. E., Beemer, F. A., Haan, M. C., Boer, J. A. H., Mellenbergh, G. J., & Wolters, W. H. G. (2001). Facial attractiveness and facial impairment ratings in children with craniofacial malformations. *Cleft Palate-Craniofacial Journal, 38*, 336–392. https://doi.org/10.1597/1545-1569_2001_038_0386_faafir_2.0.c

Oswald, F., Hughes, S., Champion, A., & Penderson, C. L. (2022). In search of the appeal of the 'DILF'. *Psychology & Sexuality, 13*, 283–301. https://doi.org/10.1080/19419899.2020.1769164

Padawer, R. (2009). *Keeping up with being kept.* https://www.nytimes.com/2009/04/12/magazine/12sugardaddies-t.html

Pegoraro, L. (2014). Second-rate victims: The forced sterilization of indigenous peoples in the USA and Canada. *Settler Colonial Studies, 5,* 161–173. https://doi.org/10.1080/2201473X.2014.955947

Peñaloza, M. (2020, September 19). *A firefighter is killed in California wildfire sparked by gender reveal party.* National Public Radio. https://www.npr.org/2020/09/18/914368098/a-firefighter-is-killed-in-california-wildfire-sparked-by-gender-reveal-party

Peper, J. S., & Dahl, R. E. (2013). The teenage brain: Surging hormones–brain–behavior interactions during puberty. *Current Directions in Science, 22,* 134–139. https://doi.org/10.1177/0963721412473755

Pereto, A. (2018, May 16). *Patients over 60? Screen for STIs.* https://www.athenahealth.com/knowledge-hub/clinical-trends/over-60-stis-may-not-be-done-you

Perry, C. (2020). *How gender reveal parties reinforce a harmful binary.* https://www.verywellfamily.com/how-gender-reveal-parties-reinforce-a-harmful-binary-5077547

Reis, M., Ramiro, L., de Matos, M. G., & Diniz, J. A. (2011). The effects of sex education in promoting sexual and reproductive health in Portuguese university students. *Procedia-Social and Behavioral Sciences, 29,* 477–485. https://doi.org/10.1016/j.sbspro.2011.11.266

Robinson, K. H. (2012). 'Difficult citizenship': The precarious relationships between childhood, sexuality and access to knowledge. *Sexualities, 15,* 257–276. https://doi.org/10.1177/1363460712436469

Rosenfield, R. L., Bachrach, L. K., Chernausek, S. D., Gertner, J. M., Gottschalk, M., Hardin, D. D., . . . Saenger, P. (2000). Current age of onset of puberty. *Pediatrics, 106,* 622. https://doi.org/10.1542/peds.106.3.622

Rucinski, C. L., Sutton, E., Carlton, R., Downer, J., & Brown, J. L. (2021). Classroom racial/ethnic diversity and upper elementary children's social-emotional development, *Applied Developmental Science, 25,* 183–199. https://doi.org/10.1080/10888691.2019.1576524

Sheridan, K. J. (2020). Premature and delayed sexual maturation in children with cerebral palsy. *Cerebral Palsy,* 985–1002. https://doi.org/10.1007/978-3-319-74558-9_75

Short, M. B., & Rosenthal, S. L. (2008). Psychosocial development and puberty. *New York Academy of Sciences, 1135,* 36–42. https://doi.org/10.1196/annals.1429.011

Smet, N., & Lucas, C. B. (2020). Occupational therapy view of child development. In J. C. O'Brien & H. Kuhaneck (Eds.), *Case-Smith's occupational therapy for children and adolescents* (8th ed., pp. 76–121). Elsevier.

Smith, T. W., Davern, M., Freese, J., & Morgan, S. L. (2019). *General social surveys, 1972–2018.* NORC at the University of Chicago.

Stern, A. M. (2005). Eugenics and historical memory in America. In *Eugenic Nation: Faults and frontiers of better breeding in modern America* (2nd ed., pp. 1–11). Blackwell.

Stuewig, J., Tangney, J. P., Kendall, S., Folk, J. B., Reinsmith Meyer, C., & Dearing, R. L. (2015). Children's proneness to shame and guilt predict risky and illegal behaviors in young adulthood. *Child Psychiatry and Human Development, 46,* 217–227. https://doi.org/10.1007/s10578-014-0467-1

Syme, M. L., Klonoff, E. A., Macera, C. A., & Brodine, S. K. (2012). Predicting sexual decline and dissatisfaction among older adults: The role of partnered and individual physical and mental health factors. *Journal of Gerontology: Series B. Psychological Sciences and Social Sciences, 68,* 323–327. https://doi.org/10.1093/geronb/gbs087

Szucs, L. E., Lowry, R., Fasula, A. M., Pampati, S., Copen, C. E., Hussaini, K. S., . . . Steiner, R. J. (2020). Condom and contraceptive use among sexually active high school students—Youth Risk Behavior Survey, United States, 2019. *MMWR, 69*(1), 11–18. https://www.cdc.gov/healthyyouth/data/yrbs/pdf/2019/su6901-H.pdf

Taouk, L. H., Fialkow, M. F., & Schuolkin, J. A. (2018). Provision of reproductive healthcare to women with disabilities: A survey of obstetrician-gynecologists' training, practices, and perceived barriers. *Health Equity, 2,* 207–215. https://doi.org/10.1089/heq.2018.0014

Thirumalai, A., & Page, S. T. (2019). Recent developments in male contraception. *Drugs, 79,* 11–20. https://doi.org/10.1007/s40265-018-1038-8

Tilley, E., Walmsley, J., Earle, S., & Atkinson, D. (2012). 'The silence is roaring': Sterilization, reproductive rights and women with intellectual disabilities. *Disability and Society, 27,* 413–426. https://doi.org/10.1080/09687599.2012.654991

Torpy, S. J. (2000). Native American women and coerced sterilization: On the trail of tears in the 1970s. *American Indian Culture and Research Journal, 24*(2), 1–22. https://doi.org/10.17953/aicr.24.2.7646013460646042

van Lankveld, J. D. M., Dewitte, M., Verboon, P., & van Hooren, S. A. H. (2021). Associations of intimacy, partner responsiveness, and attachment-related emotional needs with sexual desire. *Frontiers in Psychology, 21,* 1–13. https://doi.org/10.3389/fpsyg.2021.665967

Walker, B., Otte, K., LeMond, K., Hess, P., Kaizer, K., Faulkner, T., & Christy, D. (2020). Development of the Occupational Performance Inventory of Sexuality and Intimacy (OPISI): Phase one. *Open Journal of Occupational Therapy, 8,* 1–18. https://doi.org/10.15453/2168-6408.1694

Weber, A. M., Cislaghi, B., Meausoone, V., Abdalla, S., Mejiía-Guevara, I., Loftus, P., . . . Darmstadt, G. L. (2019). Gender norms and health: Insights from global survey data. *The Lancet, 393,* 2455–2468. https://doi.org/10.1016/S0140-6736(19)30765-2

Witten, T. M. (2008). Life course analysis—The courage to search for something more: Middle adulthood issues in the transgender and intersex community. *Journal of Human Behavior in the Social Environment, 8,* 189–224. https://doi.org/10.1300/J137v08n02_12

Workman, C. I., Humphries, S., Hartung, F., Aguirre, G., Kable, J., & Chatterjee, A. (2020). *Morality is in the eye of the beholder: The neurocognitive basis of the "anomalous-is-bad" stereotype.* https://doi.org/10.31234/osf.io/mz75u

World Population Review. (2021). *Age of consent by state 2021.* https://worldpopulationreview.com/state-rankings/age-of-consent-by-state

Worley, G., Houlihan, C. M., Herman-Giddens, M. E., O'Donnell, M. E., Conaway, M., Stallings, V. A., . . . Stevenson, R. D. (2002). Secondary sexual characteristics in children with cerebral palsy and moderate to severe motor impairment: A cross-sectional survey. *Pediatrics, 110,* 897–902. https://doi.org/10.1542/peds.110.5.897

Wu, J. P., McKee, M. M., McKee, K. S., Meade, M. A., Plague, M., & Sen, A. (2017). Female sterilization is more common among women with physical and/or sensory disabilities than women without disabilities in the United States. *Disability and Health Journal, 10,* 400–405. https://doi.org/10.1016/j.dhjo.2016.12.020

Wu, J., Zhang, J., Mitra, M., Parish, S. L., & Minama Reddy, G. K. (2018). Provision of moderately and highly effective reversible contraception to insured women with intellectual and developmental disabilities. *Obstetrics and Gynecology, 132,* 565–574. https://doi.org/10.1097%2FAOG.0000000000002777

Yazdanpanahi, Z., Beygi, Z., Akbarzadeh, M., & Zare, N. (2016). To investigate the relationship between stress, anxiety and depression with sexual function and its domains in women of reproductive age. *International Journal of Medical Research and Health Sciences, 5*(10), 223–231.

6

Sexuality and Intimacy Screening and Assessment

Beth Ann Walker, *PhD, MS, OTR, FAOTA*

CHAPTER HIGHLIGHTS

- Developing an occupation-focused approach to evaluation
- Professional responsibilities
- Theory-based assessment
- Occupational Performance Inventory of Sexuality and Intimacy
- Introducing the client to the topic of sexuality and intimacy and screening for services
- Components of a comprehensive evaluation
- Writing goals

KEY TERMS AND CONCEPTS

Family planning
Intimacy
Occupational Performance Inventory of Sexuality and Intimacy
Occupational Therapy Sexual Assessment Framework
Sexual activity
Sexual expression
Sexual health
Sexual interest
Sexual knowledge
Sexual response
Sexual self-view

This chapter discusses the role of evaluation in occupational therapy to assess aspects of client sexuality and intimacy. After reviewing the history of the development of occupation-focused assessment of sexuality and intimacy, the chapter discusses professional responsibilities, elements of comprehensive assessment, and advice for initiating the screening and evaluation process. Case examples are provided.

Developing an Occupation-Focused Approach to Evaluation

To appreciate the role of evaluation of sexuality and intimacy in occupational therapy, it is important to explore what led to the development of assessment tools in this area. A literature review indicates a resounding call to the profession regarding the role of occupational therapy in addressing the sexuality and intimacy needs of clients. In 1978, Neistadt and Baker highlighted a process to identify the major functional problems related to sex for people with physical disabilities. Since then, extensive research has highlighted the need for occupational therapy practice to address sexuality and intimacy and defined the profession's scope and direction in this area (e.g., Eglseder & Webb, 2017; Walker, Otte, et al., 2020). Research has also revealed known barriers to addressing sexuality and intimacy in occupational therapy practice (e.g., McGrath & Sakellariou, 2016; Rose & Hughes, 2018).

Occupational therapy practitioners may avoid discussing sexuality and intimacy with clients for several reasons. A review of the literature suggests that barriers tend to cluster around the themes of comfort, competence, attitude, and prioritization (Areskoug-Josefsson et al., 2016; McGrath & Sakellariou, 2016). Practitioners have noted that they often avoid discussing the topic because they are embarrassed, uncomfortable, and not sure how and when to bring up topics that may be considered taboo. Why should it be the client's responsibility to address sexuality with the practitioner? Clients are more likely to discuss sex when they are directly asked (Valvano et al., 2014). Failure to recognize or address the impact of illness, injury, disability, or life stage on client sexuality, intimacy, and overall sexual health and well-being may lead to several negative outcomes (Exhibit 6.1).

Most discussions regarding barriers to the practice of occupational therapy in addressing sexuality and intimacy refer to the use of the PLISSIT model, developed by Annon (1976), to navigate the conversation between practitioners and clients. The PLISSIT model is frequently referred to in the literature for use by health care professionals of all specialties to help introduce and assist in discussing sexual matters within clinical settings. The model comprises four levels—*p*ermission, *l*imited *i*nformation, *s*pecific *s*uggestions, and *i*ntensive *t*herapy—and was originally designed for sexuality counseling and education. It is useful in understanding the different levels of addressing sexuality and intimacy with clients and serves as a guide for how to request clients' permission to address sexual concerns, provide clients with general information about their concerns, give specific suggestions regarding their questions, and offer intensive therapy as needed. Therapists who do not feel equipped to address clients' sexual concerns or who have not had the appropriate training may refer clients to a specialized sexuality therapist.

The focus of the PLISSIT model is to help practitioners introduce the topic of sexuality and intimacy, establish that clients can discuss these issues with them, and determine the level of counseling needed. Once the client grants permission to discuss sexuality and intimacy, the practitioner must rely on the client to initiate the conversation, readily identify known deficits in occupational performance, and provide general information about the concerns that the client feels comfortable addressing. This model can be problematic, because although practitioners can create a positive atmosphere for the discussion, not all clients are able to readily identify, articulate, or understand the scope of possible performance issues applicable

EXHIBIT 6.1
Potential Outcomes Associated With Failure to Address the Sexuality and Intimacy Needs of Clients

- Lower quality of life
- Decreased life satisfaction
- Higher levels of depression and anxiety
- Lowered self-esteem
- Poor body image
- Decreased satisfaction in gender-based role identity and performance
- Feelings of dissociation from one's sexual identity
- Lowered self-confidence
- Hampered or impaired sexual expression
- Confusion about the impact of conditions on sexuality and intimacy
- Incorrect assumptions that the client is asexual
- Reduced access to available resources
- Decline in engagement in sexual activity
- Lowered sexual satisfaction
- Difficulty performing acts required to engage in sex, such as transfers, dressing, and positioning safely
- Decreased arousal levels, sexual interest and desire, and sexual response associated with sexual activity
- Social isolation
- Lowered self-efficacy in pursuit of new relationships
- Disruption in roles and routines associated with intimate relationships
- Strained intimate or sexual relationships, or dissolution of those relationships
- Difficulties with physiological arousal
- Difficulty achieving an orgasm
- Inadequate sexual education
- Increased risk for sexually transmitted infections

to occupational therapy services or know that occupational therapy practitioners address these topics (Walker, 2020b).

As occupational therapy practitioners, how do we expect a client in an occupational therapy session to respond to an impromptu question asking whether they have any concerns regarding aspects of sexuality and intimacy? Most clients would *not* respond as follows:

> *As a matter of fact, my partner and I haven't had sex since my accident a year ago, I live in constant fear that my colostomy bag is going to bust, foreplay is a challenge because my hand goes numb when I try to massage my clit or my partner's clit, and it's getting harder and harder to reach orgasm. I wonder if my medication interferes with my desire to participate in sexual activities. I was strong—a protector and a provider. My partner and I really valued that about each other, and now they probably see me as a burden. I never know who I can talk to in this ultraconservative health care environment. You've been so candid and open with me about sex. Thank you for being a sexuality-affirming occupational therapist, because I felt like there was no one who would understand or be able to help me.*

In addition, the details clients feel comfortable sharing are often only the tip of the iceberg. More structure and guidance are needed to facilitate the conversation and comprehensively assess the client's occupational performance needs (Walker, LeMond, et al., 2020).

Professional Responsibilities

According to the *Occupational Therapy Code of Ethics* (American Occupational Therapy Association [AOTA], 2020a), under Principle 1, Beneficence, "[o]ccupational therapy personnel shall demonstrate a concern for the well-being and safety of persons" (p. 3). Sexuality affects how people see themselves and others and how they approach relationships. People are social beings with an innate desire to relate to and connect with other people. Without intimacy on some level, health and wellness are compromised.

The *Code of Ethics* further outlines the Standards of Conduct for Occupational Therapy Personnel. The fourth standard, Service Delivery, states that "[o]ccupational therapy personnel strive to deliver quality services that are occupation based, client centered, safe, interactive, culturally sensitive, evidence based, and consistent with occupational therapy's values and philosophies" (p. 7). In addition, occupational therapy personnel are responsible for providing appropriate evaluation and a plan of intervention for recipients of occupational therapy services specific to their needs. If practitioners do not address their clients' concerns, who will? Although many professions address aspects of sexuality and intimacy with clients, occupational therapy practitioners are the experts in understanding the impact of client factors, environment, and activity demands on participation in valued occupations (Walker, 2020b).

The *Occupational Therapy Practice Framework: Domain and Process* (4th ed.; *OTPF–4;* AOTA, 2020b) states that evaluation is a key component in the occupational therapy process. The purpose of evaluation in occupational therapy is to collaborate with clients to determine what they want and need to do; understand their occupational history; and identify their capabilities, supports, and barriers to optimal health, well-being, and participation within their contexts. It is important for occupational therapy practitioners to use valid and reliable measurements that clearly capture, identify, and measure occupational performance to support the need for skilled occupational therapy services.

Occupational therapy practitioners have also been called to be more deliberate in using theory-based and occupation-centered assessments (Gillen & Hinojosa, 2015; Walker, Otte, et al., 2020). Taking an occupation-centered perspective toward evaluation will more likely lead to occupation-based or occupation-focused intervention and guide clinical reasoning (Fisher, 2014). Gill et al. (2011) suggested that a comprehensive analysis of factors, including gender identity, sexual orientation, relationship status, age, physical health, and strengths and barriers to relationships, would enhance the evaluation and intervention process regarding sexuality and intimacy.

Introducing the Client to the Topic of Sexuality and Intimacy and Screening for Services

It is important to establish, early in the therapeutic relationship, that sexuality and intimacy are appropriate and acceptable topics to be addressed during therapy. Occupational therapy practitioners should express to clients that it is normal for them to have questions or concerns about how their condition or life stage may affect sexuality and intimacy. They should also indicate that many clients would like more information regarding this topic but do not know whom or what to ask. The earlier the topic of sexuality and intimacy is introduced, screened, assessed, and addressed, the greater the likelihood is that the client will receive skilled services that positively influence their ability to participate in sexuality and intimacy.

Through a discussion of the role of occupational therapy with people of all ages, clients can be informed that sex and intimacy are considered important and valued ADLs. Telling clients that it is understandable for them to be apprehensive about discussing the topic (and that they should not feel obligated to do so) assures them that the topic is appropriate to broach with the practitioner. It also helps assure them that they have permission to talk and learn about the impact their condition may have on sexuality and intimacy. Practitioners should be sure to convey that any information the client provides or discusses will be strictly confidential.

Components of a Comprehensive Evaluation

Once a need for service has been established, a comprehensive evaluation of sexuality and intimacy should follow. This evaluation should be occupation centered rather than diagnosis centered and address all aspects of the various occupational dimensions of sexuality and intimacy. It should determine how a person's client factors, body structures, and body functions influence performance of relevant occupations that occur within the client's context. Occupational therapists are encouraged to use standardized occupational therapy assessments, which enable practitioners to articulate how the findings from the assessment relate to the practice of occupational therapy (Gillen & Hinojosa, 2015).

Comprehensive assessment should also take into consideration the client's present condition or diagnosis, symptoms, limitations, strengths, past medical history, precautions, prognosis, and clinical pathway. The use of multiple assessments may be necessary to provide the most accurate picture of the factors influencing occupational performance. For example, occupational therapists may also incorporate any of the following as part of a well-rounded assessment: manual muscle testing and assessment of range of motion, tactile sensation, pain scales, perceived exertion, fatigue, cognitive skills, or psychosocial factors. According to Soros and Reese (2019), other formal assessments include the Canadian Occupational Performance Measure (Law et al., 2019), the Adolescent/Adult Sensory Profile (Brown & Dunn, 2002), and the Patient-Reported Outcomes Measurement Information System (PROMIS) Sexual Function and Satisfaction Measure (Weinfurt et al., 2015).

Contextual Considerations

During the evaluation process, occupational therapy practitioners should strive to fully appreciate the context in which their clients' sexuality and intimacy occurs to gain "insights into the overarching, underlying, and embedded influences on engagement" in this area (AOTA, 2020b, p. 9). Physical, technological, social, attitudinal, and accessible resources play an essential role in communicating sexuality or participation in activities relevant to sexuality and intimacy. Physical environments incorporate natural and built surroundings as well as the objects that are in them. Practitioners should consider elements within a person's physical environment that may influence optimal performance in related activities. They should also pay attention to the social atmosphere and co-occupations of their clients and recognize the availability and expectations of those who are significant to clients, such as partners, friends, and caregivers (AOTA, 2020b).

According to Walker, Otte, et al. (2020), personal factors of context, age, socioeconomic status, gender, and educational status are all part of the way people internally and externally view their sexual identity and how they express themselves. The values and beliefs within a person's cultural context dictate accepted sexual practices and norms that influence personal sexual expression, identity, and activity. These factors also influence the availability of a person's sexual partners and the avenues in which they have the opportunity to gain sexual knowledge and experience. The experience of sexuality and intimacy is also shaped by a person's temporal context, given that perceptions, expectations, participation, and performance change over time and across the life course. How people identify and express themselves as sexual beings and participate in activities pertaining to sexuality and intimacy are heavily influenced by their virtual context, whether through smartphones, computers, or social media.

Theory-Based Assessment

Walker, Otte, et al. (2020) developed the ***Occupational Therapy Sexual Assessment Framework*** (OTSAF) to define the occupational nature of sexuality and intimacy; depict how the theoretical constructs intertwine with the domain of occupational therapy; and further guide scale development, intervention design, and measurement of outcomes. A clear conceptualization of the construct being measured is vital to instrument development. Development of the OTSAF involved delineating, defining, and determining the breadth of the occupational nature of sexuality and intimacy.

According to the OTSAF, sexual activity, sexual expression, intimacy, sexual health, and family planning are valued occupations. Like all occupations, performance of these occupations is influenced by client factors, body functions, body structures, and performance skills and patterns needed for optimal participation within the context of the client. More specifically, the main client factors related to sexuality and intimacy consist of body functions (including sexual interest and sexual response); body structures; and values, beliefs, and spirituality (including sexual knowledge and sexual self-view).

Occupational Performance Inventory of Sexuality and Intimacy

The ***Occupational Performance Inventory of Sexuality and Intimacy*** (OPISI©; Walker, 2020a, 2020b)* was created to comprehensively screen, assess, and measure performance related to the complex occupational nature of sexuality and intimacy; it is based on the OTSAF. The OPISI was designed for use by occupational therapy practitioners as part of a skilled service for clients of occupational therapy. It consists of an initial screen and an in-depth self-assessment of the main client factors related to sexuality and intimacy, as described in the OTSAF.

OPISI Development

Phase 1 in the development of the OPISI was informed by Devellis's (2017) guidelines for scale development and included the following steps: mapping the construct, reviewing 31 existing tools associated with the topic of sexuality and intimacy, categorizing existing items into constructs of the OTSAF, modifying items to reflect terminology consistent with the *OTPF*, creating new items until theoretical saturation was achieved, and determining indicators and scale of measurement. The last step of Phase 1 was a pilot study to review the initial item pool (Walker et al., 2020).

Phase 2 (Walker et al., 2021) used a modified Delphi technique to further develop and validate the OPISI; this process consisted of three iterative rounds with the purpose of gaining consensus between a panel of experts. Each round focused on

* The OPISI tools and resources are public domain documents that may be downloaded following registration at http://opisi.uindy.edu. Although items of the OPISI are included within this chapter and used with permission, the OPISI is protected by copyright under U.S. copyright laws and is the property of Beth Ann Walker and the University of Indianapolis. Readers may not copy, reproduce, distribute, publish, display, modify, create derivative works, transmit, or in any way exploit any such content as it pertains to the items of the OPISI included within this book.

gathering feedback concerning the clarity, relevance, importance, and inclusion of each item within the final tool. Through iterative rounds, researchers added, modified, and removed items until all items reached 80% agreement among the expert panel members.

OPISI Administration: Initial Screen and In-Depth Assessment

The OPISI screening tool consists of 13 items in a check-all-that-apply format. One item addresses the importance of the topic to the client, 8 items address the different constructs of the OTSAF, and 4 items concern preferences for service delivery. The purpose of the initial screen is to assure the client that sexuality and intimacy are appropriate and acceptable topics to be addressed during therapy and to gather and review information about the client to determine the need for continued evaluation and intervention. The screening tool may be presented to a client at any point during occupational therapy services. In addition, physicians have administered the OPISI screening tool when related topics are brought up during appointments to determine the need for referral for occupational therapy services.

The OPISI in-depth self-assessment was designed to provide a greater understanding of the client factors and body functions that influence performance of occupations associated with sexuality and intimacy within the client's context. It presents a list of possible concerns in each OTSAF dimension of sexuality and intimacy and asks the client to identify those that are problematic. For the dimensions in which a client has concerns, occupational therapists can work with the client to develop goals, plan interventions, and make necessary referrals.

Each dimension includes a four-item performance measure to quantify the client's perception of occupational performance regarding ability, satisfaction with ability, understanding of how their condition affects performance (sexual knowledge), and confidence in their skills and ability to make necessary modifications to change performance (self-efficacy). The client rates each component of the performance measure on a scale of 1 to 10, where 1 represents the lowest rating.

Importance of Sexual Knowledge

Sexual knowledge is a client factor that refers to what a person knows, understands, believes, and values regarding sexuality and intimacy (Walker, Otte, et al., 2020). A person's understanding of how their condition, disability, illness, or injury may influence their participation in intimate activities, expression of sexuality, and overall health and well-being is an aspect of sexual knowledge. Occupational therapy services that aim to address the OTSAF dimensions of sexual activity, sexual interest, sexual response, sexual expression, sexual self-view, intimacy, sexual health, and family planning will add to the client's overall sexual knowledge. In addition, it is imperative that occupational therapy practitioners gather enough information from their clients during the evaluation process to collaboratively determine where knowledge gaps may exist.

Dimensions of the Occupational Performance Inventory of Sexuality and Intimacy

The sections that follow describe each dimension of the OPISI (sexual activity, sexual interest, sexual response, sexual expression, sexual self-view, sexual health, and family planning). Each section includes detailed information on the dimension and a case example to illustrate how the dimension might present with a client. With all dimensions, it is important for the occupational therapy practitioner to attend to the client's ratings on the four performance measures, because these ratings will help guide intervention.

Sexual activity

The occupation of ***sexual activity*** involves a person's ability to safely engage in sexual or intimate activities (alone or with others). Sexual activities may include caressing, kissing, foreplay, masturbation, oral sex, anal sex, vaginal sex, and the use of sexual toys or devices (Walker, Otte, et al., 2020). Evaluation in this area should seek to identify all the client's relevant concerns and to understand the client's perception of not only their ability to participate in sexual activities of their choice, whether performed alone for self-pleasure or with a partner, but also their satisfaction with their performance. Possible client concerns regarding sexual activity in the OPISI are listed in Exhibit 6.2.

The concerns in Exhibit 6.2 are not the only ones a person might have in the area of sexual activity, but they serve as a place to start and should open up opportunities for the client to discuss any other issues. Next, the occupational therapy practitioner should seek to determine how well the client understands the influence of their condition or life stage on their participation in sexual activities. The practitioner should also ask the client how confident they are in their skills and abilities to make necessary changes to improve their participation in sexual activities. Case Example 6.1 presents an evaluative scenario that includes screening, self-assessment, and measurement of performance for a client who recently had a myocardial infarction.

Sexual interest

Sexual interest is a client factor that encompasses a person's psychological and physiological drive, motivation, desire, or libido related to participation in sexual activities, whether alone or with another person (Walker, Otte, et al., 2020). It is often associated with a body function. Evaluation in this area should seek to identify the client's relevant concerns and attempt to understand the client's perception of their sexual interest and their satisfaction with their current sexual interest or

EXHIBIT 6.2
Client Concerns in the OPISI Regarding the Occupation of Sexual Activity

1. I am not sexually active, and this concerns me.
2. I am not satisfied with the quality of my sex life.
3. My symptoms prevent me from enjoying or participating in sexual activities.
4. My condition prevents me from engaging in sexual activities as frequently as I would like.
5. I am not satisfied and/or comfortable with cuddling and/or physical intimacy.
6. I have not had enough sexual experience to know what my sexual activity preferences are.
7. I have not established sexual boundaries or do not know how to determine my sexual boundaries.
8. I would like to explore alternative options to increase the variety of ways I participate in sexual activities.
9. I experience pain during foreplay or sexual activities that do not include penetration.
10. I experience discomfort or pain with penetration.
11. I avoid participation in sexual activities that include penetration due to pain.
12. I avoid participation in sexual activities for fear that my symptoms will get worse.
13. I am not sure how to modify sexual activity to accommodate for my limitations or symptoms.
14. I have difficulty positioning myself adequately or safely during sexual activities.
15. I worry about my ability to control my bladder and/or bowel or urinary and/or bowel symptoms during sexual activity.
16. I am worried about how my catheter, colostomy bag, tubes, wires, or other medical device interferes with sexual activity.
17. I have limited knowledge of or ability to use alternative methods of giving or receiving pleasure.
18. I have limited knowledge or ability to use sex toys.
19. Lack of privacy in my daily life interferes with my ability to engage in intimate and/or sexual activities.
20. I experience limited or absent hand function, which makes participating in sexual activities a challenge.
21. Tremors or shaking in my hands or body hinders my engagement in sexual activity.
22. I worry that I do not have the strength, energy, or endurance to adequately participate in sexual activity.
23. I worry about getting dizzy during sexual activity.
24. I worry about losing my balance during sexual activity.
25. I do not think my body is flexible enough to participate in sexual activity.
26. I lack the coordination needed to engage in certain sexual activities.
27. Impaired sense of touch and pressure interferes with my ability to enjoy certain sexual activities.
28. I am concerned that limited vision or hearing interferes with my sexual activity.
29. I become anxious and find it hard to relax during sexual activities.
30. I worry that my medications will affect my performance during sexual activity.
31. My limited ability to attend to my appearance and hygiene in preparation for sexual activities is a problem.
32. I experience difficulty dressing/undressing myself or my partner in preparation for sexual activities.
33. I experience difficulty opening, putting on, or removing a condom, inserting or removing a diaphragm, and/or applying lubrication during sexual activities.

Source. From *Occupational Performance Inventory of Sexuality and Intimacy (OPISI),* by B. A. Walker, 2020a (https://opisi.uindy.edu). Copyright © 2020 by Beth Ann Walker and University of Indianapolis.

CASE EXAMPLE 6.1. STEFON: SEXUAL ACTIVITY CONCERNS AFTER MYOCARDIAL INFARCTION

Stefon is a 67-year-old male pediatrician who recently had a myocardial infarction. Although he had a good understanding of his cardiac condition, he was not sure of its impact on his sexual activity. Before discharge from the hospital, his occupational therapist mentioned that many people have concerns regarding their participation in sexual activities. After a screen, the hospital occupational therapist referred Stefon to an outpatient occupational therapy clinic for further evaluation using the OPISI.

Stefon identified the following concerns pertaining to sexual activity:

- I avoid participation in sexual activities for fear that my symptoms will get worse.
- I worry that I do not have the strength, energy, or endurance to adequately participate in sexual activity.
- I would like to explore alternative options to increase the variety of ways I participate in sexual activities.

Stefon noted that because of his fear of having another heart attack, he rated his ability to participate in sexual activities with his partner as 0/10. He also rated his satisfaction with his ability as 0/10. Stefon rated his understanding of how his heart condition influenced his participation in sexual activities as an 8/10, because he knew that he needed to avoid getting his heart rate up, but he assumed that meant he could no longer have sex with his partner. He rated his confidence in his skills and ability rather high (8/10), noting that he was willing to make necessary accommodations if doing so would enable him to regain participation in sexual activities.

desire. Possible client concerns regarding sexual interest in the OPISI are listed in Exhibit 6.3.

Once concerns regarding sexual interest are identified, the practitioner should seek to determine how well the client understands how their condition or life stage influences their sexual interest. In addition, it is important for the practitioner to ask the client how confident they are in their skills and ability to make necessary changes to change their sexual interest. Case Example 6.2 presents an evaluative scenario, including screening, self-assessment, and measure of performance for a person with multiple sclerosis (MS) who is recovering from a recent severe exacerbation of symptoms.

EXHIBIT 6.3
Client Concerns in the OPISI Regarding the Client Factor of Sexual Interest

1. I am dissatisfied with my desire to engage in sexual activities.
2. I worry that my condition interferes with my overall level of sexual interest, drive, or desire.
3. My condition interferes with feeling aroused or excited in preparation for or during sexual activities.
4. It takes me longer to get "turned on" or aroused for participating in sexual activities.
5. Limited energy interferes with my desire to participate in sexual activities.
6. The amount of physical and/or emotional effort required to participate in sexual activities diminishes my sexual interest or desire.
7. My sexual interest is low because I am sad or depressed.
8. I do not fully understand what turns me on or off sexually.
9. I avoid situations that arouse me sexually.
10. I am not interested in sexual activity at the same time as my partner(s).
11. Pain, or anticipation of pain, interferes with my desire to participate in sexual activities.
12. Lack of sleep interferes with my interest in participating in sexual activities.
13. Lack of spontaneity interferes with my sex drive.
14. Stress between myself and my partner(s) interferes with my sex drive.
15. Limited control of body movements interferes with my sex drive.
16. Anger and/or resentment interferes with my sex drive.
17. I worry that I rely on the use of drugs or alcohol to enhance my desire for sexual activity.
18. Lack of time to participate in sexual activities interferes with my sex drive.
19. Inability to perform my previous or preferred role (leader or follower) interferes with my interest in engaging in sexual activity.
20. I am concerned that my medications interfere with my interest in engaging in sexual activity.
21. Previous physical, sexual, or emotional abuse interferes with my sex drive.
22. Fear of pregnancy interferes with my interest in sex and intimacy.
23. The pressure to start a family interferes with my desire to participate in sexual activities.
24. Fear of sexually transmitted infections interferes with my interest in sex and intimacy.
25. I experience sexual desire, but I do not initiate sexual activity.
26. I worry that my interest in sex is excessive.

Source. From *Occupational Performance Inventory of Sexuality and Intimacy (OPISI),* by B. A. Walker, 2020a (https://opisi.uindy.edu). Copyright 2020 by Beth Ann Walker and University of Indianapolis.

Sexual response

Sexual response is a client factor that consists of the body's physical response associated with sexual activity, including physiological arousal, response to erogenous zones, nipple erection, clitoral excitation, erection, vaginal lubrication, prostate release, ejaculation, and orgasm (Walker, Otte, et al., 2020). Similar to sexual interest, sexual response is considered a body function that influences performance of desired occupations. Evaluation in this area should aim to reveal concerns the client has regarding their body's sexual response. Possible client concerns regarding sexual response in the OPISI are listed in Exhibit 6.4.

Once concerns are identified and discussed, the occupational therapist should document the client's perception of their body's ability to respond sexually and how satisfied the client is with their body's current sexual response. The therapist

CASE EXAMPLE 6.2. SARAH: SEXUAL INTEREST CONCERNS AFTER EXACERBATION OF MULTIPLE SCLEROSIS SYMPTOMS

Sarah is a 57-year-old woman with multiple sclerosis (MS) who is recovering from a recent severe exacerbation of symptoms, which lasted for 2 months. Sarah is currently receiving occupational therapy in an outpatient setting 3 times a week. She also has been taking antidepressant medication for about 6 months. Sarah was presented with the OPISI screen as part of the standard evaluation process at the clinic. Once her categorical concerns were identified, she completed the in-depth self-assessment, which identified the following concerns relevant to sexual interest:

- Limited energy interferes with my desire to participate in sexual activities.
- I am concerned that my medications interfere with my interest in engaging in sexual activity.
- Inability to perform my previous or preferred role (leader or follower) interferes with my interest in engaging in sexual activity.

Sarah reported times when she would feel excited during the day thinking about sexual activities she had planned for later in the evening with her girlfriend, but that once evening arrived, she was always wiped out and just did not feel like she had the energy to participate. She often asked her girlfriend for a "raincheck." A friend posted on social media about how their antidepressant interfered with their sexual desire, and Sarah wondered whether the decline in her libido over the past few months might be related to her own antidepressant medication.

Sarah also shared that historically, she has usually been the one who initiates and is more dominating during sexual encounters and reported that "being a more passive participant just does not seem as appealing to me." She rated her sexual interest as 3/10 and her satisfaction with that level as 3/10. She indicated that she knew her MS was the culprit and felt like she had a pretty good understanding of how her condition was affecting her sexual interest (8/10), but she did not feel very confident in her skills and ability to make changes to improve outcomes (3/10).

should aim to determine how well the client understands the influence their condition has on their body's sexual response. Thorough evaluation also includes a measurement of self-efficacy to determine how confident the client is in their ability to make necessary adjustments to change their body's sexual response. Case Example 6.3 describes an evaluative pathway that includes screening, self-assessment, and measure of performance for a person who sustained bilateral above-the-knee amputations 2 years prior to seeing the occupational therapy practitioner.

EXHIBIT 6.4
Client Concerns in the OPISI Regarding the Client Factor of Sexual Response

1. My body's physical response associated with sexual activity has changed as a result of my condition and this is a problem.
2. I experience difficulty becoming aroused during foreplay or when erogenous zones are touched.
3. It is taking me longer than it has in the past to become sexually aroused.
4. I experience pain during foreplay, which interferes with my body's ability to become aroused.
5. Although I am aroused mentally, nothing happens physically.
6. I experience delay or difficulty achieving orgasm with masturbation.
7. I experience delay or difficulty achieving orgasm during sexual activity with a partner.
8. I am unable to feel satisfied with sexual activity due to lack of orgasm.
9. I would like to find other means of experiencing sexual satisfaction to compensate for lack of orgasm.
10. I experience loss of feeling or numbness in my genitals.
11. I struggle with vaginal dryness.
12. I struggle obtaining an erection or maintaining it once I have initiated sexual activity.
13. I worry about being aroused at inappropriate times.
14. Age-related changes interfere with my participation in sex and intimacy.
15. I struggle to relax during sexual activity.
16. I worry that side effects of my medication may be interfering with my body's sexual response.

Source. From *Occupational Performance Inventory of Sexuality and Intimacy (OPISI),* by B. A. Walker, 2020a (https://opisi.uindy.edu). Copyright 2020 by Beth Ann Walker and University of Indianapolis.

CASE EXAMPLE 6.3. JASON: SEXUAL RESPONSE CONCERNS 2 YEARS POST BILATERAL ABOVE-THE-KNEE AMPUTATIONS

Jason is a 27-year-old man who sustained bilateral above-the-knee amputations after a traumatic car accident 2 years ago. He lives with his girlfriend of 5 years. During a wellness visit with his physician, he expressed some concerns about the impact his amputations were having on his sex life. The physician had Jason review the OPISI screen, and a referral to occupational therapy was made. When completing the in-depth self-assessment on sexual response, Jason identified the following concerns:

- My body's physical response associated with sexual activity has changed as a result of my condition, and this is a problem.
- I experience difficulty becoming aroused during foreplay or when erogenous zones are touched.
- I experience pain during foreplay, which interferes with my body's ability to become aroused.

When the occupational therapist discussed Jason's concerns with him, additional information was revealed. Jason explained that he had trouble with prostate release and obtaining and maintaining an erection while being stimulated anally, which he had not experienced before the accident. Jason also mentioned

(Continued)

CASE EXAMPLE 6.3. JASON: SEXUAL RESPONSE CONCERNS 2 YEARS POST BILATERAL ABOVE-THE-KNEE AMPUTATIONS *(Cont.)*

struggling with phantom limb pain, which was often unexpected and difficult to work through in the heat of the moment. Difficulty positioning his body comfortably without excess pressure and pain also seemed to interfere with his body's ability to become aroused and caused him to tighten his anus on his partner's fingers or on her strap-on dildo. The therapist also learned that Jason felt exposed, anxious, and uncomfortable when he removed his prostheses during foreplay. He explained that it was difficult to relax, particularly his anal sphincter, when his partner caressed his "stumps." Jason reported that the combination of pain and his inability to become aroused distracted him during foreplay when trying to focus on stimulating his partner's clitoris.

He rated his satisfaction with his sexual response as 2/10 and his body's ability to obtain and maintain an erection as 5/10. He rated his understanding of how his condition was influencing his sexual response as 7/10. Jason indicated that he was not very confident (3/10) in his skills and ability to make necessary changes to improve the outcome because he did not see how his situation would change; he expressed that these were just symptoms he needed to live with.

Sexual expression

The IADL of ***sexual expression*** is the ability to express oneself as a sexual being; it involves expressing sexuality, including gender identity, through behaviors, mannerisms, preferences, appearance, pronouns, political engagement, acquired tendencies, daily routines, symbolic actions, and preferred roles (Walker, Otte, et al., 2020). Evaluation of sexual expression should aim to understand the client's concerns regarding occupational performance. Possible client concerns regarding sexual expression in the OPISI are listed in Exhibit 6.5.

EXHIBIT 6.5
Client Concerns in the OPISI Regarding the IADL of Sexual Expression

1. I worry that I no longer appear as masculine/feminine/other as I would like.
2. I do not feel that I am able to fulfill the roles that I associate with my gender identity.
3. I worry that I am too passive or not assertive enough about sexual aspects of my life.
4. I struggle talking about my sexuality.
5. I am no longer comfortable expressing my sexual identity.
6. I am concerned about my ability to play an active role in my sexuality.
7. I feel that depression may be interfering with my ability to express my sexuality.
8. I feel that anxiety may be interfering with my ability to express my sexuality.
9. My ability to participate in community-based activities where I openly express my sexuality has changed.
10. My ability to express pride in who I am as a sexual being has changed.

Source. From *Occupational Performance Inventory of Sexuality and Intimacy (OPISI),* by B. A. Walker, 2020a (https://opisi.uindy.edu). Copyright 2020 by Beth Ann Walker and University of Indianapolis.

Once concerns have been identified and discussed, the occupational therapy practitioner should seek to fully understand how the client perceives their ability to express themselves as a sexual being and their level of satisfaction associated with their performance in this area. Seeking to understand how well the client understands the influence of their condition on their sexual expression will serve the practitioner well in determining which information and resources would be the most appropriate to provide. Determining the client's self-efficacy for making the changes needed to produce meaningful modifications in their ability to express themselves as a sexual being provides an avenue to determine the best approach to client-centered care. Case Example 6.4 presents an evaluative scenario regarding sexual expression concerns for a person who sustained a spinal cord injury.

CASE EXAMPLE 6.4. GAEL: SEXUAL EXPRESSION CONCERNS 6 MONTHS POST C6 SPINAL CORD INJURY

Gael is a 24-year-old man who sustained a C6 spinal cord injury (SCI) 6 months ago. He was discharged to home with his husband 4 months ago and currently receives occupational therapy three times per week at an outpatient clinic. During his initial evaluation, the occupational therapist reviewed with Gael that many people who have had an SCI have concerns about how their injury may affect sexuality and intimacy.

The occupational therapist gave the OPISI screening tool to Gael and explained that he could take it home and review it on his own, with or without his husband. They made a plan to review the screen at the next visit.

Gael's screening results indicated a concern about sexual expression, so the therapist gave him the Sexual Expression portion of the OPISI in-depth inventory to be completed as homework before the next session. Gael identified the following concerns:

- I worry that I no longer appear as masculine/feminine/other as I would like.
- I do not feel that I am able to fulfill the roles that I associate with my gender identity.
- My ability to participate in community-based activities where I openly express my sexuality has changed.

When Gael discussed his concerns with the therapist, he mentioned feeling that his wheelchair personified weakness. He had always worn blue jeans and tucked-in button-up shirts, and now he typically wore elastic-waist pajama pants and a sweatshirt because they were easiest to don. Gael also described that before the accident he was an active leader in the local gay community and spent a lot of time participating in advocacy efforts, marches, and peaceful protests at the state capital. He no longer felt able to participate in those activities.

(Continued)

CASE EXAMPLE 6.4. GAEL: SEXUAL EXPRESSION CONCERNS 6 MONTHS POST C6 SPINAL CORD INJURY *(Cont.)*

Gael had worked as a construction site manager and had been the breadwinner of the family. At home, he typically performed what he considered "manly" duties, such as yardwork and home maintenance, whereas his husband primarily worked at home and did most of the cooking and cleaning. Now, the roles seemed to be reversed. Gael further explained that this role reversal also extended into the bedroom, because he no longer felt able to express assertiveness during sexual activities and felt unable to take on a dominating role. He rated his current ability to express himself as a sexual being as 3/10 and his satisfaction with this ability as 2/10. He rated his understanding of how his SCI interfered with his ability to express himself as a sexual being as 8/10, and he rated as 5/10 his confidence in his skills and ability to make necessary changes.

Sexual self-view

Sexual self-view, a client factor, involves a person's self-perception as a sexual being. It includes aspects of sexual identity, gender identity, sexual self-esteem (i.e., comfort and confidence with one's sexual self-view), and body image (i.e., mental representation of how they picture themselves and their body; Walker, 2020b). Possible client concerns regarding sexual self-view in the OPISI are listed in Exhibit 6.6.

EXHIBIT 6.6

Client Concerns in the OPISI Regarding the Client Factor of Sexual Self-View

1. I feel less confident in my sexuality.
2. My condition leaves me feeling less masculine/feminine/other.
3. I feel that my low sexual self-esteem interferes with my ability to have a satisfying intimate/sexual relationship.
4. The extent of care and assistance I need leaves me feeling powerless, which impacts my sexual self-esteem.
5. I feel that my guilt or my partner's(s') guilt regarding my condition interferes with our ability to enjoy intimacy and sexual activity.
6. I do not think the people around me see me as a sexual being.
7. I am afraid of being rejected sexually.
8. I am not sure I understand my feelings regarding my sexuality, gender identity, or sexual orientation.
9. I worry that my insecurities with my sexuality interfere with my ability to have a satisfying intimate/sexual relationship.
10. I worry that my sexual desires now interfere with my religious/spiritual beliefs.
11. I do not feel that my sexual identity is accepted by people I interact with on a daily basis.
12. I worry that I am not sexually attractive or appealing to my partner(s) or potential partner(s).

Source. From *Occupational Performance Inventory of Sexuality and Intimacy (OPISI),* by B. A. Walker, 2020a (https://opisi.uindy.edu). Copyright 2020 by Beth Ann Walker and University of Indianapolis.

When a client identifies concerns about sexual self-view, the occupational therapy practitioner should refer to the OPISI performance measure, ask the client the extent to which they feel their condition has affected this view, and then determine their satisfaction with their current sexual self-view. A thorough discussion should aim to reveal how well the client understands the impact their condition may have on their sexual self-view and their capacity to make necessary changes to modify outcomes. Case Example 6.5 presents an evaluative scenario that includes screening, self-assessment, and measure of performance for a woman who is recovering from a stroke and has concerns relevant to Sexual Self-View.

CASE EXAMPLE 6.5. MAYA: CONCERNS ABOUT SEXUAL SELF-VIEW 6 MONTHS AFTER STROKE

Maya is a 59-year-old woman who had a hemorrhagic stroke about 6 months ago. She lives with her husband of 42 years and needs 24-hour supervision because of severe left hemiparesis necessitating moderate to maximum assistance with ADLs. After her stroke, Maya spent 5 months at a long-term care facility for rehabilitation and recently was discharged to home with home health services. Although someone stays with Maya while her husband is at work, that person does not perform toileting tasks, so Maya's spouse comes home twice a day to assist with intermittent catheterization. In the evenings, her husband prepares meals, waits on her, helps with her bowel management program and her shower, and gets her ready for bed.

The occupational therapist gave Maya the OPISI screen during her initial evaluation at Maya's home. The screen revealed concerns related to sexual activity, intimacy, and sexual self-view. The OPISI in-depth self-assessment was administered in the next session. Maya identified the following concerns regarding sexual self-view on the in-depth inventory:

- The extent of care and assistance I need leaves me feeling powerless, which impacts my sexual self-esteem.
- I feel that guilt regarding my condition interferes with my ability to enjoy intimacy and sexual activity.
- I worry that I am not sexually attractive or appealing to my partner(s) or potential partner(s).

During the interview, Maya made several comments to the occupational therapist that she felt "like a baby," incapable of doing anything for herself, and was not sure why her husband stayed with her. She missed having sex with her husband and thought about bringing it up a few times, but she felt guilty because he "works around the clock" providing for her and attending to all of her care needs.

(Continued)

CASE EXAMPLE 6.5. MAYA: CONCERNS ABOUT SEXUAL SELF-VIEW 6 MONTHS AFTER STROKE *(Cont.)*

Maya also reported being extremely self-conscious about the toll the hemiparesis has taken on her appearance and expressed that her husband would never find her sexually attractive again. Maya rated the extent to which she felt her stroke had affected her sexual self-view as 10/10 and rated her current sexual self-view as 2/10. She rated her understanding of how her stroke has influenced her sexual self-view as 4/10 and did not feel confident that she was able to make changes to improve this view (2/10).

Intimacy

The occupation of intimacy falls under the category of social participation in the *OTPF–4*. ***Intimacy*** involves a person's ability to initiate and maintain close intimate relationships, including the ability to give and receive the affection needed to successfully interact in the role as an intimate partner (Walker, Otte, et al., 2020). An important distinction that occupational therapy practitioners need to understand and convey is that their clients can be intimate with a partner without being sexual. In addition, intimacy commonly plays a complex role in a couple's sex life. Lack of intimacy can serve as a barrier to participation in intimate and/or sexual activities. Intimacy is perhaps the most complex area of assessment, given the multiple types and levels of intimate relationships. Possible client concerns regarding intimacy in the OPISI are listed in Exhibit 6.7.

When a client identifies concerns about intimacy and discusses them with the occupational therapy practitioner, the next step is to ask the client to rate their ability to give and receive the affection needed to initiate or maintain their intimate relationships. Further assessment of occupational performance would include determining the client's satisfaction with their current occupational performance related to intimacy, determining their understanding of the influence of their condition on intimacy, and ascertaining how confident they are in their ability to make necessary adjustments to change the quality of their intimate relationships. Case Example 6.6 portrays an evaluative scenario that includes screening, self-assessment, and measure of performance for a person who endured a traumatic brain injury (TBI) 8 months prior.

Sexual health

Sexual health is an aspect of the ADL of health management. ***Sexual health*** refers to a person's ability to develop, manage, and maintain routines for sexual health, including practicing safe sex and identifying, understanding, selecting, and using protection. Possible client concerns regarding sexual health in the OPISI are listed in Exhibit 6.8.

EXHIBIT 6.7
Client Concerns in the OPISI Regarding the Occupation of Intimacy

1. I am not comfortable discussing aspects of sexuality and intimacy or my sexual needs with my partner(s).
2. I am not comfortable asking my partner(s) for help during intimate activities such as dressing, undressing, positioning, condom application, applying lubrication, etc.
3. I feel that my partner's(s') limited understanding of my condition serves as a barrier in our intimate relationship.
4. My partner is my caregiver, and I feel like this interferes with our intimate relationship.
5. I am not satisfied with the amount of affection expressed in my intimate relationship(s).
6. I would like to explore nonsexual ways to be intimate with my partner(s).
7. I feel my condition prevents me from being satisfied with my intimate relationship(s).
8. I find it difficult to express my sexual interest and desires in a way that my partner(s) understands.
9. Limitations in my partner's(s') ability to show compassion or empathize with my condition interferes in our intimate relationship.
10. My symptoms/condition make it challenging to show affection to my partner or for my partner to show affection to me.
11. I often refuse to engage in sexual activities with my partner(s) or my partner(s) often refuses to engage in sexual activities with me, and this causes problems in our intimate relationship.
12. I feel my symptoms/condition limit or interfere with quality time spent with my partner(s).
13. I have difficulty regulating my emotions, which has a negative impact on my intimate relationship(s).
14. I have difficulty prioritizing or engaging in pleasant, loving, affectionate shared time with my partner(s).
15. I would like to take more initiative to engage in intimate activities with my partner(s), but I feel awkward or unsure about how to do it.
16. My symptoms/condition make it challenging to fulfill my partner's(s') intimate needs or desires or for my partner(s) to meet my intimate needs or desires.
17. My mood or behavior interferes with my ability to adequately express intimacy and/or sexual interest to my partner(s) or potential partner(s).
18. I worry that my partner(s) or potential partner(s) will not respect my boundaries within our intimate relationship.
19. My limited ability to create a romantic environment is a problem.
20. I do not have a partner, and this concerns me.
21. I am afraid to become intimately and/or sexually involved with another person.
22. I am concerned that I will be taken advantage of in relationships.
23. I do not feel safe with my current sexual partner(s).
24. I struggle finding people to date.
25. My ability to understand, access, and use social media platforms to develop intimate relationships is limited.
26. My ability to travel to meet partner(s) is limited.
27. My ability to access the physical environments linked to socializing (restaurants, bars, coffee shops) limits my ability to find a partner.
28. My ability to end a relationship with a partner when needed is limited.

Source. From *Occupational Performance Inventory of Sexuality and Intimacy (OPISI),* by B. A. Walker, 2020a (https://opisi.uindy.edu). Copyright 2020 by Beth Ann Walker and University of Indianapolis.

CASE EXAMPLE 6.6. AARAV: INTIMACY CONCERNS 8 MONTHS POST TRAUMATIC BRAIN INJURY

Aarav is a 26-year-old man who sustained a traumatic brain injury (TBI) 8 months ago while serving in the Army. He has been married for 5 years and has two small children. During his follow-up appointment at the Veterans Affairs hospital, Aarav discussed having concerns about his sex life. His physician gave Aarav the OPISI screen, which revealed concerns regarding sexual activity, sexual self-view, and intimacy. The physician ordered an occupational therapy evaluation to determine the need for occupational therapy services.

During the initial visit, Aarav preferred that his wife, Meera, be present, saying that he was not allowed to be alone in a room with a woman who was not his spouse. The occupational therapist discussed the OPISI screen and the role of occupational therapy with Aarav and Meera, established rapport, and conducted an occupational profile. The therapist included questions about culture and religion to better understand how these factors influenced presenting concerns. With the therapist, Aarav and his wife agreed on preferred terminology, a style of communication, and an approach to intervention that would feel most comfortable for them. The in-depth inventory portion of the OPISI for intimacy was assigned as homework to be completed before the next visit.

During the next visit, the following identified concerns were discussed:

- I am not comfortable discussing aspects of sexuality and intimacy or my sexual needs with my partner(s).
- My symptoms/condition make it challenging to show affection to my partner or for my partner to show affection to me.
- I have difficulty regulating my emotions, which has a negative impact on my intimate relationship(s).
- I would like to explore nonsexual ways to be intimate with my partner(s).

Aarav indicated that he knew his symptoms were affecting his relationship but felt uncomfortable discussing them when his wife brought them up, because he felt that men typically do not discuss such things with their wife. Aarav viewed any problems related to sexual dysfunction and intimacy as a sign of weakness. Symptoms that seemed to be most problematic were impulsivity, moodiness, and fixation on sexual activity. Aarav's appetite for sexual activity had increased substantially, and his wife mentioned that he was frequently propositioning her for sexual intercourse at inopportune times throughout the day; she felt it was starting to interfere with her parenting responsibilities. Aarav no longer showed her signs of affection such as hugs, kisses, romantic gestures, and foreplay. She implied that it was difficult to reciprocate affection when Aarav was moody and

(Continued)

CASE EXAMPLE 6.6. AARAV: INTIMACY CONCERNS 8 MONTHS POST TRAUMATIC BRAIN INJURY *(Cont.)*

quick tempered and noted that she felt inadequate when she could not become sexually aroused and ready for sex as quickly as Aarav.

Aarav rated his ability to give and receive the affection needed to maintain his relationship with his wife as 8/10, and his satisfaction with intimacy as 2/10. He rated his understanding of how his TBI has influenced intimacy as 6/10 and rated his confidence in being able to make changes to improve the quality of his intimate interactions as 7/10.

EXHIBIT 6.8

Client Concerns in the OPISI Regarding the Occupation of Sexual Health

1. Due to my condition, I am concerned about my ability to practice safe sex.
2. I am concerned about my ability to protect myself from unwanted sexual advances, sexual assault, or rape.
3. I have a hard time recognizing when another person does not want to participate in sexual activities with me.
4. I do not know how to choose the right method of contraception or protection to prevent sexually transmitted infections.
5. I do not know how to determine if I am experiencing symptoms of a sexually transmitted infection.
6. I am afraid to discuss or am not sure how to communicate my concerns about sexually transmitted infections with my doctor.
7. I do not know how to choose the right method of contraception to prevent pregnancy.
8. I do not know how to use, forget to use, or have physical limitations that prevent me from using contraception (including ability to open packaging) as intended to prevent pregnancy or sexually transmitted infections.
9. I worry about my ability to manage my menstrual health and hygiene during my period.
10. I do not know how to or am afraid to discuss safe sex practices with my partner(s).

Source. From *Occupational Performance Inventory of Sexuality and Intimacy (OPISI),* by B. A. Walker, 2020a (https://opisi.uindy.edu). Copyright 2020 by Beth Ann Walker and University of Indianapolis.

When concerns regarding sexual health are identified and discussed, the occupational therapist should ask the client to rate their ability to practice safe sex and their satisfaction with this ability. It is also important to determine how well the client understands the impact their condition has on their sexual health and how confident they are in being able to manage or change their sexual health. Case Example 6.7 presents an evaluative scenario, including screening, self-assessment, and measure of performance, for an adult with an intellectual disability who lives in a group home and is found to have concerns regarding sexual health.

CASE EXAMPLE 6.7. JOSIE: SEXUAL HEALTH CONCERNS OF AN ADULT WITH AN INTELLECTUAL DISABILITY

Josie is a 34-year-old woman with an intellectual disability who lives in a group home. Her guardian caught her engaging in sexual activities with another resident, panicked, and scheduled a case management meeting to discuss moving her to another facility. A referral to occupational therapy was made to determine and address Josie's sexuality and intimacy needs.

During the initial evaluation, the occupational therapist conducted an occupational profile. According to Josie, she had been secretly dating another resident, Abel, in the group home. She stated that she could not figure out why people did not want her to date Abel. Josie mentioned that her parents sat on the couch at night, asked each other about their day, held hands, and watched TV together. She implied that she wanted to do that with someone special, too, and was unsure why she was not allowed to.

Because of Josie's inability to read and fully comprehend the OPISI in written form, the occupational therapist discussed the items using simple terms followed by explanations to ensure appropriate understanding. According to the therapist, the following concerns regarding sexual health seemed most relevant to Josie:

- Due to my condition, I am concerned about my ability to practice safe sex.
- I am concerned about my ability to protect myself from unwanted sexual advances, sexual assault, or rape.
- I do not know how to choose the right method of contraception or protection to prevent sexually transmitted infections (STIs).
- I do not know how to or am afraid to discuss safe sex practices with my partner(s).

Josie reported that she understood basic sexual anatomy and had watched videos on intercourse so that she would know what to expect. She asked Abel to have sex, but he said he could not because he did not want to have a baby. Josie said she knew she needed to use condoms but did not know what they looked like or how to buy them. Her knowledge of protection was limited to pregnancy prevention, and she was not aware of the use of protection to prevent STIs.

Josie said she felt like she knew how to communicate consent but did not feel confident in her ability to say no or deny consent to someone when she did not want to have sex with them. For example, if anyone other than Abel approached her about having sex, came on to her, or flirted with her, she was unsure about how to be assertive in saying no if she felt pressured to participate in intimate activities with them.

(Continued)

CASE EXAMPLE 6.7. JOSIE: SEXUAL HEALTH CONCERNS OF AN ADULT WITH AN INTELLECTUAL DISABILITY *(Cont.)*

Josie expressed that she really wanted to have sex with Abel, but her parents had told her that she was not allowed to. She wanted to talk to her parents about her desire to have sex but did not know how. After Abel's rejection of sex with her, she also did not know how to bring up the topic again with him. She knew consent was important and did not want to pressure Abel, but she also wanted to share with him what she learned in the video on safe sex and pregnancy prevention.

The performance measure questions were presented to Josie, but she did not understand the concept of the Likert scale as it related to overall ability, satisfaction, understanding, and confidence associated with sexual health. When presented with an alternative visual analog scale using faces, her confusion with the concepts increased. She was able to discuss which concerns were the most important to her. Those concerns involved wanting to know more about practicing safe sex, how to properly talk about sex with Abel without making him uncomfortable or violating his right to refuse to have sex, and how to be assertive when communicating when she does not want to engage in sexual activity with another person.

Family planning

As a byproduct of conversations about sexuality and intimacy, practitioners will find that many clients have questions and concerns regarding their desire to start a family. ***Family planning,*** an IADL, is a person's ability to develop, manage, and maintain routines associated with fertility, pregnancy, or parenthood. Possible client concerns regarding family planning in the OPISI are listed in Exhibit 6.9.

EXHIBIT 6.9
Client Concerns in the OPISI Regarding the IADL of Family Planning

1. I do not know how to choose the right method of contraception to prevent pregnancy.
2. I do not know how to use, forget to use, or have physical limitations that prevent me from using contraception (including ability to open packaging) as intended to prevent pregnancy or sexually transmitted infections.
3. I wonder about my ability or my partner's ability to conceive a child.
4. I wonder about my body's ability to accommodate for the physical changes associated with pregnancy.
5. My partner is hesitant to create a family with me because they will take on most of the responsibility.
6. I worry about my ability or my partner's ability to manage the responsibilities associated with pregnancy.
7. In addition to my standard care needs, I am concerned about my ability or my partner's ability to manage the day-to-day tasks associated with parenting.
8. I feel my ability to provide care and supervision to support the developmental needs of a child may be limited.

Source. From *Occupational Performance Inventory of Sexuality and Intimacy (OPISI),* by B. A. Walker, 2020a (https://opisi.uindy.edu). Copyright 2020 by Beth Ann Walker and University of Indianapolis.

After discussing the client's concerns about family planning, the occupational therapist should have the client rate their ability to manage aspects of fertility and family planning as well as their satisfaction with this ability. Similar to the other constructs, the therapist should ask the client to rate their understanding of how their condition may influence aspects of family planning and their capacity to make necessary modifications to change family planning. Case Example 6.8 depicts an evaluative scenario for an individual with complex trauma and multiple amputations who has concerns related to family planning.

CASE EXAMPLE 6.8. TIANA: FAMILY PLANNING CONCERNS OF A YOUNG ADULT WITH MULTIPLE AMPUTATIONS

Tiana, a 22-year-old woman, lost her right arm above the elbow, right leg at the hip, and right ovary as a result of her pelvis being crushed on the right side after she became pinned under equipment at her job at a manufacturing plant 18 months ago. As part of an initial occupational therapy evaluation in an outpatient clinic when Tiana was fitted with new prostheses, Tiana was given the OPISI screen. Tiana indicated that she had concerns regarding her ability to develop, manage, and maintain routines associated with pregnancy and parenthood. Tiana and her spouse had been in the process of discussing when to start a family just before her accident but now had the following concerns:

- My partner is hesitant to create a family with me because they will take on most of the responsibility.
- I wonder about my ability or my partner's ability to conceive a child.
- I feel my ability to provide care and supervision to support the developmental needs of a child may be limited.

Tiana's husband was present for the next session to discuss related concerns. Tiana was taking several medications, and with only one functioning ovary, she had questions about her ability to even conceive a child. She also had concerns about her ability to change diapers or hold her baby for feeding. Tiana's husband indicated that he had taken on many responsibilities since his wife had been injured and worried that many of the physical responsibilities associated with parenting would fall to him and be more than he could handle. The couple lived in a two-story home, but Tiana was no longer able to access the second floor. Tiana was afraid that she would not be able to care for a child once the child became mobile and wondered what she would do if the child crawled behind the couch or upstairs. Tiana rated her ability to manage anticipated aspects of parenting as a 2/10 and her satisfaction with that ability as a 2/10. She had a pretty good understanding of her limitations and rated that as an 8/10. She rated her confidence in her skills and ability to make necessary modifications as a 6/10.

Writing Goals

A vital aspect of the evaluation and intervention process is the creation of well-written, client-centered, measurable, occupation-focused goals. Such goals enable occupational therapy practitioners to measure the effectiveness of related interventions and identify changes from baseline skills that are expected as a result of skilled services (Sames, 2014). Goals commonly used in occupational therapy include rehabilitation, habilitation, maintenance, modification, prevention, and health promotion. Regardless of the intervention focus, goals should aim to quantify the client's perception of occupational performance on the four OPISI performance measures: ability, satisfaction with ability, understanding of how their condition affects performance (sexual knowledge), and confidence in their skills and ability to make necessary modifications to change performance (self-efficacy).

Summary

Assessment is a vital aspect of the occupational therapy process. It is important to establish early in the therapeutic relationship that sexuality and intimacy are appropriate and acceptable topics to be addressed during therapy. Occupational therapy clients should be presented the opportunity to identify relevant dimensions of the OTSAF that pertain to them for further evaluation as needed. Through comprehensive assessment, client-centered and occupation-focused goals can be developed.

Beth Ann Walker, PhD, MS, OTR, FAOTA, is an associate professor for the School of Occupational Therapy at the University of Indianapolis. She is best known for breaking the silence in addressing sexuality and intimacy in occupational therapy worldwide through the development of the OTSAF and OPISI. She also served on the World Health Organization Development Group for the creation of a Package of Rehabilitation Interventions for People with Chronic Obstructive Pulmonary Disease.

References

American Occupational Therapy Association. (2020a). AOTA 2020 occupational therapy code of ethics. *American Journal of Occupational Therapy, 74,* 7413410005. https://doi.org/10.5014/ajot.2020.74S3006

American Occupational Therapy Association. (2020b). Occupational therapy practice framework: Domain and process (4th ed.). *American Journal of Occupational Therapy, 74*(Suppl. 2), 7412410010. https://doi.org/10.5014/ajot.2020.74S2001

Annon, J. (1976). The PLISSIT model: A proposed conceptual scheme for the behavioral treatment of sexual problems. *Journal of Sex Education and Therapy,* 2(1), 1–15. https://doi.org/10.1080/01614576.1976.11074483

Areskoug-Josefsson, K., Larsson, A., Gard, G., Rolander, B., & Juuso, P. (2016). Health care students' attitudes towards working with sexual health in their professional roles: Survey of students at nursing, physiotherapy and occupational therapy programmes. *Sexuality and Disability, 34*, 289–302. https://doi.org/10.1007/s11195-016-9442-z

Brown, C., & Dunn, W. (2002). *Adolescent/Adult Sensory Profile*. Psychological Corporation.

DeVellis, R. F. (2017). *Scale development: Theory and applications* (4th ed.). Sage Publications.

Eglseder, K., & Webb, S. (2017). Sexuality education and implications for quality of care for individuals with adult onset disability: A review of current literature. *American Journal of Sexuality Education, 12*, 409–422. https://doi.org/10.1080/15546128.2017.1407980

Fisher, A. G. (2014). Occupation-centred, occupation-based, occupation-focused: Same, same or different? *Scandinavian Journal of Occupational Therapy, 21*, 162–173. https://doi.org/10.3109/11038128.2012.754492

Gill, C., Sander, A., Robins, N., Mazzei, D., & Struchen, M. (2011). Exploring experiences of intimacy from the viewpoint of individuals with traumatic brain injury and their partners. *Journal of Head Trauma Rehabilitation, 26*, 56–68. https://doi.org/10.1097/HTR.0b013e3182048ee9

Gillen, G., & Hinojosa, J. (2015). He said—He said: A scholarly conversation about assessment. *Open Journal of Occupational Therapy, 3*(3). https://doi.org/10.15453/2168-6408.1198

Law, M., Baptiste, S., Carswell, A., McColl, M., Polatajko, H., & Pollock, N. (2019). *Canadian Occupational Performance Measure* (5th ed., rev.). COPM, Inc.

McGrath, M., & Sakellariou, D. (2016). The Issue Is—Why has so little progress been made in the practice of occupational therapy in relation to sexuality? *American Journal of Occupational Therapy, 70*, 7001360010. https://doi.org/10.5014/ajot.2016.017707

Neistadt, M., & Baker, M. F. (1978). A program for sex counseling the physically disabled. *American Journal of Occupational Therapy, 32*, 646–647.

Rose, N., & Hughes, C. (2018). Addressing sex in occupational therapy: A coconstructed autoethnography. *American Journal of Occupational Therapy, 72*, 7203205070. https://doi.org/10.5014/ajot.2018.026005

Sames, K. M. (2014). *Documenting occupational therapy practice* (3rd ed.). Pearson.

Soros, J., & Reese, K. (Hosts). (2019, July 12). Putting the ASS in assessment (No. 8) [Audio podcast episode]. In *OT After Dark*. Anchor. https://anchor.fm/ot-after-dark/episodes/Episode-8-Putting-the-ASS-in-Assessment-e4ju22

Valvano, A., Penwell-Waines, L., Stepleman, L., West, L., Wilson, C., Macapagal, K., & Waller, J. (2014). Health professions students' perception of sexuality in patients with physical disability. *Sexuality and Disability, 32*, 413–427. https://doi.org/10.1007/s11195-014-9347-7

Walker, B. A. (2020a). *Occupational Performance Inventory of Sexuality and Intimacy (OPISI)*. https://uindy.edu/health-sciences/ot/opisi

Walker, B. A. (2020b). *Occupational Performance Inventory of Sexuality and Intimacy (OPISI): Technical manual*. Beth Ann Walker and University of Indianapolis.

Walker, B. A., Conner, G., Mckay, L., Heckert, C., Cole, M., & Dhani, V. (2021). *Development of the Occupational Performance Inventory of Sexuality and Intimacy: Phase Two* [Unpublished manuscript]. School of Occupational Therapy, University of Indianapolis.

Walker, B. A., LeMond, K., Otte, K., Hess, P., Conner, G., Bem, L., & Walker, J. (2020, April 22). *Measuring occupational performance of sexuality and intimacy with comfort, competence, and confidence: An introduction to the OPISI* [Webinar]. American Occupational Therapy Association's 2020 Virtual Conference Series/Ideas and Connections. https://myaota.aota.org/shop_aota/product/OL8113

Walker, B. A., Otte, K., LeMond, K., Hess, P., Kaizer, K., Faulkner, T., & Christy, D. (2020). Development of the Occupational Performance Inventory of Sexuality and Intimacy (OPISI): Phase one. *Open Journal of Occupational Therapy, 8,* 1–18. https://doi.org/10.15453/2168-6408.1694

Weinfurt, K. P., Lin, L., Bruner, D. W., Cyranowski, J. M., Dombeck, C. B., Hahn, E. A., . . . Flynn, K. E. (2015). Development and initial validation of the PROMIS® sexual function and satisfaction measures Version 2.0. *Journal of Sexual Medicine, 12,* 1961–1974. https://doi.org/10.1111/jsm.12966

7

Intimate Partnerships

Judith G. Rogers, *OTR/L, and* **Elizabeth K. Schmidt,** *PhD, OTR/L*

CHAPTER HIGHLIGHTS

- Barriers affecting intimate relationships
- Relationship types
- The role of occupational therapy in supporting intimate relationships

KEY TERMS AND CONCEPTS

ADLs
Attitudinal barriers
Bias
Civil union
Communication
Conception
Congenital disorder
Consent
Cultural humility
Dating
Disability pride
Discrimination
Domestic partnership
Emotional regulation
Family planning
Hook-up culture
IADLs
In vitro fertilization
Interdependence
Marriage
Neurodiversity paradigm
Parenting
Physical barriers
Polyamory
Pregnancy
Prejudice
Respect
Self-advocacy
Sexual self-advocacy
Social interaction skills

Many factors affect intimate partnerships for people with disabilities.[1] For example, the time of onset of a disability (e.g., at birth, during childhood or adulthood) can influence a person's self-image. Perhaps the greatest

[1] When a person uses the term *disabled person,* instead of *person with a disability,* it emphasizes the disability, making it the most important aspect of the person, instead of being a single characteristic of the person's total identity. Some people with a disability, however, prefer to emphasize their disability as a part of their identity. The authors have chosen to use person-first language, except for specific communities that have clearly indicated a preference for identity-first language (i.e., autistic and deaf communities).

barrier to successful partnerships for people with disabilities, however, is the societal stereotypes that erroneously promote the idea that people with disabilities are asexual and have no desire for a sexual or intimate relationship. This message needs to be eliminated.

Most people have sexual desire and a sexual drive regardless of whether they have a disability. People with disabilities have short- and long-term intimate relationships and are sexual beings. Their relationships may be with people with or without disabilities, and they may be fleeting or last a lifetime.

Disability, however, may lead to difficulty in finding a partner or dating. ***Dating*** refers to the act of engaging in activities (i.e., "going on dates") with someone else to get to know them better and determine whether they may be a compatible partner. People with disabilities may also face ***discrimination*** (unjust treatment on the basis of the group, class, or category to which that person belongs), ***prejudice*** (negative attitudes toward others), or ***bias*** (preferences toward other people) from potential partners, many of whom have ingrained biases against dating someone with a disability. Additionally, potential partners may not have an accurate understanding of how someone with a disability can live an independent life. If someone with a disability desires a long-term relationship, moving beyond these initial preconceived ideas is paramount.

The objective of this chapter is to highlight the experiences of people with disabilities in various intimate partnerships, that is, meeting potential partners, dating, partnership, growing their family (e.g., pregnancy, adoption, parenting), and family separation. By understanding the experiences of people with a variety of disabilities and how perceptions of those disabilities, among other issues, may affect intimate relationships, occupational therapy practitioners can better support such clients.

Occupational therapy practitioners can facilitate intimate partnerships for people with disabilities across the life course by addressing safety, consent, self-advocacy, social interaction skills, emotional regulation, sensory differences, participation in ADLs and IADLs, family planning, and parenting. It is also imperative that occupational therapy practitioners recognize and acknowledge how their own and other people's biases affect people with disabilities as they engage in intimate partnerships. Practitioners must continuously challenge their own and other people's biases to have a positive impact on clients and promote occupational justice.

As authors, we believe it is important to acknowledge our experiences, because they may influence the information we share in this chapter. We are both White, straight, and cisgender. One of us grew up having a disability, and the other did not. We acknowledge the level of prejudice that people with disabilities face, and this chapter provides case examples that describe instances in which discrimination, attitudinal biases, and barriers have affected intimate relationships. The case examples in this chapter use pseudonyms, but the stories are from interviews with real people with disabilities and are shared with their permission.

Barriers Affecting Intimate Relationships

The intimate relationships of people with disabilities are affected by physical barriers, emotional and attitudinal barriers, and disability-specific barriers. In addition, a person's life stage can influence their intimate relationships (see Chapter 5, "Sexual and Intimate Occupations Across the Lifespan," for information about the differences of life stage on intimate partnerships).

Physical Barriers

Physical barriers are structural in nature and are commonly understood as the cause of accessibility issues within a community or building. People with disabilities face a variety of physical barriers to intimate relationships, too. For example, people who use a motorized wheelchair often face significant accessibility barriers and limitations on their ability to explore their environment alone or in a group. Friends and acquaintances of people with disabilities often do not ask if a venue is accessible to them. It is not uncommon for people to assume that people who use wheelchairs cannot walk, when they are often able to walk short distances. Many homes are inaccessible, and transportation barriers are common. The use of a wheelchair-accessible van is limited to those who can afford one. In addition, many people have limited access to public transportation (e.g., those living in rural or suburban areas).

A recent *New York Times* article (Beery, 2020) describes the isolation that can occur from physical barriers. **Ms. Sotnikova,** a 33-year-old data scientist in Atlanta, uses a power wheelchair, and "for years, people have admitted to excluding her from parties, picnics and other gatherings that they assumed, often incorrectly and always patronizingly, that she wouldn't be able to attend." The article indicates that Ms. Sotnikova was not invited to events because her coworkers and friends assumed she could not get into their homes because of inaccessibility.

All of these factors can limit people with disabilities from meeting potential partners, hooking up, or dating. For example, **Nirvana** has a neuromuscular disability. She has experienced difficulty in dating because of the limited routes available using mass transit. Nirvana uses dating apps and, for first dates, she uses mass transit to meet people at cafés or at other locations that might not be close to her home. Using mass transit can also make it difficult if Nirvana and a partner want to get away for a long weekend or go to another venue.

Emotional and Attitudinal Barriers

People with disabilities often encounter several emotional and attitudinal barriers that can affect their ability to develop and maintain intimate partnerships. ***Attitudinal barriers*** are impediments to relationships associated with the person with disabilities or with another person's attitude. These barriers involve decreased self-worth, underestimated abilities, and assuming responsibility for problems out of their control. For example, someone with decreased self-worth might stay in an abusive relationship because they do not feel worthy of a healthier relationship.

Differences in self-image can be found among people with disabilities who have or do not have ***disability pride.*** People who have disability pride acknowledge disability culture and take pride in being a part of it. For example,

> people with disabilities have forged a group identity. We share a common history of oppression and a common bond of resilience. We generate art, music, literature, and other expressions of our lives, our culture, infused from our experience of disability. Most importantly, we are proud of ourselves as people with disabilities. We claim our disabilities with pride as part of our identity. We are who we are: we are people with disabilities. (Brown, 2003, pp. 80–81)

People who embrace disability culture are eager to see everyone with disabilities and their allies embody this sense of pride. Those who do not embrace this culture may feel both self-conscious and apologetic about being disabled instead of recognizing their self-worth.

Feelings that people with disabilities, especially teenagers and young adults, have about themselves may also be influenced by others' emotions, such as those of their parents, peers, or partners. For example, a teenager with a disability may be taught in school to use public transportation and then want to use public transportation to meet potential partners. If the parents cannot become comfortable with the teen using public transit by herself, their own fears may limit the teen's independence and potential for intimate partnerships (Codd & Hewitt, 2020). This isolation and limited experience can, in turn, affect the teen's feelings of self-worth. Having control over their environment can improve these feelings and may lead to feeling empowered.

Family members who hold negative societal attitudes about disabilities may hinder a teen's development of intimate relationships. For example, many parents discourage dating altogether because they do not recognize their child as a sexual being or they fear that their child will be taken advantage of (English et al., 2018; Pownall et al., 2012; Schmidt et al., 2021). As a result, teens with disabilities may feel that they cannot date or have long-term intimate relationships. In addition, these attitudes can lead to people remaining in unfulfilling or even abusive relationships out of fear that they will not find anyone else. Moreover, youth with disabilities are less likely to receive sex education than their nondisabled peers (Barnard-Brak et al., 2014), which can affect their readiness to engage in safe dating and intimacy practices. Doren et al. (2012) reported that when parents broaden their expectations of whom their teenagers with disabilities can date and where they can go to meet potential partners, it can foster teenagers' ability to develop intimate relationships.

Similarly, people with disabilities may face discrimination or negative societal attitudes about their disability from nondisabled peers. In high school, it is common for people to feel pressured to fit in with a larger group and avoid people who do not fit within a norm. As people age, however, they begin to hold more expansive views of themselves and others.

Experiencing these negative outlooks during the teen years can have several detrimental effects, contributing to unhealthy relationships and limiting opportunities to meet potential partners. For example,

- **Claire,** who has hemiplegic cerebral palsy, had a nondisabled boyfriend who told her that the only reason she had friends was because she had disabilities and they felt sorry for her. Claire stayed with him another 3 months despite his negative behavior.
- Likewise, **Carter,** who has cerebral palsy and a minor speech impairment, walked during high school but switched to a wheelchair during college to more easily get around campus. He tried dating during high school but was unsuccessful because of attitudinal bias (e.g., he was not invited to parties). Carter believed he was not invited to these parties because his classmates felt uncomfortable with his disability. Carter's social life improved in college because people were less concerned with fitting into a group or norm and more willing to get to know others. He meets partners at parties and has been able to date during college. He also has used a dating app to find a long-term girlfriend.
- **Camilla** did not know any other people with disabilities while growing up. She was born with cerebral palsy and has a mild limp. Although she made friends easily, she did not date in high school. However, she still desired some sexual experiences and worried she would never date or marry. While in high school, she and her nondisabled friends would often go cruising so they could meet guys and make out (but not "hook up"—i.e., have sex).

People with disabilities who also have disadvantaged identities (those based on, for example, race, sexual orientation, gender, geographic location, immigration status, and age) often face additional attitudinal barriers and discrimination, limiting their ability to develop and maintain intimate relationships. Abelson (2014, p. 57) suggested that disability is "a complex variable when examining intersectionality" because the perception of a person's disability can change based on the situation or the day, and it can evolve over time. Abelson studied transgender men's experiences of discrimination and violence as well as the ways in which gendered violence is influenced by race, class, social location, and ability. Case Example 7.1 presents Abelson's story of Michael, a transgender man, and how his disability affected his experiences with gender, sexuality, and violence.

Disability-Specific Barriers

People with disabilities may face barriers to intimate relationships specific to their type of disability. Note that the disabilities and barriers discussed here are not an exhaustive list. Case Example 7.2 provides cases covering several of the disabilities discussed in this section.

CASE EXAMPLE 7.1. MICHAEL: ATTITUDINAL BARRIERS

Michael, a 40-year-old, White transgender man, was a student and educational worker and about 3 years into his gender transition at the time of the interview. He was raised in a working-class family and earned working-class wages, but he expected to have higher wages upon completion of his degree. Michael has a disability for which he has to use a wheelchair or walking aids to get around.

Michael described a sense of invisibility regarding gender and sexuality: He felt that when he used a wheelchair, most people saw him only as disabled. "There's this strange thing when you're in a wheelchair. Where is that everybody sees you? Everyone recognizes you, or thinks they do—and no one actually looks at your face. . . . Part of what was really interesting is that I was seen as such an asexual being. . . . I started transitioning, and it's like a lot of people weren't looking close enough to notice. Because they see the wheelchair. They see the chunk of steel under my ass instead of seeing my face" (Abelson, 2014, p. 57). Although gender and sexuality were central to this experience, it was the way they intersected with his disability that stood out most to Michael.

Congenital disabilities: cognitive and physical

A ***congenital disorder*** is a medical condition that is present at or before birth. Congenital disorders can be acquired during fetal development or from the genetic makeup of the parents (Veritas Health, n.d.). Many physical disabilities are known at birth, whereas cognitive disabilities may not be diagnosed until later. When the disability is diagnosed early, some parents feel overwhelmed and may decide to give up their child for adoption at birth or may be overprotective of their child, while others become fighters for their child's rights. Some parents become overprotective because of their own fears and limit their child's independence (Codd & Hewitt, 2020), but others go on to become champions of disability rights and pride. Case Example 7.2, Natalia and Barbra Anne, describes how congenital physical disabilities affect intimate relationships.

Intellectual or cognitive disabilities

The experience of sexual abuse is common among people with disabilities (Jones et al., 2012; Spencer et al., 2005; Sullivan & Knutson, 2000). For people with intellectual or developmental disabilities, it is particularly common (Pecora et al., 2019) and it may lead to added difficulties with long-term partnerships. It is not unusual for many parents or other caregivers to worry about abuse (English et al., 2018; Pownall et al., 2012; Schmidt et al., 2021). As a result, the person with cognitive differences may be less likely to receive much needed support from the community in meeting potential partners and establishing intimate relationships.

Facial anomalies

Although it can be difficult for people with an obvious physical disability to start dating and build relationships, people with facial anomalies often encounter even greater prejudice. Research has suggested that people prefer symmetrical faces and bodies and are less likely to respond positively to people with facial anomalies (Grammer et al., 2003; Workman et al., 2020). Thus, people with facial anomalies, like Felicia in Case Example 7.2, are more likely to encounter stigma.

Sensory disability

Sensory disabilities include blindness or low vision, deafness or hard of hearing, and sensory differences common in autism or other neurodevelopmental disorders. This section discusses common barriers in establishing and maintaining intimate partnerships for people with these conditions. Although most sensory disabilities occur during adulthood, the blind and deaf people interviewed for this section were born with these disabilities.

Blind or low vision. Before technology was widely available, most people with visual impairment met their dates through in-person social interactions. People who went to a school for the Blind commonly dated people who also were vision impaired. Currently, people use a variety of techniques to meet potential partners, such as social interactions and dating websites, whether apps for people in general or for people who are blind or have low vision (see Badiah and Babar in Case Example 7.2).

Deaf or hard of hearing. Ninety percent of deaf children are born to hearing families; 10% are born to deaf families (National Institute on Deafness and Other Communication Disorders [NIDCD], 2016). Many deaf people use American Sign Language (ASL) as their first and primary language (Start ASL, 2020). Many hard-of-hearing people may also use hearing aids or cochlear implants (NIDCD, 2016), which has expanded the options for how deaf people are taught. Because there is more integration of deaf children into full-inclusion classes at school, they may be taught in a combination of ASL and speech. Even before the cochlear implant was used, ASL was and continues to be taught in junior colleges and universities. Thus, more hearing people know and use ASL.

The increased use of ASL in hearing communities, along with the use of technology, has expanded opportunities for social relationships for deaf and hard-of-hearing people. Dating apps that serve the Deaf community, including ones specifically for LGBTQIA+[2] people, are available. Before these developments, deaf people typically met each other in schools or at Deaf clubs and other social venues. As more

[2] The term *LGBTQIA+* refers to the diverse and unique communities formed by lesbian, gay, bisexual, transgender, queer, intersex, asexual, and additional sexual and gender-minoritized people. As greater awareness, social acceptance, and safety improve for these individuals and communities, new terms may emerge as language evolves to describe identities that exist outside of societal recognition and acceptance.

deaf people are integrated into mainstream culture and education, more opportunity exists for hearing and deaf people to meet, date, and establish long-term intimate relationships.

Many examples exist of deaf people partnering with hearing people, particularly hearing people who know ASL or have been raised in Deaf culture. For example, Debra is profoundly deaf and wears hearing aids. She previously attended a school program that used ASL and speech. In high school, she met a hearing student with whom she has had a lifelong partnership. David is profoundly deaf and wears hearing aids. He signs ASL and speaks English. He met and has been a lifelong partner with an ASL interpreter, who is a child of deaf parents.

Sensory differences. Unlike people with mobility disabilities, who may find improved dating opportunities after high school, teenagers who are autistic or have sensory dysregulation can experience challenges throughout life, including fitting in and dating in settings that are noisy or bright or have adverse smells (see Anna in Case Example 7.2). As a result, the prospect of dating may feel impossible to them.

CASE EXAMPLE 7.2. SPECIFIC DISABILITIES AND THEIR EFFECTS ON INTIMATE RELATIONSHIPS

Congenital physical disability

Natalia has muscular dystrophy, a progressive neuromuscular disability. She walked until middle school but has used a wheelchair since then. She had a "date" when in the third grade, and that person is still her friend. As Natalia aged, she met and dated a boy from a camp for children with muscular dystrophy. Later, she dated both people with disabilities and nondisabled people. When Natalia wanted sexual relations, she needed to be transferred into bed. Sometimes her date could do that, or she scheduled a personal care attendant. At one point, she tried different dating apps, but they were unsuccessful. She met her spouse on a date that a friend arranged for her. Natalia's experience illustrates that a specialized camp provides opportunities for dating at an earlier age than most people with disabilities have and can strengthen confidence and resolve to continue to date long after camp has ended.

Barbra Anne has a rare disability called upper bilateral amelia and lower bilateral hemimelia, which means that she is missing both her upper and lower extremities. Barbra Anne was generally interested in dating and had sexual desire, but she was unsuccessful in finding dates. She enjoyed watching sports, and she found a few local sports bars that she could access in her wheelchair and became friends with the staff there. Because Barbra Anne was comfortable at these bars, she found meeting men there easier and safer. She later met her future husband

(Continued)

CASE EXAMPLE 7.2. SPECIFIC DISABILITIES AND THEIR EFFECTS ON INTIMATE RELATIONSHIPS *(Cont.)*

at a hotel pool while they were both attending different professional meetings. When they went out for the first date, Barbra Anne's attendant was seated at a nearby table to provide assistance when needed. They enjoyed their conversations and eventually committed to a long-term partnership.

Facial anomaly

Felicia has Nager syndrome, which can include facial anomalies and life-threatening breathing problems (Medline Plus, 2017). Felicia dated during college. Felicia and her then-boyfriend, Barry, wanted to marry. Barry wanted to have children, but Felicia decided she did not want to have children because of the high probability of passing on a more severe form of Nager syndrome to the child. Felicia decided to end the relationship with Barry over this difference. She later married Hank, who supported her choice to not have children.

Blindness

Badiah and Babar are siblings and totally blind. Despite being raised by the same parents, they had different occupational goals regarding intimate partnerships, which their occupational therapy practitioner took into consideration when working with each of them. Although Badiah had the desire to date, her parents did not allow it during high school, despite allowing Babar to do so. The occupational therapy practitioner at Badiah's school taught her to use mass transit, and she used this skill to meet her dates in secret outside of school and her home. Babar had permission from his parents to date, but he did not want to, so the occupational therapy practitioner did not develop goals for him related to intimate partnerships.

Autism

Anna is a 19-year-old autistic woman. She is interested in dating, but her parents are afraid that she will be taken advantage of. In high school, they would not allow her to attend events that were not school sanctioned and supervised. Therefore, Anna had no dating experience when she entered college, despite a strong interest in intimate partnerships. This situation negatively affected her quality of life and depression. In college, however, she was able to attend both school-sanctioned and other events with peers she meets in her classes. She also visited a university health clinic that provided her with access to sexual health classes taught by an autistic sexual self-advocate and a certified occupational therapy assistant from the community. These opportunities and education allowed Anna to safely meet her first partner outside of school. She felt very comfortable making sexual decisions when exploring a relationship for the first time.

Relationship Types

Occupational therapy practitioners need to be respectful and cognizant of the wide variety of relationship structures or goals while working with their clients. In recent years in the United States, there has been an increase in acceptance of ***hook-up culture,*** or an emphasis on sexual contact free of commitment or emotional intimacy (Reiling et al., 2018). Hook-up culture has also diversified the types of relationships and intimate partnerships available. Many partners consider themselves to be not exclusive or not committed solely to one another initially. Before relationship status is fully defined, the partners involved may go through different processes to form their relationships, such as talking or dating. People with disabilities also experience these stages of meeting potential partners and dating.

In addition to variations in the status of relationships, various types of partnerships exist. For example, most Western culture values monogamy or commitment to one partner at a time as the norm (Ferrer, 2019). However, some people in Western culture have an interest in ***polyamory*** (i.e., multiple simultaneous romantic or life partners) despite conforming to social norms of monogamy (Ferrer, 2019). After a stage of talking, hooking up, or dating, some people may choose to solidify their commitment to each other through domestic partnership, civil union, or marriage. ***Domestic partnership*** is sharing a residence with an intimate partner and may or may not include a legal union, depending on the state of residence. ***Civil union*** and ***marriage*** are terms for the legal union of a partnership. Civil unions were widely used by same-sex couples before the legalization of same-sex marriage and are still common in Western countries where same-sex marriage is not yet legal (Felter & Renwick, 2021).

Health care providers are often biased about patients' relationship structures and romantic or sexual behavior. Occupational therapy practitioners need to confront their biases and be prepared to incorporate advocacy for clients' health management goals that involve sexual health, even in health care settings that are not accepting of a client's relationship structure or sexual behavior (e.g., polyamory). This advocacy for client sexual health may be especially important for people with disabilities, because health care providers' biases (e.g., assumptions that people with disabilities are not sexually involved) may prevent these patients from receiving timely diagnoses of sexually transmitted infections and appropriate sexual health care (Greenwood & Wilkinson, 2013; Havercamp & Scott, 2015). For example, **Cayla** has athetoid quadriplegic cerebral palsy and became sterile because she did not get a timely diagnosis of pelvic inflammatory disease, which can be caused by gonorrhea or chlamydia. Her providers never asked her if she was sexually active as a part of the examination.

Role of Occupational Therapy in Supporting Intimate Relationships

Intimate relationships are an important element of social participation. This section discusses cultural humility as a significant component of occupational therapy in supporting intimate relationships. It also covers meeting, dating, and building partnerships, which involve various activities within the scope of the *Occupational Therapy Practice Framework: Domain and Process* (4th ed.; American Occupational Therapy Association [AOTA], 2020). These activities include safe participation and consent; self-advocacy; social interaction and emotional regulation; sensory considerations; ADLs and IADLs; and communication. Finally, the section concludes with a discussion of family planning, including the decision to become a parent, conception and pregnancy, parenting, and family separation.

Cultural Humility

Because societal and attitudinal bias are associated with discrimination, it is important for occupational therapy practitioners to practice cultural humility. ***Cultural humility*** is defined by a "lifelong, learning-oriented approach to working with people with diverse cultural backgrounds and a recognition of power dynamics in health care" (Agner, 2020, p. 1). It means "having an interpersonal stance that is other-oriented rather than self-focused, characterized by respect and lack of superiority toward an individual's cultural background and experience" (Hook et al., 2013, p. 361). It is not enough to think about one's own values, beliefs, and social position within the context of the present moment. "To practice true cultural humility, a person must [be cognizant of] preconceived ideas and must be aware of and sensitive to historic realities like legacies of violence and oppression against certain groups of people," including people with disabilities (Sufrin, 2019). When health care professionals do not have cultural humility, it can be catastrophic (see Chapter 3, "Guided Self-Reflection of Self as a Sexual Being," for more information). Cultural humility is integral to working with clients who are exploring or enhancing their intimate partnerships, regardless of their choice of partner or partners.

Like anyone else, people with disabilities have a variety of sexual roles and interests, and occupational therapy practitioners should never make assumptions about their clients' sexual roles and activities. Instead, they should ask questions during evaluation or as they get to know their client. Practitioners need to be mindful that not every client will want to discuss relationships or social participation with them. Chapter 10, "Personal Narratives of Sex, Intimacy, and Meaning," and Chapter 11, "Interventions for Sexual and Intimate Occupations," cover clients' personal experiences and interventions and expand on the interaction between the occupational therapy practitioner and the client.

Meeting, Dating, and Building Partnerships

Occupational therapy practitioners can guide clients through the process of meeting potential partners and assist them with the communication necessary for successful dating and partnerships. Meeting and dating a variety of people may lead to finding compatibility with a person, which may then result in a long-term intimate partnership.

More avenues than ever are available for potential partners to meet, including social settings, work or school, and online. Practitioners can assist clients with communication and participation in both virtual and physical contexts. As previously stated, dating may look different depending on the client's challenges (e.g., physical barriers and attitudinal barriers, discrimination against various identities), dating goals, and interests. Practitioners can support their clients by promoting safe participation and consent, self-advocacy, social interaction and emotional regulation, sensory considerations, ADLs and IADLs, and communication. Moreover, education is essential for intimacy, consent, and sexual activities.

Safe participation and consent

Cognitive and emotional stability is important for safe and healthy partnerships. ***Consent*** is the agreement between two or more people about the specific expressions of sexual activity they are comfortable with and desire. Consent requires the cognitive processes of "shaping content" within social interactions, including questions, replies, disclosures, expressing emotions, and disagreement (AOTA, 2020). These processes are important in obtaining, giving, and negotiating consent. "Every person has the right to exercise choices regarding sexual expression and social relationships" (American Association of Intellectual and Developmental Disabilities [AAIDD], 2013). Occupational therapy practitioners can support their clients by facilitating their social interaction skills to ensure that they have the capacity to obtain, provide, or decline consent.

Self-advocacy

Self-advocacy is "the action of representing oneself or one's views or interests" (Oxford English Dictionary, 1989). Self-advocates "exercise their rights as citizens by communicating for and representing themselves and others, with whatever supports they need. Self-advocates must have a meaningful role in decision making in all areas of their daily lives and in public policy decisions" (AAIDD, 2020).

Friedman and colleagues (2014) interviewed self-advocates with various neurodevelopmental disabilities to define sexual self-advocacy and identified three themes: choice, respect, and interdependence. The self-advocates described the central component of ***sexual self-advocacy*** as "my choices" (Friedman et al., 2014, p. 519). Many people with a variety of disabilities experience a loss of choice (e.g., how to find dates, where to date, who to date, when to date), which may be the result of challenges with guardianship, privacy, accessibility, or other factors. However, self-advocates reported that autonomy, decision making, and choice over their relationships and sexuality were crucial to sexual self-advocacy (Friedman et al., 2014). To make healthy choices, they reported needing communication skills, which they defined as having

- the ability to speak up and use their voice to advocate for themselves and others and
- access to reproductive health information.

Occupational therapy practitioners can support their clients by making sexual health information accessible and by assisting their clients in developing the skills to effectively communicate their needs and rights for education, relationships, intimate partnerships, and sexual preferences and desires with partners (Schmidt et al., 2019).

Self-advocates defined *respect* as the next component necessary for sexual self-advocacy. ***Respect*** refers to "knowing and respecting myself, respect for others, and respect for my rights" (Friedman et al., 2014, p. 523). Occupational therapy practitioners should respect their clients' sexual autonomy and decisions around sexuality and intimacy as well as advocate for their rights associated with sexuality and intimacy when needed. Practitioners must understand that clients may choose not to address various tendencies (e.g., avoiding eye contact) because they are perceived as an integral part of who they are. This viewpoint is in line with the neurodiversity paradigm[3] and is an important consideration for all practitioners working with clients with disabilities. Instead of focusing on changing or "fixing" certain tendencies, practitioners can support their clients in developing sexual self-advocacy skills.

Finally, Friedman et al. (2014) identified ***interdependence*** (i.e., completing a task with another person instead of independently) as an overarching theme in sexual self-advocacy. Interdependence is an important consideration for occupational therapy practitioners when addressing occupations associated with sexuality and intimacy. People do not function as isolated units; they rely on one another for support and assistance. Many people with a disability prefer a partner who understands their body's unique way of moving so that they can comfortably engage in sexual activity.

For example, **Candace** is a woman with quadriplegic cerebral palsy who can feed herself but is more limited in other ADLs. She needs to be transferred on and off the toilet and needs help with dressing. One of Candace's first boyfriends was her neighbor. Because he was a frequent visitor and watched Candace give instructions to her attendants for how to transfer her, he understood how she preferred to have her body moved. When they had sexual relations, he knew what to do to assist her and make her comfortable in bed. Candace now insists on partners who are astute and invested in learning how to touch her body. Occupational therapy practitioners can help their clients gain the sexual self-advocacy skills necessary to seek the support they need and effectively communicate those needs with health professionals, their partners, and their support providers.

Social interaction and emotional regulation

Occupational therapy practitioners can support their clients in interacting with current or future partners and identify and facilitate strategies to regulate their

[3] The ***neurodiversity paradigm*** is the idea that neurological differences are a normal part of human diversity and there is no one "right" way of neurological functioning. Moreover, the neurodiversity paradigm posits that when neurological variations are accepted and embraced, everyone is stronger for it.

emotions for successful partnerships. Specifically, they can support their clients in developing positive social interactions with partners and by helping them learn to regulate their emotions for more positive interactions. ***Social interaction skills*** are the ability to interact with another person through verbal and nonverbal language in ways that are considered appropriate within certain cultures and societal norms. ***Emotional regulation*** is a person's ability to regulate their emotions to respond appropriately to a given situation, given the cultural and societal norms (Case Example 7.3).

Sensory considerations

A variety of sensory considerations may affect people with disabilities. For example, people with low vision may have different needs regarding lighting. Some prefer to be in a well-lit environment, and others prefer a dimly lit environment. Occupational therapy practitioners should encourage clients to share their lighting preferences with their dates and intimate partners. Similarly, those who are deaf or hard of hearing may need various accommodations to support intimate partnerships.

Sensory differences, common among neurodiverse people, can be a problem when trying to engage with potential partners through dating and sexual activity. Sensory stimuli that can be potentially overwhelming include noisy environments such as bars, dance clubs, and concerts, all of which are commonly part of dating activities. Stimuli such as perfume odors and flashing lights can also be

CASE EXAMPLE 7.3. TY: EMOTIONAL REGULATION

Ty is a 35-year-old man with posttraumatic stress disorder (PTSD) and mild traumatic brain injury (TBI) sustained in combat in Afghanistan. Before his deployment, Ty was committed to Monica, and they lived together. After 6 months at home, Ty was referred to occupational therapy to address his PTSD and TBI manifestations. He presented with mild depression, limited empathy, and emotional regulation challenges. Monica described him as easily angered or brought to tears. Ty reported becoming quickly angered when plans changed or when Monica changed her mind. Ty also said he frustrates Monica when he "spaces out" when they are arguing or discussing something of importance. The couple had been in marriage and family therapy for a few weeks at the time Ty started occupational therapy.

The occupational therapy practitioner and Ty worked on developing sensory-based strategies to enhance emotional regulation when frustrated and to sustain auditory attention during conversations. Additionally, the practitioner, Ty, and Monica explored occupations the couple could do together that would allow them to practice the intimacy-building skills they learned in marriage and family therapy.

an issue. Occupational therapy practitioners can assist clients using standardized assessments, interviews, or direct observations to identify sensory processing differences. In this way, clients can identify their sensory triggers and learn to effectively communicate them to intimate partners.

ADLs and IADLs

When self-care is an activity demand of dating or sex, occupational therapy practitioners may provide support in ***ADLs,*** which are "activities oriented toward taking care of one's own body and completed on a routine basis" (AOTA, 2020, p. 30). For example, if a client cannot cut food and is going on a date that includes a meal, the practitioner can support the client in asking the restaurant kitchen to cut the food before serving or suggesting that their date feed them, framing it as an intimate and sensual experience. When practitioners are working with either a teenager or someone newly disabled, they may need to teach them how to check venues for the accessibility of the entrance and bathroom as well as the distance to the entrance from parking or transit. In addition, the practitioner and client can collaborate to find ways for support to be performed in a way that encourages intimacy.

If the client has difficulty dressing or undressing, the practitioner can include goals of finding clothes that are easier to don or doff or new techniques to aid in donning and doffing clothing. In addition, practitioners can assess a client's need to work on assertive communication for directing others, such as partners or personal attendants, to undress them. If the client identifies this task as a need, practitioners can include scripting and role playing assertive communication.

IADLs are activities that support engagement in the home and community (AOTA, 2020); they also can be goals of therapeutic intervention for intimate relationships. Occupational therapy practitioners can support their clients in developing the skills needed for shopping; meal preparation, including ensuring that all supplies are available; and home management to foster a welcoming environment for dates. Assessing the client's financial management skills, such as the ability to budget for groceries, meals out, or entertaining, can be useful for both dating and independent living.

Sexuality relates to many areas of occupation, particularly play and leisure. In another example, if a client wants to prepare for amateur night at a local strip club, the occupational therapy practitioner can help the client work on the occupation of dancing and address anxiety as a barrier for dancing in front of people. The practitioner can discuss physical barriers such as fatigue and decreased hip movement that limit a 4-minute dance routine as well as plan ahead for how the client will access the stage. The client and the practitioner can discuss certain dance styles or techniques that are less fatiguing and require little hip movement, such as a seated burlesque-inspired routine. Additionally, the treatment can include cognitive reframing of anxieties about performing and positive affirmations to enhance self-concept. Case Example 7.4 illustrates how an occupational therapist helped an autistic youth with ADL and IADL tasks for dating.

CASE EXAMPLE 7.4. AIDEN: ADLs AND IADLs

Aiden is a 20-year-old autistic man in ongoing occupational therapy for issues related to autism and transition from school to the workforce. He went out to dinner on a date with Tom, who is also age 20 years. After the date, Aiden talked with his occupational therapist about the problems he experienced during the date, such as challenges with accurately paying for the meal and the tip using the correct bills and change. The therapist also learned that Aiden ultimately wanted to make a meal for Tom at home. After using the Canadian Occupational Performance Measure (Law et al., 2019), the therapist and Aiden set a short-term goal to manage his finances for another date. The long-term goal was to prepare a full meal. Aiden planned a dinner date at a restaurant with Tom for 2 weeks after the occupational therapy session and was excited about making him a meal in the near future.

Communication

Communication includes listening skills, processing of difficult conversations, tone, and being aware of needs and preferences and asserting those needs. It is one of the most important and universal skills necessary to support successful dating and healthy intimate partnerships. Occupational therapy practitioners can educate clients on effective communication and support them in role playing to practice communication skills. For example, a practitioner and client can practice the conversation the client might have when meeting for a first date.

Family Planning

As defined in the Occupational Therapy Sexual Assessment Framework (OTSAF; Walker et al., 2020), ***family planning***[4] is "a person's ability to develop, manage and maintain routines associated with fertility, pregnancy, and/or parenthood" (p. 10), which includes preventing unwanted or unplanned pregnancies through contraception. Families are composed in many ways (e.g., married partners without children, polyamorous constellations, cohabitating siblings), but the focus of this section is the OTSAF-specific construct of family planning as focused on fertility, pregnancy, and parenthood.

Even with a disability, clients can become successful parents and carry out child care tasks. Occupational therapy practitioners should understand how the issues around parenting and growing a family influence individual decisions about sex

[4] The definition of *family planning* in the OTSAF is not inclusive of all families. This definition can be problematic for a variety of reasons, such as omitting cases of unplanned or nonconsensual pregnancies and excluding or devaluing some family structures (e.g., people who are uninterested in or unable to bear children). This term is used here strictly as described in the OTSAF and is not intended to include all family constellations or other forms of planning a family.

and intimate relationships. Parenting, conception, surrogacy, adoption, and the fear of family separation all are important factors for people with disabilities who are deciding whether they want to become parents. Additionally, stigma exists about whether people with disabilities are capable of becoming pregnant and parenting. Some of these stereotypes depend on the disability and include being unable to reproduce or being violent, uncaring, or lacking empathy as parents. Regarding autism, "despite research showing these claims toward their children or spouses to be inaccurate, they persist in guidance provided to family law professionals" (National Council on Disability, 2012, p. 119).

Occupational therapy practitioners can provide resources and support to ensure that their clients have comprehensive and medically accurate information. Clients' goals regarding parenting and their perception of their ability to parent affect their sexual and intimate occupational engagement. As a result, it is important for practitioners to understand clients' goals so that they can support clients' decisions on parenting, adoption, conception, and family separation.

Contraception

Before deciding to start a family, many people will choose to use contraception to avoid unplanned pregnancy. Contraception for people with disabilities can be complex. For example, some forms of birth control are contraindicated for use by people with certain disabilities. Additionally, certain contraceptives require particular cognitive and physical skills to use. Occupational therapy practitioners can play a role in skill development or modifications to help clients effectively use prescribed contraceptives. Practitioners may also need to work with their clients and their providers to identify appropriate contraceptives.

Becoming parents

In the United States, couples have historically encountered significant social pressure to conceive or adopt children after marriage. Yet, recent research shows a steady decline in people choosing to have children, and many couples are waiting longer to have children than in the past (Miller, 2018; Stahl, 2020). Variations of the typical family unit have become increasingly common (Nicol, 2018). Some differences in family types are related to socioeconomic status (Bloome, 2017).

According to Rogers (2006), married people with disabilities often face social pressure to not have children. "The forces of social disapproval and, often, their own fears, work against many disabled women having children" (Rogers, 2006, p. 33). Nevertheless, many people with disabilities still want to become a parent.

For example, **Leslie** has triplegia cerebral palsy and was in a long-term relationship. She wanted to have her own child even though her partner did not want to parent. So, Leslie and her partner broke up and she researched donor insemination to have her own baby. She was determined to have a baby despite not getting emotional support from her mother and other family members. This lack of support struck Leslie as unusual because her family supported her endeavors educationally, in dating, and in any other arena. Leslie thinks "that parenting is the final frontier for people with disabilities" (L. Heller, personal communication, January 17, 2021). Leslie worked with an occupational therapy practitioner to identify strategies she could use to parent without the support of her family members.

Limited information exists about specific disabilities and becoming pregnant, carrying a child, and experiencing labor and delivery, leading to anxiety and fear among prospective parents and inaccurate recommendations from physicians, which may result in worse care for the person with disabilities (Rogers, 2006). Examples abound:

- **Sharon** is paraplegic and was questioned by her gynecologist about whether she was going to keep her baby (Rogers, 2006, p. 33). Despite her gynecologist's biases and assumptions, Sharon carried her son to term, delivered him, and parented him. Her son went on to successfully graduate from college.
- **Sabine** has spina bifida and works as a health professional in the medical field. Despite working in the medical field, she "ran into ignorance from her new doctor, who told her, before examining her, that she could not carry a child to term. In fact, the doctor was wrong about this" (Rogers, 2006, p. 33).
- **Sophia Amelia** has sacral agenesis. She is missing her sacrum and coccyx and twelve vertebrae in her back. She encountered prejudice early in her first pregnancy when signing up for the Special Supplemental Nutrition Program for Women, Infants, and Children. She said, "I was told by the technician that she would not file the paperwork until I filed rape charges against the father. She thought there was no way I could have a consensual sexual relationship, to which I replied, 'I need to talk with your supervisor'" (Rogers, 2006, p. 33).

Many women like Sharon, Sabine, and Sophia Amelia have worked with occupational therapy practitioners to identify strategies to support independence in self-care tasks despite their changing bodies associated with pregnancy. Moreover, they may work with practitioners to identify strategies to care for their baby independently.

In addition, abortions have historically been consensually and nonconsensually performed on people with disabilities, and although that is less common now, people with disabilities who are pregnant still face prejudice and recommendations to abort their pregnancy. According to Rogers (2006), "bias against people with disabilities becoming parents is the inability to visualize how the person with the disability can physically parent" (p. 33).

Conception and pregnancy

Many people with disabilities can conceive and become pregnant, including through sexual intercourse and in vitro fertilization (IVF). ***Conception*** refers to sperm entering an egg to create a fetus, whereas ***pregnancy*** refers to a fetus growing in a uterus. ***IVF*** is the process of extracting eggs, retrieving a sperm sample, and then manually combining an egg and sperm in a laboratory to then transfer to the uterus (American Pregnancy Association, 2019). IVF with egg and sperm donation is used for a variety of reasons, such as when a woman is unable to become pregnant through sexual intercourse, the person who wants to become pregnant does not have a partner, the couple is in a same-sex relationship and/or is using a surrogate, or one of the people in the couple is infertile.

Parenting

An area that has recently emerged in occupational therapy practice is assisting with ***parenting,*** which is defined as the responsibility of raising and caring for a child. Occupational therapy practitioners can help facilitate clients' parenting by creating adaptive equipment, teaching baby care techniques, promoting parent–child attachment, and supporting interpersonal communication (Case Example 7.5).

Through the Looking Glass (https://www.lookingglass.org) is a resource for occupational therapy practitioners working with parents with disabilities or people with disabilities interested in parenting. In 1994, it became the first National Center for Parents With Disabilities and Their Families, receiving federal funding to conduct research. The organization has spent more than 2 decades researching and documenting the many issues faced by people with disabilities in the realm of parenting and has disseminated information about adaptive techniques and equipment both nationally and internationally.

CASE EXAMPLE 7.5. SOLUTIONS TO PARENTING CHALLENGES

Sam has a C6 spinal cord injury that left him quadriplegic. Shortly after his injury, he harvested his sperm for future use. He married his high school sweetheart, and they had a child about a year later. Sam was able to obtain specific adaptive equipment to help him bond with the baby. For example, he worked with an occupational therapy practitioner to design a seat that was attached to his wheelchair. This seat allowed him to feed and play with his baby.

Dalia and **Devin** are deaf. They are both gay and good friends and wanted to coparent a child together. After they had their child, they each found partners and are now in committed relationships. The two couples coparent the child. The flashing light monitor that is easily available in the United States did not work for Dalia and Devin. To support these deaf parents in waking during the night when the baby was crying, the occupational therapy practitioner adapted a baby monitor to shake the mattress.

Although not all parents with disabilities face bias within health care around pregnancy, it still happens too frequently. Case Example 7.6 presents several examples of discrimination against parents with disabilities.

CASE EXAMPLE 7.6. PREGNANCY AND PREJUDICE

Bill and **Brooke** are a blind couple. When Brooke went into labor, they went to the hospital to deliver their baby. A labor and delivery nurse called Child Protective Services (CPS) because she could not imagine how the blind parents could safely care for their baby. Organizations in the disability community immediately geared up to protect the parents against the unfounded belief. In response to the concerned nurse calling CPS on Bill and Brooke, the hospital staff was offered training about adaptive equipment that could be implemented by parents. The staff who attended the workshop gained knowledge and comfort that people with disabilities could successfully parent, and the CPS case was closed.

Sue Anne has sacral agenesis caudal regression syndrome. When Sue Anne and her husband decided that they wanted to be parents, Sue Anne was evaluated medically to see if pregnancy was an option. When they found out it was not, they chose to adopt through an adoption agency, which required an interview by a social worker. Because of Sue Anne's disability, the social worker questioned the couple's ability to parent. Sue Anne became proactive: She contacted an agency that works with people who have disabilities and want to parent. She also worked with an occupational therapy practitioner to envision scenarios that might occur during parenting and solutions for those scenarios. The practitioner wrote a report to the adoption agency, which approved the adoption, resulting in Sue Anne and her husband becoming parents.

Peggi has post-polio, and she and her partner, Federica, wanted to be parents. They tried in vitro fertilization with no success. Many of their friends knew they were trying to have a baby, including their friend Pika, who also has post-polio and had adopted a baby with a club foot from her country of origin, Japan. Three years later, Pika was offered another baby with a disability from Japan to adopt, but she did not want to parent another child. Pika told Peggi about the baby who needed to be adopted, and Peggi and Federica decided to adopt the child. This process included going to Japan, attending parenting classes, and allowing home visits before and after the adoption. They had to pretend that they were not in a romantic relationship, because the adoption agency at that time did not allow adoption by same-gender parents. Once Peggi and Federica returned to the United States with their child, they worked with an occupational therapy

(Continued)

CASE EXAMPLE 7.6. PREGNANCY AND PREJUDICE *(Cont.)*

practitioner to identify adaptive equipment and strategies for Peggi to diaper and bathe their child.

Charlie is a transgender man who has cerebral palsy. He wanted to become pregnant and a parent. His husband, also a transgender man, was not interested in becoming pregnant but was interested in becoming a parent. Charlie's obstetrician was well trained in transgender health, but she was not as informed about the interaction between disability and pregnancy. The obstetrician was concerned about Charlie having difficulty during pregnancy. Because disability is not covered well in medical schools, it is common for many obstetricians not to know the impact of pregnancy on a preexisting disability. Charlie and his partner had difficulty finding a sperm donor willing to work with transgender people, but Charlie's obstetrician was very open and helped Charlie find a sperm bank that would work with him. After 6 months of unsuccessful attempts to get pregnant, Charlie and his husband decided to adopt. They interviewed several agencies before finding one willing to work with a transgender couple. They now have two children through adoption. One of the children has a disability. Charlie, being an occupational therapy practitioner, has been able to figure out his own strategies to support his children.

As the scenarios in Case Example 7.6 highlight, LGBTQIA+ and people with disabilities face prejudice trying to conceive, adopt, and parent. Those who are both LGBTQIA+ and have disabilities may face additional prejudices in these areas, similar to Peggi and Charlie. Occupational therapy practitioners should advocate for occupational justice and support parents with disabilities similarly to how the disability community did in the example of Bill and Brooke.

One of the authors has observed that parents with disabilities are more likely to adopt children with disabilities; however, research is lacking on the topic. The notion that only people who are disabled should adopt a disabled baby is complex. On the positive side, parents with disabilities can be wonderful role models for their child. On the negative side, caring for children with disabilities presents unique challenges under any circumstances. If the parent is also disabled, it can increase the difficulties around baby care.

Occupational therapy practitioners can recommend equipment or modifications to parents with various disabilities (e.g., an accessible crib that allows parents to transfer a baby into a crib). Other examples are as follows:

- **Leslie,** who has triplegia cerebral palsy, has raised her child as a single mother. She says, "adaptive baby care equipment is everything." She worked with an occupational therapy practitioner who advised her on adaptive equipment and baby care techniques. In addition, Leslie invented her own techniques (e.g., doubling up on diapers in the middle of the night so she could pull the soiled one off, leaving the clean diaper, which made it much easier; L. Heller, personal communication, January 17, 2021).

- **Betsy** became blind from diabetes soon after she gave birth. Occupational therapy practitioners worked with Betsy to place wrist and ankle straps with bells on the baby early in infancy to help the baby adapt to wearing the straps. The straps allow Betsy to use her sense of hearing to know where the baby is, and they can be adapted so that the child cannot remove the strap.

Case Example 7.7 provides additional examples of parenting adaptations.

When a baby is typically developing, the baby can help with baby care activities, such as helping with transfers by crawling into a crib or onto a diapering table. Some children with disabilities, however, may not reach the same milestones as a typical baby and therefore may not be able to assist with certain baby care activities. These situations may require the parent to obtain assistance with parenting tasks.

CASE EXAMPLE 7.7. PARENTING ADAPTATIONS AND INTERVENTIONS

Susan had a stroke affecting her nondominant side soon after giving birth and only had the use of one arm. Susan was afraid she would not be able to do all the integral tasks associated with her role as a parent. She worked with her occupational therapy practitioner to identify diapering as one of the integral tasks that would allow her to parent her child without assistance. The practitioner taught Susan how to teach her baby to raise their legs by saying "bottom up" and bouncing the baby. It has been documented that a typically developing baby can do this by 3 weeks of age, which parents with a variety of disabilities have found to be very helpful. Once the baby has learned the technique, they can lift their legs to aid the parent in cleaning and changing their diaper. The practitioner also taught Susan how to use the palm of her hand to hold the diaper in place while using two fingers to unfasten or fasten the diaper tabs. The practitioner taught Susan's partner to use the same technique, so that the baby would learn it over various other approaches.

Ilene has an intellectual disability and has one child, Bonnie. Ilene had trouble caring for Bonnie initially, so she was referred to the Department of Child and Family Services (DCFS). Ilene needed help navigating various bureaucracies when Bonnie was a baby, such as learning to obtain food stamps and medical insurance. Ilene worked on a regular basis with her occupational therapy practitioner

(Continued)

CASE EXAMPLE 7.7. PARENTING ADAPTATIONS AND INTERVENTIONS *(Cont.)*

to help with bureaucracies, coping skills, and baby care techniques. For example, Ilene had a hard time knowing what Bonnie needed and coping when she cried nonstop. She learned to make sure that Bonnie was not hungry, had a clean diaper, and had her pacifier. Ilene also learned to put Bonnie in the crib, then put on music and wait 15 minutes to see if Bonnie fell asleep. If Bonnie hadn't fallen asleep after 15 minutes, Ilene would return, console her, and then give her another 15 minutes to see if she would fall asleep. Ilene used what she learned, gained confidence in facing new challenges, and demonstrated to DCFS that she was fully capable of parenting her child.

Family separation

Parents with intellectual disabilities may face biases from others about their abilities to parent. Without proper support, such as ongoing guidance and supervision, parents with intellectual disabilities are more than twice as likely to experience termination of parental rights than parents without such a disability (LaLiberte et al., 2016). Parents with intellectual disabilities also have higher rates of termination of parental rights than parents with other disabilities (LaLiberte et al., 2016). With proper support, termination of parental rights seems less likely (see Case Example 7.7).

Occupational therapy practitioners who teach parents with disabilities how to care for their child both physically and emotionally can help to reduce concerns from providers and prevent termination of parental rights. Specifically, practitioners can support parents by providing strategies to promote engagement in caregiving tasks based on parents' needs and abilities. They can also provide education about developmental milestones and activities to support child development.

Summary

Most people with disabilities are interested in some type of intimate relationship, whether long or short term. Some clients of occupational therapy may look to practitioners to help establish and maintain intimate partnerships. The occupational therapy practitioner's role in helping clients navigate any level of intimate relationship cannot be overstated. Many people with disabilities dream of having a long-term intimate partnership and raising children. For practitioners, it is important to learn the desires of the client regarding relationships, dating, and family; to not assume that any of these desires are out of reach; and to understand the impact of previous experiences of discrimination or denial of these desires.

Judith G. Rogers, OTR/L, is an occupational therapy practitioner with cerebral palsy. She received her BA at Michigan State University and her BOT at San Jose State University. She has worked at Through the Looking Glass since 1990. Rogers has presented both nationally and internationally on pregnancy and parenting among people with disabilities and published multiple book chapters on the topic. She has served on a variety of committees, including those for the CP Foundation, Bright Futures for Women's Health and Wellness, Center for Research on Women with Disabilities, National Institute of Disability and Rehabilitation Research, and National Institutes of Health. Rogers has led and co-led special interest groups of occupational therapy practitioners with disabilities with the American Occupational Therapy Association, supporting practitioners with challenges they faced in school or practice. In 2002, she received the Robert Wood Johnson Community Health Leader award.

Elizabeth K. Schmidt, PhD, OTR/L, completed both her master's degree in occupational therapy and doctorate in health and rehabilitation sciences at The Ohio State University in Columbus. She completed her postdoctoral training at Boston University and is currently an assistant professor of occupational therapy at the DeBusk College of Osteopathic Medicine at Lincoln Memorial University–Knoxville. She has grant funding from the National Institute of Disability, Independent Living, and Rehabilitation Research in Washington, DC, to conduct a participatory approach research study alongside queer autistic researchers to better understand supports and barriers to community participation for queer autistic adults. Schmidt's research is primarily focused on accessibility of sexuality education for adolescents and adults with neurodevelopmental disabilities. She is passionate about occupational justice and sexual and reproductive health autonomy for people with neurodevelopmental disabilities.

References

Abelson, M. J. (2014). Night and day: Gendered safety and violence in the everyday experiences of transgender men. In C. M. Renzetti & R. Kennedy Bergen (Eds.), *Understanding diversity: Celebrating difference, challenging inequality* (pp. 53–64). Pearson.

Agner, J. (2020). Moving from cultural competence to cultural humility in occupational therapy: A paradigm shift. *American Journal of Occupational Therapy, 74,* 7404347010. https://doi.org/10.5014/ajot.2020.038067

American Association of Intellectual and Developmental Disabilities. (2013). *Sexuality: Joint position statement of AAIDD and the Arc.* https://aaidd.org/news-policy/policy/position-statements/sexuality

American Association of Intellectual and Developmental Disabilities. (2020). *Self-advocacy and leadership: Joint position statement of AAIDD and the Arc.* https://www.aaidd.org/news-policy/policy/position-statements/advocacy

American Occupational Therapy Association. (2020). Occupational therapy practice framework: Domain and process (4th ed.). *American Journal of Occupational Therapy, 74*(Suppl. 2), 7412410010. https://doi.org/10.5014/ajot.2020.74S2001

American Pregnancy Association. (2019). *IVF—in vitro fertilization.* https://americanpregnancy.org/getting-pregnant/infertility/in-vitro-fertilization-70966

Barnard-Brak, L., Schmidt, M., Chesnut, S., Wei, T., & Richman, D. (2014). Predictors of access to sex education for children with intellectual disabilities in public schools. *Intellectual and Developmental Disabilities, 52,* 85–97. https://doi.org/10.1352/1934-9556-52.2.85

Beery, Z. (2020). *When the world shut down, they saw it open.* https://www.nytimes.com/2020/08/24/style/disability-accessibility-coronavirus.html?smid=em-share%22%20%5Ct%20%22_blank

Bloome, D. (2017). Childhood family structure and intergenerational income mobility in the United States. *Demography, 54,* 541–569. https://doi.org/10.1007/s13524-017-0564-4

Brown, S. E. (2003). *Movie stars and sensuous scars: Essays on the journey from disability shame to disability pride.* iUniverse.

Codd, J., & Hewitt, O. (2020). Having a son or daughter with an intellectual disability transition to adulthood: A parental perspective. *British Journal of Learning Disabilities, 49,* 1–13. https://doi.org/10.1111/bld.12327

Doren, B., Gau, J. F., & Lindstrom, L. E. (2012). The relationship between parent expectations and postschool outcomes of adolescents with disabilities. *Exceptional Children, 79,* 7–23. https://doi.org/10.1177/001440291207900101

English, B., Tickle, A., & dasNair, R. (2018). Views and experiences of people with intellectual disabilities regarding intimate relationships: A qualitative metasynthesis. *Sexuality and Disability, 36,* 149–173. https://doi.org/10.1007/s11195-017-9502-z

Felter, C., & Renwick, D. (2021, December 10). *Marriage equality: Global comparisons.* Council on Foreign Relations. https://www.cfr.org/backgrounder/same-sex-marriage-global-comparisons

Ferrer, J. N. (2019). From romantic jealousy to sympathetic joy: Monogamy, polyamory, and beyond. *International Journal of Transpersonal Studies Advance Publication Archive, 38*(1), 185–202. https://doi.org/10.24972/ijts.2019.38.1.185

Friedman, C., Arnold, C. K., Owen, A. L., & Sandman, L. (2014). "Remember our voices are our tools": Sexual self-advocacy as defined by people with intellectual and developmental disabilities. *Sexuality and Disability, 32,* 515–532. https://doi.org/10.1007/s11195-014-9377-1

Grammer, K., Fink, B., Moller, A. P., & Thornhill, R. (2003). Darwinian aesthetics: Sexual selection and the biology of beauty. *Biological Reviews, 78,* 385–407. https://doi.org/10.1017/S1464793102006085

Greenwood, N. W., & Wilkinson, J. (2013). Sexual and reproductive health care for women with intellectual disabilities: A primary care perspective. *International Journal of Family Medicine, 2013,* 642472. https://doi.org/10.1155/2013/642472

Havercamp, S. M., & Scott, H. M. (2015). National health surveillance of adults with disabilities, adults with intellectual and developmental disabilities, and adults with no disabilities. *Disability and Health Journal, 8,* 165–172. https://doi.org/10.1016/j.dhjo.2014.11.002

Hook, J. N., Davis, D. E., Owen, J., Worthington, E. L., Jr., & Utsey, S. O. (2013). Cultural humility: Measuring openness to culturally diverse clients. *Journal of Counseling Psychology, 60,* 353–366. https://doi.org/10.1037/a0032595

Jones, L., Bellis, M. A., Wood, S., Hughes, K., McCoy, E., Eckley, L., . . . Officer, A. (2012). Prevalence and risk of violence against children with disabilities: A systematic review and meta-analysis of observational studies. *Lancet, 380,* 899–907. https://doi.org/10.1016/s0140-6736(12)60692-8

LaLiberte, T., Piescher, K., Mickelson, N., & Lee, M. H. (2016). Child protection services and parents with intellectual and developmental disabilities. *Journal of Applied Research in Intellectual Disabilities, 30,* 521–535. https://doi.org/10.1111/jar.12323

Law, M., Baptiste, S., Carswell, A., McColl, M., Polatajko, H., & Pollock, N. (2019). *Canadian Occupational Performance Measure, 5th edition revised.* COPM Inc.

Medline Plus. (2017). *Nager syndrome.* https://medlineplus.gov/genetics/condition/nager-syndrome/

Miller, C. C. (2018, July 5). Americans are having fewer babies. They told us why. *The New York Times.* https://www.nytimes.com/2018/07/05/upshot/americans-are-having-fewer-babies-they-told-us-why.html

National Council on Disability. (2012). *Rocking the cradle: Ensuring the rights of parents with disabilities and their children.* https://www.ncd.gov/sites/default/files/Documents/NCD_Parenting_508_0.pdf

National Institute on Deafness and Other Communication Disorders. (2016). *Quick statistics about hearing.* https://www.nidcd.nih.gov/health/statistics/quick-statistics-hearing

Nicol, A. (2018). The newclear family: The broadening recognition of non-traditional families and where to draw the line. *Journal of Inequality Inquiry, 5,* https://scholarship.law.umn.edu/jii/5

Oxford English Dictionary. (1989). Self-advocacy. In *The Oxford English Dictionary* (2nd ed.). Clarendon Press.

Pecora, L. A., Hancock, G. I., Mesibov, G. B., & Stokes, M. A. (2019). Characterizing the sexuality and sexual experiences of autistic females. *Journal of Autism and Developmental Disorders, 49,* 4834–4846. https://doi.org/10.1007/s10803-019-04204-9

Pownall, J. D., Jahoda, A., & Hastings, R. P. (2012). Sexuality and sex education of adolescents with intellectual disability: Mothers' attitudes, experiences, and support needs. *Intellectual and Developmental Disabilities, 50,* 140–154. https://doi.org/10.1352/1934-9556-50.2.140

Reiling, T. T., Barton, M. S., Becker, S., & Valasik, M. A. (2018). Rape myths and hookup culture: An exploratory study of U.S. college students' perceptions. *Sex Roles, 78,* 501–514. https://doi.org/10.1007/s11199-017-0813-4

Rogers, J. (2006). *Disabled women's guide to pregnancy and birth.* Demos Medical Publishing.

Schmidt, E. K., Faieta, J., & Tanner, K. (2019). Scoping review of self-advocacy education interventions to improve care. *OTJR: Occupational Therapy Journal of Research, 40,* 50–56. https://doi.org/10.1177/1539449219860583

Schmidt, E. K., Hand, B. N., Havercamp, S., Sommerich, C., Weaver, L., & Darragh, A. (2021). Sexual education practices for people with intellectual and developmental disabilities: A qualitative study. *American Journal of Occupational Therapy, 75,* 7503180060. https://doi.org/10.5014/ajot.2020.044859

Spencer, N., Devereux, E., Wallace, A., Sundrum, R., Shenoy, M., Bacchus, C., & Logan, S. (2005). Disabling conditions and registration for child abuse and neglect: A population-based study. *Pediatrics, 116,* 609–613. https://doi.org/10.1542/peds.2004-1882

Stahl, A. (2020). *New study: Millennial women are delaying having children due to their careers.* https://www.forbes.com/sites/ashleystahl/2020/05/01/new-study-millennial-women-are-delaying-having-children-due-to-their-careers/?sh=49118583276a

Start ASL. (2020). *American Sign Language.* https://www.startasl.com/american-sign-language

Sufrin, J. (2019). *3 Things to know: Cultural humility.* Hogg Foundation for Mental Health. https://hogg.utexas.edu/3-things-to-know-cultural-humility

Sullivan, P. M., & Knutson, J. F. (2000). Maltreatment and disabilities: A population-based epidemiological study. *Child Abuse and Neglect, 24,* 1257–1273. https://doi.org/10.1016/s0145-2134(00)00190-3

Veritas Health. (n.d.). *Spine health.* https://www.spine-health.com/

Walker, B. A., Otte, K., LeMond, K., Hess, P., Kaizer, K., Faulkner, T., & Christy, D. (2020). Development of the Occupational Performance Inventory of Sexuality and Intimacy (OPISI): Phase one. *The Open Journal of Occupational Therapy, 8,* 1–18. https://doi.org/10.15453/2168-6408.1694

Workman, C. I., Humphries, S., Hartung, F., Aguirre, G. K., Kable, J. W., & Chatterjee, A. (2021). Morality is in the eye of the beholder: The neurocognitive basis of the "anomalous-is-bad" stereotype. *Annals of the New York Academy of Sciences, 1494,* 3–17. https://doi.org/10.1111/nyas.14575

8

Sexual Activity as an ADL

Jenn Soros, *PhD, OTR/L, and* **Karla D. Reese,** *DHSc, OTR/L*

CHAPTER HIGHLIGHTS

- Understanding sexual pleasure
- Sexual activity through the lens of the *Occupational Therapy Practice Framework*

KEY TERMS AND CONCEPTS

Ageism
Arousal
Attitudes
Body functions
Body image
Body structures
Client factors
Contexts
Endurance
Environmental factors
Habits
Implicit bias
Motor skills
Orgasm
Performance patterns
Performance skills
Personal factors
Process skills
Resolution
Rituals
Roles
Routines
Sex work
Sexual activity
Sexual desire
Sexual interests
Sexual pleasure
Sexual response
Sexual response cycle
Social interaction skills
Spirituality

Sexual activity is part of the human experience that falls under the occupational therapy scope of practice. The *Occupational Therapy Practice Framework: Domain and Process* (4th ed.; *OTPF–4*) lists ***sexual activity*** as an ADL and defines sexual activity as "engaging in the broad possibilities for sexual expressions and experiences with self or others" (American Occupational Therapy Association [AOTA], 2020, p. 30). Walker et al. (2020) further delineated occupations related to sexuality and intimacy within the Occupational Therapy Sexual Assessment Framework (OTSAF), defining *sexual activity* as "a person's ability to safely engage in sexual and/or intimate activities (alone or with another person)" (p. 4). Through the lens of the *OTPF–4*, occupational therapy practitioners can gain a unique perspective on sexual activity and the factors that may support or hinder participation in it. This chapter focuses on applying the *OTPF–4* to the analysis of sexual activity.

Understanding Sexual Pleasure

Occupational therapy practitioners need a foundational understanding of sexual pleasure to be able to assess the impact of disability on a client's sexual activity. Practitioners also need to understand that sexual activity is not exclusive to partnered activity but also applies to self-pleasure. Practitioners must consider the physical and psychosocial needs of each client and how those needs relate not only to the client's doing of sexual activity but also to their sexual being, sense of belonging, and ongoing process of becoming (Wilcock, 1998; Wilcock & Hocking, 2015; see also the discussion of these constructs in Chapter 1, "Pleasure, Eroticism, and Occupational Therapy"). Understanding the physical and emotional responses associated with sexual activity and their connection to sexual pleasure can help practitioners gain a better understanding of how these responses can affect their clients' sexual activity.

Sexual Interests

Sexual interests are defined in the OTSAF as the drive to participate in sexual activities (Walker et al., 2020); they directly relate to the constructs of doing, being, becoming, and belonging (Wilcock, 1998; Wilcock & Hocking, 2015). Sexual interests transcend the doing component of sexual activity because they also relate to a person's sense of identity, connection to others, and body image and self-concept. ***Body image*** can be defined as the internalized feelings a person has about their body (Connell et al., 2013). Physical changes that occur as a result of injury or physical disability can negatively affect body image, which, in turn, can adversely affect sexual interests (Connell et al., 2013). A negative body image may also be seen in people who have disabilities that are not physically observable by others (Shpigelman & HaGani, 2019). Sexual interests will vary widely from client to client; they need to be explored in interventions and respected by the clinician.

Sexual Response

Sexual response refers to the body's physiological reactions to sexual desire and activity. Reactions may include increased heart rate, breathing changes, skin flushing, response to erogenous zones, nipple hardening, increased blood flow to the genitals (causing clitoral and penile engorgement), vaginal lubrication, prostate release, ejaculation, and orgasm (Cleveland Clinic, 2017; Walker, 2020).

Occupational therapy practitioners need a foundational understanding of the phases of the ***sexual response cycle*** to be able to assess the impact of disability on a client's sexual activity. The sexual response cycle involves the physiological responses to sexual stimuli and has been examined over the years by noted scientists and sex therapists. The first to define this cycle was Masters and Johnson (1966), who described four phases of sexual response: excitement, plateau, orgasm, and resolution. In 1979, Kaplan expanded on this definition to include desire as a distinct phase of the sexual response cycle, developing a three-phase model: desire, excitement, and orgasm. The sections that follow elaborate on aspects of these two definitions of the sexual response cycle.

Desire

Sexual desire refers to being interested in activities or objects that produce feelings of wanting to engage in sexual activity. Psychological responses to sexual desire can include beginning to think about sex, planning and organizing for sex, flirting with a partner, and searching for a potential partner through use of virtual supports. Factors that may influence desire, such as imagination, hormones, age, and energy levels, should be considered in occupational therapy practice assessment. For example, practitioners need to evaluate the influence that injury or disability may have on a person's imaginative or creative outlets as they relate to participation in sexual activity. Hormonal changes, as a result of typical development, aging, or a medical condition, may affect a person's sexual desire and therefore may be an important factor in the occupational therapy process. Additionally, attention must be given to how sexual desire evolves across the lifespan, with practitioners recognizing that the sexual desire a person experienced in their youth may have changed over the course of their lived experience. Another consideration is how fluctuations in energy levels as a result of injury or medical condition, disability, or aging can influence sexual desire.

A person's sexual being may inform the occupational doing of sex. As such, it is important to explore factors that stimulate and stifle desire, an extremely personal aspect of a person's being. Note that although desire was initially proposed as the initial phase of Kaplan's (1979) sexual response cycle, not all sexual activity is preceded by desire. In addition, for some, desire is experienced as a response to arousal (Crooks & Baur, 2021).

Arousal

Excitement, or ***arousal,*** encompasses physiological changes that bring a person to the verge of orgasm and involves an increased intensity of the changes that occur during the desire phase and during sexual activity (Cleveland Clinic, 2017). Occupational therapy practitioners should gain a thorough understanding of a client's unique sensory preferences for arousal and how they connect to the doing of sexual activity. They should also be aware that these preferences can involve all areas of the body and encompass all eight senses: tactile, gustatory, olfactory, auditory, visual, proprioceptive, vestibular, and interoceptive. As previously stated, sexual desire may be accompanied by sexual arousal; however, arousal is not a necessary outcome of desire.

Orgasm and resolution

The sexual response cycle includes orgasm and resolution, although these phases are not a necessary outcome of sexual activity. The ***orgasm*** phase may involve contractions in the vaginal canal or uterus, rhythmic contractions at the base of the penis, spasms in the feet, ejaculation of semen, and an overall release of sexual tension. During the ***resolution*** phase, the body slowly returns to its typical level of functioning and may include a sense of well-being as well as fatigue (Cleveland Clinic, 2017). Occupational therapy practitioners should consider the effect of injury or disability on the orgasm and resolution phases of sexual response.

Sexual Pleasure

The understanding of sexual activity must go beyond sexual desire and sexual response and include consideration of ***sexual pleasure.*** The Global Advisory Board for Sexual Health and Wellbeing (2016) has proposed the following definition of sexual pleasure:

> Sexual pleasure is the physical and/or psychological satisfaction and enjoyment derived from solitary or shared erotic experiences, including thoughts, dreams and autoeroticism.
>
> Self-determination, consent, safety, privacy, confidence and the ability to communicate and negotiate sexual relations are key enabling factors for pleasure to contribute to sexual health and wellbeing. Sexual pleasure should be exercised within the context of sexual rights, particularly the rights to equality and non-discrimination, autonomy and bodily integrity, the right to the highest attainable standard of health and freedom of expression. The experiences of human sexual pleasure are diverse and sexual rights ensure that pleasure is a positive experience for all concerned and not obtained by violating other people's human rights and well-being.

This definition gives occupational therapy practitioners a framework for examining sexual pleasure as an important component of sexual activity. However, a desire to be sexual, coupled with the body's physical response to being sexual, does not always result in experiencing pleasure. In addition, Jones (2019) has reported that contemporary sexual science research has de-emphasized sexual pleasure, despite its role in sexual experiences. It is imperative that practitioners not lose sight of the important connection between sexual pleasure and occupations of sexual activity. This awareness will provide practitioners with a better understanding of their clients' needs and, in turn, the ability to improve clients' overall quality of life.

Sexual Activity Through the Lens of the *Occupational Therapy Practice Framework*

The doing aspect of sexual activity can be thoroughly analyzed through the lens of the *OTPF–4*. Occupational therapy practitioners are experts in examining the elements of the occupational therapy domain, recognizing the interrelationships between these elements and their influence on occupational performance. The domain established by the *OTPF–4* includes occupations, contexts, performance patterns, performance skills, and client factors (AOTA, 2020). The *OTPF–4* can serve as a foundation for analyzing all factors that influence occupational performance of sexual activity.

Occupations

Although sexual activity is an occupation and an ADL, as outlined in the *OTPF–4*, many other occupations connect to sexual activity and intimacy. Therefore, occupational therapy practitioners should consider not only sexual activity itself but also occupations related to sexual activity, such as sexual expression, sexual self-view, intimacy, sexual health, and family planning (Walker, 2020). Exhibit 8.1 summarizes how other occupations relate to sexual activity. This list is not exhaustive; it is meant to provide examples and encourage critical thinking about the connection of other occupations to sexual activity and intimacy.

EXHIBIT 8.1
Occupations and Their Relation to Sexual Activity

Occupation	Relation to Sexual Activity
	ADLs
Bathing, showering	• Performing hygiene tasks in preparation for sexual activity • Bathing or showering as part of sexual activity • Bathing or showering after sexual activity as part of the clean-up process
Toileting and toilet hygiene	• Emptying bladder and performing hygiene after sexual activity • Emptying bowels and performing hygiene in preparation for anal sex • Managing devices, such as catheters or ileostomy bags, during sexual activity
Dressing	• Wearing clothing to enhance sexual expression and sexual self-view • Donning clothing for a date • Doffing clothing, both self and others, for sexual activity • Donning breast binders, packers to create bulge in pants, breast enhancers, or gaff underwear
Eating, swallowing, and feeding	• Having a meal as part of a date • Manipulating and/or swallowing of bodily fluids during oral sex • Feeding self or others as part of sexual activity
Functional mobility	• Transferring from one surface to another in preparation for sexual activity • Taking a walk with a partner

(Continued)

EXHIBIT 8.1
Occupations and Their Relation to Sexual Activity *(Cont.)*

Occupation	Relation to Sexual Activity
Personal hygiene and grooming	• Removing body hair; performing hair care, skin care, or nail care; or applying makeup as part of sexual self-expression and sexual self-view • Wearing cologne or perfume when out with a partner
Sexual activity	• Engaging in desired sexual activities, including, but not limited to, hugging, foreplay, kissing, masturbation, oral sex, anal sex, vaginal sex, fingering, breast play, and use of sex toys and devices (Walker, 2020)
	IADLs
Child rearing	• Discussing sexual health, safety, and boundaries with children
Communication management	• Texting a partner, including sending sexual messages to a consenting partner (i.e., sexting) • Using augmentative and alternative communication devices during intimate occupations or sexual activity • Using digital communication (e.g., phone, text, email) in a long-distance relationship
Driving and community mobility	• Navigating through the community environment to meet or date partners, going to the store to purchase supplies related to sexual activities, or going to community events
Meal preparation and cleanup	• Cooking dinner for a date • Preparing a meal to have with a partner to celebrate an anniversary
Safety and emergency maintenance	• Having a safety plan when meeting a new partner from a dating app • Using prophylaxis to prevent sexually transmitted infections
Shopping	• Purchasing contraception or other family planning tools • Purchasing sex devices or toys • Purchasing clothing or accessories related to sexual self-expression and sexual self-view
	Health management
Social and emotional health promotion and maintenance	• Expressing sexual self-view • Identifying personal boundaries with others to manage emotional health • Pursuing occupations to support sexual health and wellness • Developing sexual identity through self-reflection
Symptom and condition management	• Recognizing optimal times for sexual activity based on energy conservation needs • Managing pain within sexual activity • Using coping strategies related to sexual trauma
Communication with health care system	• Communicating health-related needs about a disability or condition to health care professionals to address sexual health or activity • Communicating with health care professionals about sexual health to determine best prophylaxis for sexual activity

(Continued)

EXHIBIT 8.1
Occupations and Their Relation to Sexual Activity *(Cont.)*

Occupation	Relation to Sexual Activity
Medication management	• Managing medications to address sexual function such as desire, arousal, orgasm, or pain • Using hormone replacement therapy • Managing medications for family planning
Personal care device management	• Using, cleaning, and maintaining sex devices such as sex toys, positioning devices, prosthetics, and contraception
	Rest and sleep
Rest	• Engaging in sexual activities as a restorative occupation • Engaging in relaxing activities before or in preparation for sexual activity
Sleep preparation	• Saying goodnight to others (AOTA, 2020) • Engaging in sexual activities, such as masturbation, as a part of preparation for sleep • Setting up the sleep environment as an intimate act between partners
Sleep participation	• Taking care of the needs of others during sleep, including partner and children, which may include caregiving or breastfeeding (AOTA, 2020) • Negotiating with a partner on interacting with others to care for needs during sleep (AOTA, 2020)
	Education
Formal education	• Participating in formal sex education classes in a school district • Participating in community sex education classes for people with disabilities • Participating in formal education classes conducted by national or local organizations regarding sexual health, sexual activity, or intimacy
Informal education or interest exploration	• Seeking out information to learn about gender identity from websites or at the local library • Reading literature on dating after divorce • Completing a BDSM checklist (Discerning Specialist, 2016) • Reading magazines for advice on dating, sexual positions and techniques, and so forth
	Work
Employment	• Working for organizations such as GLAAD, Planned Parenthood or other clinics focusing on sexual health, or The Trevor Project • Working in jobs such as sex work, professional or amateur pornography, or sexual surrogacy
Retirement	• Pursuing interests in retirement related to intimate activities with a partner, dating, sexual activity, and so forth
Volunteer	• Volunteering at local organizations related to HIV education and prevention • Volunteering at community LGBTQIA+ centers • Volunteering at the National Sexual Assault Hotline (RAINN)

(Continued)

EXHIBIT 8.1
Occupations and Their Relation to Sexual Activity *(Cont.)*

Occupation	Relation to Sexual Activity
	Leisure
Leisure exploration/participation	• Pursuing leisure activities with a partner to intimately connect with one another • Pursuing leisure activities to connect to the community, which may relate to sexual expression or sexual self-view
	Social participation
Community participation	• Fundraising event for a local sexual health center • Going to LGBTQIA+ Pride events • Dating events at a local religious center
Intimate partner relationships	• Engaging in a variety of occupations with an intimate partner to maintain a close relationship (AOTA, 2020)

Note. AOTA = American Occupational Therapy Association; BDSM = bondage and discipline, domination and submission, sadism and masochism; GLAAD = U.S.-based LGBTQ media advocacy organization, the world's largest; LGBTQIA+ = lesbian, gay, bisexual, transgender, queer, intersex, asexual, and additional sexual and gender-minoritized people; RAINN = Rape, Abuse & Incest National Network.

Contexts

Contexts include the environmental and personal factors that influence a person's participation in occupations (AOTA, 2020). It is essential for practitioners to closely examine contexts and recognize their effect on clients' participation in sexual activity. A thorough analysis of contexts in relation to sexual activity can lead to clients' improved quality of performance and satisfaction during engagement in sexual activity.

Environmental factors

Environmental factors are the physical, social, and attitudinal aspects of a person's daily life (AOTA, 2020). More specifically, environmental factors include

- Natural and human-made changes to the environment;
- Products and technology;
- Support and relationships;
- Attitudes; and
- Services, systems, and policies.

Natural and human-made changes to the environment. Consideration of the natural and human-made aspects of the environment and their relation to sexual activity is important. Occupational therapy practitioners have the skills required to determine environmental barriers and design an environment that supports sexual activity. They may assess the space available for sexual activity, considering preparation and clean-up needs; analyze the height or firmness of surfaces where sexual activity may occur; and determine how lighting, sounds, and smells support or impede participation in sexual activity.

Another consideration is time-related aspects of sexual activity. Gaining an understanding of the rhythm and routines surrounding sexual activity for clients can help improve their participation in sexual activity. For example, the time of day can influence ability to participate in sexual activity; a client dealing with fatigue issues might choose to engage in sexual activity in the morning, when energy levels are higher. It is also important to evaluate the accessibility of environments that support meeting prospective sexual partners. These are just a few examples of aspects of the environment that should be examined when addressing sexual activity.

Products, equipment, and technologies. Products, equipment, and technologies that support or hinder sexual activity need to be evaluated throughout the therapy process. A client's prescribed and recreational drugs need careful attention when addressing sexual activity. As part of the process of evaluating sexual intimacy, occupational therapy practitioners should consider recommending that a physician review all medications.

Some drugs enable clients to participate in sexual activity. For example, muscle relaxants or antispasticity medications may be necessary for some clients with cerebral palsy or spinal cord injury. In addition, some medications address sexual dysfunction, such as hormone creams, sildenafil and tadalafil for erectile dysfunction, and flibanserin and bremelanotide for hypoactive sexual desire disorder in women (Cleveland Clinic, 2021). Occupational therapy practitioners need to be aware of these drugs and also determine whether support is needed for their administration. For example, a client may need a medication injected before sexual activity or assistance with managing a pill dispenser.

Side effects of drugs can affect sexual interest and the sexual response cycle. Therefore, a review of medications to identify side effects such as drowsiness, dizziness, diarrhea, nausea, and fatigue is important because knowledge of these side effects will lead to a better understanding of their potential influence on participation in sexual activity. Medications can also affect physical appearance, resulting in body image concerns. For example, prednisone can cause facial swelling, often referred to as "moon face."

Assistive technology, adaptive equipment, and medical devices also are important to evaluate when addressing sexual activity. Medical devices such as ostomies, catheters, and oxygen tubing need to be managed during sexual activity. Mobility devices such as walkers, canes, crutches, transfer boards, and mechanical lifts can influence a client's access to and safe participation in sexual activities. Additionally, the role of augmentative and alternative communication devices, such as communication boards or switches, needs to be assessed. Attention should also be paid to adaptive equipment that can support undressing of the client and their partners.

Assistive technology that specifically supports engagement in sexual activity is an important factor for occupational therapy practitioners to consider. This technology can be in the form of sex toys, positioning devices, or other sexual equipment. Sex toys can be incorporated into solo and partnered sexual experiences. For someone with a disability, toys can improve access to masturbation or sexually pleasurable sensations during partnered sex. Practitioners must recognize that although sex toys can be used as a support to sexual activity, their use is also a component of sexual experiences. Therefore, practitioners should analyze a client's ability to use preferred sex toys and explore other options that meet client needs.

Another essential element in addressing clients' sexual activity is recognizing that this activity is not limited to physical environments. Virtual environments have become more prevalent in recent years. In a 2019 survey, 30% of adults in the United States say they have used an online dating service (Anderson et al., 2020). Virtual environments, however, go beyond platforms specific to dating. For example, social media platforms such as Facebook, Instagram, Reddit, TikTok, and Twitter, as well as online communities such as Gaia Online and IGN, play a role in how people meet and interact.

In addition, the virtual context has expanded people's access to employment, including sex work. ***Sex work*** is an umbrella term for providing sexual services or performances in exchange for money, goods, or services (Sawicki et al., 2019). Various online platforms allow sex workers to engage in a controlled, virtual environment. Occupational therapy practitioners need to be aware of how clients use virtual environments to engage in sexual activity.

Because of the increased use of virtual environments, occupational therapy practitioners need to understand the potential benefits of these services for their clients and be aware of potential barriers to online platform access, including software and hardware challenges. They should examine their clients' ability to access cell phones, computers, and tablets as well as ensure that clients have the means to communicate with these devices in a variety of formats, including voice chat, direct messaging, and social media posting or commenting. Practitioners should also assess how a client uses virtual platforms and understands safety and boundaries in the virtual world.

Support and relationships. Occupational therapy practitioners need to take into account all client relationships, even nonsexual ones, and how they support or hinder clients' sexual activity. For example, people who provide assistance to a person with a disability, including paid and unpaid caregivers, may need to be part of the client process of dating and engaging in sexual experiences. If a client requires assistance with functional mobility or community transportation, it could be a barrier to dating and sexual activity. Practitioners should assess the ability to have and maintain privacy for clients who live with family or caregivers or in a long-term care residence. Any dependence on parents or a partner for care can limit a person's desire for and ability to engage in sexual activity (Kattari, 2014; Wiegerink et al., 2011).

Caregivers may require education on the importance of supporting sexual activity as an occupation. Education could include how implicit bias affects engagement in sexuality. ***Implicit bias*** consists of the unconscious, or uncontrollable, processes that influence our judgment (FitzGerald & Hurst, 2017). Implicit bias accounts for the disconnect between what a person believes and wants to do and the unconscious influence of negative associations about a person or group of people (FitzGerald & Hurst, 2017). Implicit bias is responsible for societal attitudes that view people with disabilities as asexual; this bias also may affect individual abilities to engage in sexual activity; (Morales et al., 2016; Sakellariou & Simó Algado, 2006; Sellwood et al., 2017; Vaughn et al., 2014; Wiegerink et al., 2011). Education could also include discussions on setup needs for participation in sexual activity and needs for cleanup after engagement in sexual activity. School-based personnel may need education on interventions in place regarding masturbation, including appropriate places to masturbate and clean-up strategies for the student.

An unpaid caregiver may be a significant other who engages in sexual activity with the client. In this situation, occupational therapy practitioners should seek to understand the unique dynamic in which a person provides care to and engages in sexual activity with a client. Attention should be given to the stressors that may come with providing personal care to the person with whom one is in a sexual relationship. The psychosocial implications of this relationship need to be considered during the occupational therapy process (see Chapter 6, "Sexuality and Intimacy Screening and Assessment"). Nevertheless, the partner–caretaker can have a positive influence on engagement in sexual activity through communication and helping with problem solving around challenges (Kattari, 2014). The psychosocial implications of this relationship, as well as relationship factors that affect engagement in sexual activity, need to be considered during the occupational therapy process.

Attitudes. ***Attitudes*** include the "observable evidence of customs, practices, ideologies, values, norms, factual beliefs, and religious beliefs held by people other than the client" (AOTA, 2020, p. 11). One potential attitude to be aware of is the stereotype that people with disabilities are asexual and not interested in intimacy and sexual activity (Esmail et al., 2010; Morales et al., 2016; Sellwood et al., 2017; Vaughn et al., 2014). Conversely, the view of people with disabilities as asexual strengthens the perception of them as hypersexual or kinky if they do express an interest in sex (Mona et al., 2017). These polar and stigmatizing views of asexual and hypersexual may create provider bias that affects client care. Occupational therapy practitioners must also be aware that clients may face stigma about their sexuality from family, friends, and community members, again resulting in limited access to resources needed for participation in sexual activity and to accurate sexual health information. Education and advocacy on sexual rights and their relationship to human rights should be part of the occupational therapy process to address this stigma.

Heteronormative views are prevalent in society and can lead to bias in health care practices (Enson, 2015). Occupational therapy practitioners must be aware of potential societal biases regarding sexual activities, sexual orientations, and gender identities so that they can move beyond a frame of reference that encompasses only heterosexual, cisgendered, monogamous relationships. This awareness should involve actively exploring their own understanding of the lives of LGBTQIA+[1] people and critically examining heteronormativity, cisnormativity, and monogamy. Understanding and addressing one's own biases are essential to addressing sexual activity in a culturally competent manner that is inclusive of all client populations (see Chapter 3, "Guided Self-Reflection of Self as a Sexual Being," and Chapter 4, "Sexuality, Bias, and Impact: Preventing Clinician Harm").

Another potential attitude that needs to be considered when addressing sexual activity is societal stigmas regarding specific practices or beliefs. Practices that may elicit stigma include engaging in kink, covering certain body parts when in public for modesty, and saving sex for marriage. Other stigmatized beliefs may include nonmonogamy or polyamory. Various aspects of a person's life that are related to a sense of belonging and to the doing aspect of sexual activity may be susceptible to stigma, such as preference for virtual sex or sex workers. Occupational therapy practitioners must understand not only societal views of these practices and beliefs but also their own implicit biases that may affect their relationship with clients.

Ageism, or discrimination based on age, is another attitude that needs to be considered when addressing sexual activity. Heywood et al. (2019) observed that the portrayal of older adults as having reduced physical or cognitive abilities can result in assumptions about their sexual interest and activity. For example, it is often assumed that older adults have decreased sexual interest and decreased engagement in sexual activity, but the reality is that many older adults have pleasurable and fulfilling sex lives. Understanding the implications of ageism in sexual activity is particularly important in long-term-care facilities, where staff may make incorrect assumptions about the sexual interest of residents, causing decreased interest and engagement in sexual activity (Heywood et al., 2019; see also Chapter 5, "Sexual and Intimate Occupations Across the Lifespan").

Services, systems, and policies. Services, systems, and policies can support engagement in sexual activity or be a barrier to it. Analysis of their potential effects on sexual activity should not be ignored. As previously discussed, stigma regarding people with disabilities and older adults not being interested in sexual activity is prevalent. This stigma may lead to, for example, institutional rules requiring doors to be open or not allowing for private time, limiting engagement in sexual activity. In addition, agency policies may restrict what a paid caregiver can do to support sexual activity, possibly precluding them from assisting with setup or cleanup required to support sexual activity.

Sex education policies should also be examined. The level of sex education that a client has received may affect their ability to safely engage in sexual activity. Again, awareness of the role of stigma can be helpful, particularly for clients with

---

[1] The term *LGBTQIA+* refers to lesbian, gay, bisexual, transgender, queer, intersex, asexual, and additional sexual and gender-minoritized people. As greater awareness, social acceptance, and safety improve for these individuals and communities, new terms may emerge as language evolves to describe identities that exist outside of societal recognition and acceptance.

disabilities and for older adults. For example, students with disabilities may not have received the same education as their nondisabled peers, even in the same school. Understanding a client's current level of sexual knowledge is an important aspect of addressing sexual activity during the occupational therapy process.

Personal factors

Personal factors are "the particular background of a person's life and living . . . the unique features of the person that are not part of the health condition or health state" (AOTA, 2020, p. 40). Such factors include age, sexual orientation, gender identity, race and ethnicity, cultural identification, and life experiences (AOTA, 2020). Personal factors may influence clients' engagement in sexual activity, so occupational therapy practitioners should consider

- sexual development across the lifespan (see Chapter 5, "Sexual and Intimate Occupations Across the Lifespan"),
- sexual positioning needs outside of heteronormative penetration,
- how a transgender client's experience and context influences their intimate partnerships and social participation,
- how a client's life experience has influenced their intimacy, and
- potential implications of intersectional identities on participation in sexual activity.

Other personal factors may come into play. It is important for practitioners to thoroughly examine all client personal factors and examine their influence on participation in sexual activity.

Performance Patterns

Performance patterns involve the habits, routines, roles, and rituals that support or hinder engagement in occupations (AOTA, 2020). ***Habits,*** or specific and automatic behaviors, need to be developed that will support engagement in sexual activity (AOTA, 2020). An example for occupational therapy clients is confirming the timing of medication administration for birth control or erections. ***Routines*** are patterns of behaviors that provide a structure for engagement in occupation (AOTA, 2020). Occupational therapy practitioners need to work with clients to create routines that support sexual activity. Examples include being able to empty an ostomy bag or self-catheterize before sexual activity. ***Roles*** are sets of behaviors shaped by society, culture, and context (AOTA, 2020). Practitioners need to understand the effect that roles and role changes, such as those resulting from an acquired disability, have on sexual activity (see Chapter 3, "Guided Self-Reflection of Self as a Sexual Being"). Additionally, caregiver roles need to be assessed, particularly when a client's personal care is part of a typical routine and the caregiver has the additional role of intimate partner. ***Rituals*** are symbolic actions that tie to a person's identity (AOTA, 2020). It is important that occupational therapy practitioners recognize and respect client rituals regarding sexual activity.

Performance Skills

According to the *OTPF–4*, ***performance skills*** are "observable, goal-directed actions that result in a client's quality of performing desired occupations" (AOTA, 2020, p. 43). Performance skills include motor skills, process skills, and social interaction skills (AOTA, 2020) and play an integral role in occupational performance regarding sexual activity.

Motor skills

Motor skills include the ability of a person to move their body or to move and interact with objects (AOTA, 2020). Motor skills as they pertain to sexual activity include how people position their body, obtain and hold objects, move themselves and objects, and sustain performance (AOTA, 2020).

The positioning of the body is how a person moves through the environment and arranges and aligns themselves to other people or objects related to the occupation (AOTA, 2020); it is an essential component of sexual activity. A person may need to move throughout the environment to get to the location of desired sexual activity, either within a home or community environment. The position of the body during sexual activity can affect performance. It is therefore important to consider how a position influences sexual functioning, sexual pleasure, and sexual satisfaction. For example, for a person who has just had a hip replacement, it is vital to consider hip precautions during sexual activity. Similarly, it may be beneficial for another person with limb differences to use a suction cup dildo while in the shower to position themselves to masturbate effectively. A person may feel passive or less engaged in sex when they are lying flat on their backs but more engaged when propped up and able to access their partner's nipples with their mouth. People may independently position themselves into desired positions for sexual activity or use positioning devices such as wedges, bolsters, pillows, leg spreaders, slings or swings, or other props to achieve the desired position for sexual activity.

How a person obtains and holds objects, including how they reach, bend, grip, and manipulate objects, can affect the performance of sexual activities (AOTA, 2020). The ability to reach is essential for a person to obtain items needed for sexual activity, such as prophylaxis, contraception methods, lubricants, sex devices and toys, and garments, as well as to make contact with a partner. If difficulty with grip or object manipulation (i.e., dexterity) prevents sexual satisfaction, certain sex devices or toys such as masturbation sleeves, dildos or vibrators with extended handles, finger vibrators, or hands-free devices (e.g., suction cup dildos, vibrators or dildos in pillows, remote-controlled vibrators) may be beneficial. These devices can be used when engaging in masturbation or sexual activity with a partner or partners.

As with positioning, the ability of a person to move their body or objects is an essential component of sexual activity and can affect engagement in sexual activity, both with or without a partner or partners. This motor skill includes how a person coordinates, moves, lifts, walks, transports, uses force, and uses smooth fluid movements and may include sex devices or toys, contraception, prophylaxis, or a partner (AOTA, 2020). Different sexual positions and the use of devices or toys may require coordination. When engaging in sexual activity with a partner, a person might have to coordinate oral–motor movements to kiss while simultaneously coordinating finger and wrist movements for penetration. During masturbation, a person may coordinate different movements to stimulate different areas of the body at the same time.

Finally, it is critical to take into consideration endurance and pace during sexual activity. ***Endurance*** is the ability to complete the tasks without physical fatigue or stopping to rest or catch one's breath (AOTA, 2020). Occupational therapy practitioners may explore principles of energy conservation and incorporate them in therapy for clients with chronic conditions that affect endurance such as multiple sclerosis, fibromyalgia, or cardiac conditions. In addition, the ability to maintain a consistent pace or tempo throughout sexual activity can affect performance and engagement.

Process skills

Process skills are skills that relate to selecting, interacting, and using objects; carrying out actions and steps; and preventing problems from occurring or recurring related to occupational performance (AOTA, 2020). Process skills include applying knowledge, organizing time, organizing space and objects, and adapting performance (AOTA, 2020).

How people apply knowledge may affect their occupational performance of or engagement in sexual activity. They will choose not only the desired sexual activity but also objects or other people required to engage in the activity. People also apply knowledge about how objects are used, such as the appropriate use of prophylaxis, including pre-exposure prophylaxis for HIV (commonly referred to as PrEP) and contraceptive methods; lubricants; positioning devices; and sex devices or toys. Applying knowledge may include reading labels on medication or instruction manuals to ensure safe use.

To successfully engage in sexual activity, a person may need to organize the activity's timing, including initiation, sequencing, and termination of the activity (AOTA, 2020).

Participation in sexual activities requires that the space be organized. One critical component to organizing space is the setup of the environment. The environment can include the physical environment, the sensory environment, and the social environment (AOTA, 2020). Setting up the physical environment may include arranging equipment or devices (e.g., wedges, bolsters, pillows, sling or swing) to provide safe and effective positioning for sexual activity. Devices and equipment meant to increase participation in other areas of occupation (e.g., hospital bed, wheelchair, assistive devices, catheters, ostomy bags) often become barriers for sexual activity (Taylor, 2011). Thus, people may need to consider how these devices could affect sexual activity and the need to modify the physical environment to allow for participation in sexual activity.

Setting up the sensory environment may include selection of lighting; scented candles, perfumes or colognes, or lubricants; satin sheets or other materials; music (or reducing other environmental sounds); and taste sensations. The social environment may also be considered if sexual activity includes a partner or partners, both in the physical and virtual contexts. After the environment has been organized, people must navigate through the environment. The ability to navigate through virtual environments plays a critical role in modern sexual activity. It may include online dating platforms, pornography websites and virtual communities, and video chatting and sexting. Finally, the environment must be restored, including cleaning up after the sexual activity has concluded.

Throughout sexual activity, people adapt to their own performance. They notice how they feel during sexual activity, including what does and does not feel good, and then they adjust accordingly. The response to sexual activity may be a physical response in moving their body into a different position or space or a communicative response in which the person tells a partner their requests for adjustment during the activity. The need for communication and response and adjustment is important for each participant during sexual activity, and even more so for those who engage in kink or BDSM,[2] to ensure a pleasurable and safe experience for all involved (Tellier, 2017).

Social interaction skills

Social interaction skills and communication during sexual activity are essential throughout sexual activity with a partner or partners. Social interaction skills that occur during sexual activity include initiating and terminating social interactions, communication, problem solving, and ongoing consent. The ability to initiate social interaction, as well as terminate social interaction, is important not only for engagement in sexual activity but also for obtaining consent from all parties involved during the activity.

Communication between partners and having a supportive partner or partners can increase sexual satisfaction for some people (Rose & Hughes, 2018). People with disabilities have a greater need for sexual communication regarding boundaries, pain, physical needs, emotional needs, and planning (Tellier, 2017). Partner connection may increase communication and confidence, allowing people to share their wants and desires (Kattari, 2014). Having a supportive, communicative, and creative partner or partners to help problem solve through challenges with sexual activity can also enhance the engagement in sexual activity (Kattari, 2014). Social interaction skills can influence communication and affect sexual activity performance. Occupational therapy practitioners should consider the intimate relationship and may suggest activities that build connections and strategies to enhance effective communication (see Chapter 6).

[2] *BDSM* is bondage and discipline, domination and submission, sadism and masochism.

Client Factors

Client factors are aspects of the person that are central to who they are. They affect occupational performance and include values, beliefs, and spirituality; body functions; and body structures (AOTA, 2020). A person's values, beliefs, and spirituality can significantly influence the types of sexual activity in which they engage (see Chapter 3, "Guided Self-Reflection of Self as a Sexual Being"). A person's values consist of beliefs about what is right and wrong and what is essential (AOTA, 2020). Whereas one person may value commitment in a relationship and engage in sexual activities with only one person, another person may have different values related to relationships and may engage in consensual nonmonogamous relationships with multiple partners. It is essential to be cognizant of various relationship types and how values can influence different relationships.

Spirituality is another aspect of the person that may have a significant influence on sexual activity. ***Spirituality*** is sometimes defined as the process of developing an inner sense of self through reflection and thought (Vaughn et al., 2014). Some people experience spirituality through religious practices, whereas others express spirituality through their relationship with nature, music, the arts, or a set of philosophical beliefs (Sulmasy, 2002). Spirituality can offer a person a profound sense of who they are and provide them with connection to self-esteem, desire, and sexuality (Vaughn et al., 2014). A person's experience with pleasure and sexual activity can relate to their spirituality and sense of self.

Spirituality may influence engagement in activities. For example, a person may not engage in practices such as masturbation because of their religious beliefs, or a person may experience feelings of guilt if they engage in practices that their religion views as wrong, such as gay relationships (Cella et al., 2010; Morales et al., 2016). Eastern spirituality traditions, such as Tantrism and Taoism, view sexuality and spirituality as connected, and self-discovery is viewed as a sexual ideal (Sakellariou & Simó Algado, 2006). Each person has unique values, beliefs, and spirituality that help create unique meaning in the engagement of sexual activity.

Body functions and body structures are also a factor in engagement in sexual activity. ***Body functions*** are the physiological and psychological functions of the body (AOTA, 2020). ***Body structures*** are the anatomical parts of the body that support body function (AOTA, 2020). Exhibit 8.2 summarizes how body functions and structures relate to sexual activity.

Summary

Sexual activity is an essential and personal occupation that provides different meanings for different people. From an occupational justice perspective, all people have the right to engage in occupations that are meaningful to them, including engaging in sexual activity. As discussed throughout this chapter, numerous occupations are related to sexual activity, sexual expression, sexual self-view, intimacy,

Exhibit 8.2
Body Function and Structures and Their Relation to Sexual Activity

Body Function and Structure	Relation to Sexual Activity
	Mental functions
Memory	• Remembering partners' names • Remembering to give consent and receive consent
Sensory perception	• Preferring deep pressure versus light pressure • Using flavored or scented lubricants • Playing background music • Using low lighting
Emotional	• Having an emotional connection or disconnection to sexual partners • Having an emotional response to sexual experiences
Experience of self	• Developing sexual self-esteem and expressing gender identity and sexual orientation
Consciousness or orientation	• Being able to provide consent (especially important for people with cognitive disabilities, dementia, or brain injuries)
Psychosocial	• The development and integration of mental functions leading to creating personal and interpersonal skills for social interactions, including social and interpersonal skills required for dating, maintaining a relationship, or managing conflict within intimate relationships
Energy	• Having the energy required for sexual activity • Having motivation to engage in sexual activities
	Neuromuscular function and movement
Joint mobility and stability during sexual activity	• Having reduced range of motion and structural integrity of joints may limit certain sexual positions or activities
Muscle endurance and tone	• Having limitations in muscle endurance and tone that requires increased support or the use of assistive devices
Motor reflexes, involuntary movements, control of voluntary movement	• Positioning during sexual activities that elicits or inhibits motor reflexes or involuntary movements • Using modified positioning or devices to compensate for a change in mobility
	Cardiovascular, hematological, immunological, and respiratory functions
Heart rate, blood pressure, respiration	• Requiring monitoring of heart rate, blood pressure, and respiration to ensure they remain at safe levels during sexual activity
	Voice and speech functions; digestive, metabolic, and endocrine system functions; genitourinary and reproductive functions
Voice and speech functions	• Using AAC devices to communicate with partners • Having limited ability to access sexual health services because some AAC devices do not have the vocabulary for sexual health (Retznik et al., 2017)
Digestive, metabolic, and endocrine systems	• Wearing lingerie and undergarments that are designed for use with ostomies

(Continued)

Exhibit 8.2
Body Function and Structures and Their Relation to Sexual Activity *(Cont.)*

Body Function and Structure	Relation to Sexual Activity
Genitourinary and reproductive function	• Managing catheters during sexual activity • Selecting and using appropriate contraception methods to assist with family planning • Engaging in sexual activity during menstruation • Managing menstruation, including using and removing devices to be able to engage in sexual activity • Experiencing menopausal changes in sexual function, including sexual interest, psychological responses, and emotional responses to sexual activity • Managing erectile dysfunction medication or using assistive devices such as penis pumps or strap-on devices • Exploring sexual activities that do not require an erect penis • Having an injury or illness that caused trauma to the genitals, affecting sexual activity
	Skin and related structure functions
Skin functions and integrity	• Assessing skin integrity, including pressure ulcers, burns, scar tissue, and wounds, and its effect on sexual activity and positioning

Note. AAC = augmentative and alternative communication device.

sexual health, and family planning. Through the lens of the *OPTF–4*, occupational therapy practitioners can explore with their clients the complexity of these occupations. In addition, practitioners must take into consideration context, performance patterns, performance skills, and client factors to address sexual and intimate occupations. Through a comprehensive analysis of sexual activity, occupational therapy practitioners have the tools to ensure that clients can engage in meaningful occupations and, in turn, improve their overall quality of life.

Jenn Soros, PhD, OTR/L (she/her), is an assistant professor at Cleveland State University in the Department of Occupational Therapy in Cleveland, Ohio. Dr. Soros's area of research focuses on sexuality and intimacy from an occupational perspective.

Karla D. Reese, DHSc, OTR/L (she/her), is a clinical assistant professor at Cleveland State University in the Department of Occupational Therapy in Cleveland, Ohio. She is the co-creator and co-host of OT After Dark, a podcast focusing on sexuality and intimacy for individuals with disabilities.

References

American Occupational Therapy Association. (2020). Occupational therapy practice framework: Domain and process (4th ed.). *American Journal of Occupational Therapy, 74*(Suppl. 2), 7412410010. https://doi.org/10.5014/ajot.2020.74S2001

Anderson, M., Vogels, E., & Turner, E. (2020, Oct. 2). *The virtues and downsides of online dating.* https://www.pewresearch.org/internet/2020/02/06/the-virtues-and-downsides-of-online-dating

Cella, D., Riley, W., Stone, A., Rothrock, N., Reeve, B., Yount, S., . . . Hays, R. (2010). Initial health item banks and first wave testing of the Patient–Reported Outcomes Measurement Information System (PROMIS) network: 2005–2008. *Journal of Clinical Epidemiology, 63,* 1179–1194. https://doi.org/10.1016/j.jclinepi.2010.04.011

Cleveland Clinic. (2017). *Sexual response cycle.* https://my.clevelandclinic.org/health/articles/9119-sexual-response-cycle

Cleveland Clinic. (2021). *How is sexual dysfunction treated?* https://my.clevelandclinic.org/health/diseases/9121-sexual-dysfunction#management-and-treatment

Connell, K. M., Coates, R., Doherty-Poirier, M., & Wood, F. M. (2013). A literature review to determine the impact of sexuality and body image changes following burn injuries. *Sexuality and Disability, 31,* 403–412. https://doi.org/10.1007/s11195-013-9321-9

Crooks, R., & Baur, K. (2021). *Our sexuality.* Wadsworth/Cengage Learning.

Discerning Specialist. (2016). *BDSM checklist.* https://www.discerningspecialist.com/articles/bdsm-101/34-bdsm-checklist

Enson, S. (2015). Causes and consequences of heteronormativity in healthcare and education. *British Journal of School Nursing, 10,* 73–78. https://doi.org/10.12968/bjsn.2015.10.2.73

Esmail, S., Darry, K., Walter, A., & Knupp, H. (2010). Attitudes and perceptions towards disability and sexuality. *Disability and Rehabilitation, 32,* 1148–1155. https://doi.org/10.3109/09638280903419277

FitzGerald, C., & Hurst, S. (2017). Implicit bias in healthcare professionals: A systematic review. *BMC Medical Ethics, 18,* 1–18. https://doi.org/10.1186/s12910-017-0179-8

Global Advisory Board for Sexual Health and Wellbeing. (2016). *Working definition of sexual pleasure.* https://www.gab-shw.org/our-work/working-definition-of-sexual-pleasure/

Heywood, W., Minichiello, V., Lyons, A., Fileborn, B., Hussain, R., Hinchliff, S., . . . Dow, B. (2019). The impact of experiences of ageism on sexual activity and interest in later life. *Ageing and Society, 39,* 795–814. https://doi.org/10.1017/S0144686X17001222

Jones, A. (2019). Sex is not a problem: The erasure of pleasure in sexual science research. *Sexualities, 22,* 643–668. https://doi.org/10.1177/1363460718760210

Kaplan, H. (1979). *Disorders of sexual desire.* Brunner/Mazel.

Kattari, S. K. (2014). Sexual experiences of adults with physical disabilities: Negotiating with sexual partners. *Sexuality and Disability, 32,* 499–513. https://doi.org/10.1007/s11195-014-9379-z

Masters, W., & Johnson, V. (1966). *Human sexual response.* Little, Brown.

Mona, L. R., Cameron, R. P., & Clemency Cordes, C. (2017). Disability culturally competent sexual healthcare. *American Psychologist, 72,* 1000. https://doi.org/10.1037/amp0000283

Morales, E., Gauthier, V., Edwards, G., & Courtois, F. (2016). Women with disabilities' perceptions of sexuality, sexual abuse and masturbation. *Sexuality and Disability, 34,* 303–314. https://doi.org/10.1007/s11195-016-9440-1

Retznik, L., Wienholz, S., Seidel, A., Pantenburg, B., Conrad, I., Michel, M., & Riedel-Heller, S. G. (2017). Relationship status: Single? Young adults with visual, hearing, or physical disability and their experiences with partnership and sexuality. *Sexuality and Disability, 35*(4), 415–432. https://doi.org/10.1007/s11195-017-9497-5

Rose, N., & Hughes, C. (2018). Addressing sex in occupational therapy: A coconstructed autoethnography. *American Journal of Occupational Therapy, 72,* 7203205070. https://doi.org/10.5014/ajot.2018.026005

Sakellariou, D., & Simó Algado, S. (2006). Sexuality and occupational therapy: Exploring the link. *British Journal of Occupational Therapy, 69,* 350–356. https://doi.org/10.1177/030802260606900802

Sawicki, D. A., Meffert, B. N., Read, K., & Heinz, A. (2019). Culturally competent health care for sex workers: An examination of myths that stigmatize sex work and hinder access to care. *Sexual and Relational Therapy, 34,* 355–371. https://doi.org/10.1080/14681994.2019.1574970

Sellwood, D., Raghavendra, P., & Jewell, P. (2017). Sexuality and intimacy for people with congenital physical and communication disabilities: Barriers and facilitators: A systematic review. *Sexuality and Disability, 35,* 227–244. https://doi.org/10.1007/s11195-017-9474-z

Shpigelman, C.-N., & HaGani, N. (2019). The impact of disability type and visibility on self-concept and body image: Implications for mental health nursing. *Journal of Psychiatric and Mental Health Nursing, 26,* 77–86. https://doi.org/10.1111/jpm.12513

Sulmasy, D. P. (2002). A biopsychosocial-spiritual model for the care of patients at the end of life. *The Gerontologist, 42,* 24–33. https://doi.org/10.1093/geront/42.suppl_3.24

Taylor, B. (2011). The impact of assistive equipment on intimacy and sexual expression. *British Journal of Occupational Therapy, 74,* 435–442. https://doi.org/10.4276/030802211x13153015305637

Tellier, S. (2017). Advancing the discourse: Disability and BDSM. *Sexuality and Disability, 35,* 485–493. https://doi.org/10.1007/s11195-017-9504-x

Vaughn, M., Silver, K., Murphy, S., Ashbaugh, R., & Hoffman, A. (2014). Women with disabilities discuss sexuality in San Francisco focus groups. *Sexuality and Disability, 33,* 19–46. https://doi.org/10.1007/s11195-014-9389-x

Walker, B. A. (2020). *Occupational Performance Inventory of Sexuality and Intimacy (OPISI).* University of Indianapolis. https://uindy.edu/health-sciences/ot/opisi

Walker, B. A., Otte, K., LeMond, K., Hess, P., Kaizer, K., Faulkner, T., & Christy, D. (2020). Development of the Occupational Performance Inventory of Sexuality and Intimacy (OPISI): Phase one. *The Open Journal of Occupational Therapy, 8,* 1–18. https://doi.org/10.15453/2168-6408.1694

Wiegerink, D., Roebroeck, M., Bender, J., Stam, H., Cohen-Kettenis, P., & Transition Research Group South West Netherlands. (2011). Sexuality of young adults with cerebral palsy: Experienced limitations and needs. *Sexuality and Disability, 29,* 119–128. https://doi.org/10.1007/s11195-010-9180-6

Wilcock, A. (1998). Reflections on doing, being and becoming. *Canadian Journal of Occupational Therapy, 65,* 248–256. https://doi.org/10.1177/000841749806500501

Wilcock, A., & Hocking, C. (2015). *An occupational perspective of health* (3rd ed.). Slack.

9

Trauma-Informed Care

Varleisha D. Gibbs, *PhD, OTD, OTR/L, ASDCS, FAOTA,*
and **Sameera Qureshi,** *MS, OTR*

CHAPTER HIGHLIGHTS

- Defining the various forms of trauma
- Establishing the neurophysiological connection between trauma and sexuality
- Review of trauma-informed care approaches
- Effects of trauma related to gender and gender identity
- Effects of sexual violence and trauma on sex and intimacy
- Assessment and intervention approaches that the occupational therapy practitioner can implement when addressing trauma, sexuality, and intimacy

KEY TERMS AND CONCEPTS

ACTION-from-trauma
Acute stress disorder
Adverse childhood experiences
Big-T Trauma
Body mapping
Body shaming
Checking in
Complex trauma
Contextual sensory investigation
Cultural trauma
Gender dysphoria
Genderism
Grounding
Intergenerational trauma
Little-t trauma
Mental disorders
Mental distress
Mental health
Mental health problem
Mental illnesses
Misgendered
Objectification
Purity culture
Rape culture
Sexual abuse
Sexual assault
Sexual harassment
Sexualization
Sexual violence
Slut shaming and blaming
Trauma
Trauma-informed care
Trauma response
Trauma triggers
Traumatic adverse experiences
Vicarious trauma
Victim blaming

It is paramount to acknowledge the effect of adverse experiences on a person's mental, psychological, physical, intimate, and sexual well-being. Historically, the diagnosis of trauma—posttraumatic stress disorder (PTSD) to be exact—was one reserved for war-related illnesses, but the more subtle forms of trauma, such as child abuse, generational trauma, racism, and genderism, can also have lasting effects on overall well-being and various aspects of sexuality.

A study on adverse childhood experiences (ACEs) conducted at Kaiser Permanente's 45,000-patient San Diego Health Appraisal Clinic in 1995 ignited a necessary discussion around reconceptualizing trauma (Felitti et al., 1998). ***ACEs*** include emotional, social, physical, household, and community dysfunction that have the potential to lead to toxic stress and trauma. This 2-year study (now known as the ACE Study) highlighted that more than half of the subjects presented with at least one ACE. The study helped to redefine trauma, connecting it to childhood and not limiting it to posttraumatic stress experienced by war veterans (Felitti et al., 1998). Indeed, the researchers revealed that the detrimental effects of trauma correlated not only to one's mental well-being but also to physical well-being. People reporting at least two traumatic events were 2 to 4 times more likely to have physical risk factors related to health, disease, and lifespan (Felitti et al., 1998).

Occupational therapy practitioners are likely to encounter clients who have experienced at least one adverse experience, whether as a child or as an adult, and must therefore consider the connection between trauma and client symptomatology. For example, repeated trauma and adverse experiences may result in heightened pain responses, hyperactivity, and aggression (Gibbs & Harley, 2021). In this context, the conditioned reactions can affect the client's ability to feel safe and secure, be intimate with others, and establish healthy sexual bonds.

In this chapter, we unpack the connection among PTSD, exposure to adverse life experiences, and sexuality. Before delving into this discussion, we first start by reviewing the neurological connections and the physiological manifestations of trauma.

What Is Trauma?

Trauma is

> the result of an event, series of events, or set of circumstances that is experienced by an individual as physically or emotionally harmful or life threatening and that has lasting adverse effects on the individual's functioning and mental, physical, social, emotional, or spiritual well-being. (Substance Abuse and Mental Health Services Administration [SAMHSA], 2014, p. 7)

In recent years, neuroscientific research has shaped and changed how we have come to understand trauma with regard to both determining what is considered trauma and incorporating modalities for healing based on holistic approaches (Perryman et al., 2019). When one hears about trauma, the following events—"big-T traumas"—come to mind: war, natural disasters, living in poverty, or being a victim of sexual assault. These big-T traumas certainly cause trauma. Yet, "little-t traumas" also occur and are often dismissed or misunderstood in terms of their effect on the human mind, body, and soul. These events can equally lead to experiencing trauma and have mostly been informed by the ACE Study (Centers for Disease Control and Prevention, 2021).

A ***big-T Trauma*** is a reaction to a deeply disturbing, life-threatening event or situation—for example, wars, natural disasters, violent crimes, school shootings, or serious car accidents. This form of trauma is often the most commonly recognized. In addition, the death of a parent or guardian can be a big-T trauma. This form of trauma can be acute or chronic: Acute refers to a single traumatic incident, whereas chronic indicates repeated, ongoing trauma, such as abuse or domestic violence (Barbash, 2017).

Little-t traumas are classified as stressful events that happen to all of us at one point or another. These are interpersonal stressors, such as employment changes, challenging breakups, unplanned major expenses, or the loss of a loved one. In terms of children, this form of trauma could manifest as parents experiencing divorce or multiple moves and resulting difficulties with acclimatizing to new environments. Depending on the interplay of a number of factors—including genetics, our environment, past experiences, and neurobiology—these events can lead to varying levels of traumatic responses, but they are not correlated with causing PTSD (Barbash, 2017).

Research and Neuroscience

With posttraumatic stress, the traumatic experiences remain present in the body's sensory system. For this reason, trauma related to sexuality is not isolated to the reproductive organs. Adverse experiences can affect the entire body. Moreover, nonsexual trauma can, in turn, affect one's sexuality. The autonomic nervous system becomes easily triggered, resulting in symptoms such as flashbacks, nightmares, and increased general anxiety while blocking explicit memory of the specific details in an attempt to protect the person from further harm (Maren, 2014). Generally speaking, these symptoms occur because the body fails to process the sensory aspects of the trauma. In the presence of stress, fear, or uncertainty, an unconscious response occurs that involves the primitive parts of the central nervous system rather than the higher cortices (Gibbs & Harley, 2021).

When the body senses a threat, it can go into survival mode, and the brain structures involved in this process then switch to focus on self-preservation and protection. The subconscious brain tries to make sense of the experiences. The hippocampus becomes a protector as it seeks to determine similarities in prior lived experiences. It analyzes the sensory stimuli to determine whether the present event aligns with stored emotions from the past. In doing so, it identifies whether there is a need to respond in a protective fashion, as occurred with previous stressful or threatening experiences.

Through a direct pathway to fear, the limbic system reacts, shutting down the areas for executive function in the frontal lobe. Although the amygdala plays a major role in sounding the alarm, the hippocampus attempts to encode the experience by categorizing it based on past experiences. If the various aspects of the experience match previous dangerous experiences, the hippocampus will begin consolidating the occurrence as dangerous, and then the person will produce an appropriate response to the perceived danger. If the limbic system cannot make sense of the incoming sensory stimuli, it rejects the messages from reaching the higher brain centers for processing. Instead, the primitive brain keeps the fight–flight stress response active and the body on high alert. The trauma remains "stuck" within the body as a result of the heightened sensory reactions and because traumatic memories are stored both neurologically and somatically (Gibbs & Harley, 2021).

With this disruption, the hippocampus is unsuccessful in consolidating the experience into memories because it cannot make sense of the occurrence. Therefore, memories are not stored consciously and remain as fragmented sensory ones. To this end, ***trauma triggers***—reactions to sensory or psychological stimuli that evoke a physiological reaction reminiscent of a previous traumatic event—easily elicit a response from the unconsolidated memories: the ***trauma response.***

The trauma response affects one's mental, physical, emotional, social, and spiritual well-being. It can result from isolated, pervasive, or multiple events leading to long-term distress for the person (Center for Substance Abuse Treatment, 2014). The physiological sensations of a trauma response can mimic each other: For example, an adult who was physically abused as a child may be triggered by the emerging feelings leading up to sexual intercourse, thus resulting in a trauma response and sexual dysfunction, even though the two traumas are unrelated.

Stimuli evoking the trauma response may be directly or indirectly related to the trauma (e.g., someone speaking loudly may evoke fear in an adult who experienced childhood abuse and had an aggressive parent). The result is frequent activation of the fight–flight system (i.e., sympathetic nervous system), leading to long-term implications. The exposure to prolonged levels of stress hormones (i.e., cortisol) may result in a decrease in volume of the hippocampus and an increase in size of the amygdala (Krugers et al., 2010). Moreover, the immune system is suppressed as a means of preserving energy, which increases the body's inflammatory response (Pelt, 2011).

Over time, the effects on the sympathetic nervous system can lead to physiological conditions, such as hypertension, obesity, and chronic pain. In addition, depression and anxiety may ensue. Although these symptoms can have detrimental effects on intimacy and sexuality, trauma itself can have a direct impact. The body releases norepinephrine during sexual experiences as well as during fear responses

(Yehuda et al., 2015). As a result, people experiencing posttraumatic stress may have difficulty distinguishing between the trauma response and sexual reactions.

Being Trauma Informed

SAMHSA's (2014) trauma-informed approach provides guidance for occupational therapy practitioners and survivors to address the needs of clients receiving occupational therapy services. Being trauma informed supports clients who may have lived adverse experiences that are affecting their sexuality. The strength-based approach starts with the "three Es" of trauma as a means of identifying and defining trauma:

1. *Events:* represent what actually occurred.
2. *Experiences:* acknowledge how the person interpreted the event (e.g., how it made them feel—personal meaning or significance).
3. *Effects:* understand the adverse effects of the trauma, including its short- and long-term effects on behavioral, psychosocial, and physical health (SAMHSA, 2014).

In addition to the three Es, practitioners should strive to provide ***trauma-informed care*** (TIC)—a context in which trauma is addressed or treatments are deployed that contribute to positive outcomes for trauma survivors, the people receiving services, and the people staffing the systems (SAMHSA, 2014).

TIC outlines four approaches that guide the subsequent care and intervention process:

1. Realize trauma's widespread effects on recovery
2. Recognize the signs and symptoms of trauma
3. Respond by integrating knowledge about trauma into policies, procedures, and practices
4. Resist retraumatization by identifying possible triggers and toxic environments for all involved (SAMHSA, 2014).

The first approach requires awareness and acknowledgment that traumatic events occur and can have detrimental effects on overall well-being. For the second approach, it is crucial to recognize the signs and symptoms of trauma, such as changes in behavior. Integrating knowledge, as described in the third approach, includes developing supportive and healthy practices for everyone. The third approach aligns with the fourth regarding avoidance of retraumatization (e.g., establishing policies around proactive methods instead of physically restraining someone in emotional distress).

TIC also outlines six principles, as follows:

1. *Safety:* ensuring physical and psychological safety at every level of the organization (e.g., client and staff)
2. *Trustworthiness and transparency:* being open and transparent regarding decision making and goal development
3. *Peer support:* sharing lived experiences from others with a similar trauma history
4. *Collaboration and mutuality:* sharing power and decision making
5. *Empowerment, voice, and choice:* supporting self-advocacy
6. *Cultural, historical, and gender issues:* removing stereotypes of culture and gender.

Mental Health and Traumatic Experiences

The World Health Organization (2020) defined ***mental health*** as

> a state of complete physical, mental and social well-being and not merely the absence of disease or infirmity. Mental health is a state of well-being in which an individual realizes his or her own abilities, can cope with the normal stresses of life, can work productively and is able to make a contribution to his or her community.

The effect on a person's mental health of having experienced trauma is ever present, yet nuanced. A person's genetic makeup, upbringing, environment, and many other factors contribute to the mental effects of trauma (van der Kolk, 2014). On learning about trauma, many people, including health care professionals, associate it with the presence of a mental illness, such as depression, anxiety, or PTSD. Although people who experience trauma may be diagnosed with a mental illness, that is not true in all cases; nevertheless, all clients should receive TIC (Kutcher, n.d.). In addition, when mental health is spoken about generally as referring to an aspect of health, it is often misunderstood as mental illness. For these reasons, it is important that clarity be provided regarding mental health and its related terminology (Kutcher, n.d.).

To bring nuance into how occupational therapy practitioners understand and speak about trauma, the language we use about mental health is critical. Stanley Kutcher has developed a pyramid-shaped model of mental health literacy that denotes four categories of mental health: (1) no distress, problem, or disorder; (2) mental distress; (3) mental health problem; and (4) mental disorder (Kutcher, n.d.). The first category, "no distress, problem, or disorder," is on the bottom level of the pyramid. For someone who has experienced trauma, being located in this category is exemplified by the person's ability to function meaningfully and successfully in their daily occupations, including sex and intimacy.

The next level up the pyramid is ***mental distress,*** which refers to transient experiences that cause a person's stress levels to rise over a duration of time; the person is able to reconcile and work through what is causing stress to rise, resulting in a return to its baseline level (Kutcher, n.d.). People who have experienced trauma may experience mental distress temporarily if they are reminded of their trauma or are triggered (e.g., initial nervousness when meeting a new and potentially intimate partner for the first time, concerns about how to communicate boundaries in new relationships). Although the trigger may cause distress, people experiencing mental distress are able to draw on their mental, physical, spiritual, and other capacities to work through this temporary state (Kutcher, n.d.). For example, they may use breathing techniques to ground themselves in the present moment or use sensory strategies, such as a firm hug from their partner and verbal assurance that they are safe in the present moment.

The third category, ***mental health problem,*** involves an event or events that have a greater effect on a person's occupations or functioning; the person may need professional intervention. Generally speaking, a mental health problem may affect sex and intimacy to a greater degree of severity than mental distress. A person who has experienced trauma may find it challenging to be emotionally or physically intimate in their relationship, given that sex and intimacy are often present. Or, perhaps an occupational therapy practitioner who has personally experienced trauma is constantly triggered while working with clients who also have experienced trauma, thereby affecting the practitioner's presence with the client. Professional support in these contexts may mean seeking out a trauma-informed therapist or counselor, an occupational therapy practitioner, or other service providers. Often, with the support of professionals, a person who is experiencing a mental health problem is provided with strategies and supports aimed at improving their participation and success with their occupations (Kutcher, n.d.).

The fourth category, at the top of the mental health pyramid, refers to ***mental disorders,*** sometimes known as "mental illnesses," a term covered in great detail in the *Diagnostic and Statistical Manual of Mental Disorders* (5th ed.; *DSM–5;* American Psychiatric Association [APA], 2013). ***Mental illnesses*** are mental disorders diagnosed by a mental health professional, such as a psychiatrist or psychologist. People who have experienced trauma may be diagnosed with common mental disorders including depression, anxiety, or PTSD (Kutchner, n.d.), all of which can affect sex and intimacy occupations.

The mental health literacy model does not denote a hierarchical trajectory for individual mental health (Kutchner, n.d.). Instead, it may be helpful as a means to understand the relationship between a client's trauma and their sex and intimacy occupations, which is often fluid. As occupational therapy practitioners, our insights about someone who has experienced trauma ideally comes from a thorough understanding and analysis of their occupations and environments as well as through conversations with the client.

Diagnosis of Trauma

The clinical diagnosis of PTSD in the *DSM–5* is no longer clustered within Anxiety Disorders but within Trauma- and Stressor-Related Disorders (APA, 2013). Compared with the *DSM–IV* (4th ed.; APA, 1994), which required three symptoms, the *DSM–5* requires four symptoms for a diagnosis of PTSD:

1. Intrusive thoughts and repeated memories, dreams, or flashbacks
2. Avoidance of reminders of the trauma
3. Negative thoughts and feelings
4. Arousal reactive symptoms.

The diagnosis requires symptoms for at least 1 month and being exposed to or directly witnessing the traumatic event or events, learning about trauma affecting a loved one, or being exposed to the details of the traumatic event. Such information must be received directly and not through a third party, such as a media outlet (APA, 2013).

It is crucial to recognize the criteria for PTSD to ensure proper service provision and necessary referrals. As previously mentioned, the occupational therapy practitioner must view trauma beyond the formal diagnosis. Not all levels of stress meet this clinical diagnosis. Yet, life events require the practitioner's attention specifically when addressing issues related to sexuality. Sexual violence, abuse, harassment, difficulties with intimacy, racism, genderism, sexualization, or asexualization are traumatic experiences that potentiate into symptomology that, in turn, may affect the client's well-being and occupational performance.

SAMHSA (2014) defined ***traumatic adverse experiences*** as

> [i]ndividual trauma [resulting] from an event, series of events, or set of circumstances that is experienced by an individual as physically or emotionally harmful or life threatening and that has lasting adverse effects on the individual's functioning and mental, physical, social, emotional, or spiritual well-being. (p. 7)

Given the impact of traumatic adverse experiences on functioning, it is critical for practitioners to explore a client's meaningful participation in sexuality and intimacy occupations.

Types of Trauma

Trauma occurs in many forms. This section describes acute stress, complex trauma, intergenerational trauma, and cultural trauma. People experiencing complex and intergenerational trauma may express emotional dysregulation, musculoskeletal problems, challenges with sensory perception and self-regulation, self-care skills, and cognitive deficits (Gorman & Hatkevich, 2016). Cultural trauma involves various types of harm based on collective experiences and also has implications for individual expression of intimacy and sexuality. Physical distance, emotional withdrawal, freeze, and aggressive behaviors resulting from trauma can affect the ability to engage in intimate relationships and sex. The effects of toxic stress can also lead to challenging behaviors for clients of occupational therapy practitioners.

Acute Stress

Although trauma can have a significant effect on occupation, so can acute stress. There are parallels between the clinical diagnosis of PTSD and ***acute stress disorder*** (ASD), which is a disabling psychological condition occurring immediately after an adverse physiological reaction to physical, psychological, or emotional stimuli or experiences; symptoms do not last more than 1 month (American Psychological Association, 2023). An example are the reactions people may experience after a motor vehicle accident or a fall. A person may experience fear, physiological changes, and emotional distress for a period of time, causing them to alter and adapt their behavior. Perhaps they avoid activities related to the incident for a short period of time. They eventually return to their typical behavior, however.

Although the event may have been traumatic, the onset and duration of the symptoms differ from PTSD. The symptoms of ASD are briefer in duration and do not exceed a 1-month period. Similar to the cascading effects of PTSD, the symptoms of ASD can interfere with overall functioning. Although most people will have an immediate recovery from ASD, for others, symptoms may persist. In this case, continuation of symptoms longer than 1 month may result in a diagnosis of PTSD.

Both disorders deserve attention, given their association with reduced health and well-being. Indeed, clients who have experienced acute stress may still require support and intervention to enhance their quality of life, even if they do not meet diagnostic criteria. Therefore, occupational therapy practitioners should identify additional methods to detect dysfunction.

Complex Trauma

Continued long-term exposure to traumatic events affects a person at various biopsychosocial levels. Although ***complex trauma*** is not recognized in the *DSM–V*, the term describes "exposure to multiple traumatic events, often of an invasive, interpersonal nature, and the wide-ranging, long-term impact of this exposure" (National Child Traumatic Stress Network, 2016, p. 2). Repeated trauma can lead to various deficits affecting function, and exposure to trauma during childhood can have detrimental effects on neurodevelopment and psychosocial well-being. Hence, performance in various aspects related to sexuality are hampered.

Meaningful and positive sexual experiences or the establishment of relationships could be challenging. For example, emotional dysregulation can challenge the ability to connect with others intimately and sexually.

Secondary to complex trauma can be triggers related to touch and sexual activity as the result of heightened stress and physical reactions. For example, a person might contract their pelvic muscles as a bracing protective response to touch or the anticipation of penetration. They are likely to subsequently experience increased pain during penetration or mentally check out to avoid feeling the pain. To this end, occupational therapy practitioners must be able to identify the signs of complex trauma and the maladaptive responses a client may present while receiving services.

Intergenerational Trauma

Intergenerational trauma is a type of trauma that affects generations of a specific group of people and does not require direct experience of a traumatic event (Gibbs & Harley, 2021). Although offspring may not have experienced a trauma firsthand, the trauma directly affects the children and future generations. Epigenetics and child-rearing practices—both nature and nurture—may influence the intergenerational transference of trauma (Kellermann, 2013). The projections of trauma symptoms to offspring can affect their development and psychosocial well-being (Schechter et al., 2011). Hence, posttraumatic stress hampers performance of basic ADLs, IADLs, and social participation of descendants through generations.

For example, in the United States, Black American adults may experience some of the highest rates of posttraumatic stress (Sibrava et al., 2019). Such trauma is tethered to a painful past of enslavement, colonization, and racial discrimination. Enslavers sexually assaulted enslaved women while their enslaved husbands were made to watch, and that trauma continues to affect the relational bond in Black families today. Moreover, murder, torture, and separation of families not only fill stories passed between generations but are interwoven through the DNA of the descendants. Gene expression can change secondary to people's lived experiences, affecting how descendants cope and engage with the surrounding world. For example, stress hormone levels may be altered as a result of intergenerational trauma. Bowers and Yehuda's (2016) study revealed that the epigenetics—these changes in gene expression—can affect a descendant's ability to handle stress secondary to altered levels of cortisol in descendants, leading to other health issues, such as insulin resistance and hypertension.

The Black American history of slavery and racism may lead to victimization syndrome (Lawrence et al., 2009). The "victim" may be more likely to receive forms of abuse such as physical, mental, and sexual abuse from other individuals, including romantic partners. This self-perception may be viewed as a form of survival; however, viewing oneself as a victim can lead to unhealthy relationship dynamics, including mistrust in others, codependent behavior, or low sexual self-advocacy.

Cultural Trauma

Cultural trauma is defined as collective experiences involving physical or psychological injury, emotional stress, emotional damage ancillary to discrimination, and historic marginalization (National Network to End Domestic Violence, 2017). Unfortunately, the history of racism, discrimination, and violence against various groups has continued into present day. Many marginalized communities, including people with disabilities as well as racial, ethnic, religious, and LGBTQIA+[1] communities, have experienced collective trauma. For example, today's constant exposure to violence affecting the Black American community is a contributing factor to that collective trauma. Although the media shares heartbreaking stories of racial violence, it fails to discuss the long-term effects of Black people's witnessing, through media outlets, the maltreatment and harm to other Black bodies. Occupational therapy practitioners must acknowledge the impact of cultural trauma on the provision of care as well as the implications related to intimacy, sexual identity, and sexuality.

Another factor pertaining to sexuality is interracial relationships. The partnership between people from different racial and ethnic groups has a tainted history of violent backlash in the United States. Interracial marriages did not become legalized until 1967, yet even now, the effects of racism impede on the establishment of partnerships and intimate relationships as the result of societal beliefs and discrimination. And people who are interracial, like those in other underrepresented groups, may experience trauma in the form of racism, discrimination, and confusion around self-identity (i.e., societal pressures to choose one ethnicity despite being multiethnic), which can affect their ability to establish partnerships and engage in social interactions.

Sexualization and Objectification

When people receive attention based on physical characteristics, self-expression, or gender, the result may be challenges with intimacy or viewing oneself as a sexual being. These challenges may be the outcome of aligning a negative connotation with sexual objectification. ***Sexualization***—that is, having a heightened awareness of sexuality or developing a correlation between having physical characteristics and being sexual (Merriam-Webster, n.d.-b)—prioritizes physical attributes or desirability over any of a person's other character traits, such as intelligence, strength, or humor, thus leading to a singular view of that person as only a sexual entity.

[1] The term *LGBTQIA+* communities refers to the diverse and unique communities formed by lesbian, gay, bisexual, transgender, queer, intersex, asexual, and additional sexual and gender minoritized people. As greater awareness, social acceptance, and safety improve for these individuals and communities, new terms may emerge as language evolves to describe identities that exist outside of societal recognition and acceptance.

Objectification, defined as treating someone like an object or dehumanizing them (Merriam-Webster, n.d.-a), may involve appearance-based perceptions that result in negative stereotypes and assumptions. For example, viewing someone as hypersexualized because of their physique may lead to the presumption that they lack moral character. The recipient may feel shame (body shaming) or judgment from others. They may avoid sexual encounters or flirtation from others so as not to confirm the perception of being overly sexual. These reactions can lead to mental health disorders, such as body dysmorphia, eating disorders, and depression. In addition, sexualization can lead to presumptions of being open to casual intercourse, which may increase the risk of sexual assault (Kellie et al., 2019).

Society, Culture, and Gender Roles Related to Trauma

Societal, cultural, and gender roles that prioritize one group over another (e.g., men viewed as superior to women, heterosexual people as superior to gay people) influences the prevalence of trauma, leaving those who are marginalized to feel inferior and more susceptible to toxic stress. In addition, traditional roles, cultural norms, and expectations may affect people's perceived ability to protect themselves when experiencing relationship violence. Women, for example, are twice as likely as men to develop PTSD after a traumatic event (American Psychological Association, 2017).

Trauma disproportionality affects people who are LGBTQIA+. The collective trauma experienced by the LGBTQIA+ community stems from violent attacks; fear of social rejection; and prejudice embodied in homophobia, queerphobia, transantagonism,[2] and ***genderism,*** which is the belief that gender is binary and no other forms of gender exist beyond the two rigid forms (i.e., man and woman) perpetuated by cisgender people (Neumann et al., 2021). Cisnormative society and systems feed and justify discrimination, violence, transphobia, and transantagonism. Chronic stress and traumatic experiences—large and small—greatly affect the health and well-being of a community. To this end, many LGBTQIA+ people can benefit from support in the form of mental health services.

The seeking of services in itself can lead to another level of trauma, perhaps deterring use of care. For example, Gender Identity Dysphoria is a clinical diagnosis identified in the *DSM–5*. Not all transgender people experience ***gender dysphoria*** (discomfort and dissatisfaction with the gender assigned at birth), yet those seeking medical services may require the diagnosis to access care. Transgender,[3]

---

[2] *Transantagonism* refers to hostility or discrimination toward transgender people. Transantagonism focuses on the harm and trauma inflicted on transgender people as opposed to a claim that people "fear" transgender people (i.e., "transphobia"). Claims of fear or panic have historically been used to justify violence against LGBTQIA+ people.

[3] *Transgender* describes people whose gender identity differs from the sex assigned to them at birth.

gender-nonconforming,[4] and gender-diverse[5] people also experience the repeated trauma of being ***misgendered,*** which is having one's gender incorrectly identified by others. They may also be bullied in their communities and by society at large, resulting in hypervigilance, chronic stress, and perpetually feeling unsafe. Although mental health services are necessary, finding a service provider with the proper knowledge and experience, and who perhaps identifies as an ally, may be a challenge.

Unfortunately, LGBTQIA+ people report disproportionately high rates of suicidal ideation and suicide attempts as a result of the significant trauma and violence inflicted on them from the cisnormative society and institutions with which they interact. According to Joseph Christian Ungco, chair of the Network for LGBTQIA+ Concerns in Occupational Therapy,

> simply being LGBTQIA+ isn't the cause of high rates of mental illness in our communities; it's the constant, everyday dealing with homophobia, transantagonism, cisnormativity, heteronormativity, and all the ways society tells us we don't belong and are not valued that creates the conditions for chronic stress and mental illness. We need to understand that so we can more effectively reduce trauma and create conditions that uplift LGBTQIA+ joy and thriving. (Ungco, personal communication, April, 24, 2021)

Sexual Violence

Sexual violence greatly contributes to trauma. It is broadly defined as a nonconsensual act of violence using sex and sexuality as the weapon (Rape, Abuse & Incest National Network [RAINN], n.d.). Under the umbrella of sexual violence are sexual harassment, sexual abuse, and sexual assault.

Sexual harassment is unwanted sexual attention, such as physical touch, jokes, online or digital content, or emotional attention. Homophobia, transphobia, or queerphobia can manifest as sexual harassment or pose further threats as abuse or assault. ***Sexual abuse*** is when the person committing sexual harm of any kind is in the position of leadership or authority, such as someone's manager/supervisor, teacher, family elder, or religious leader. ***Sexual assault*** is unwanted and nonconsensual sexual contact, and it is commonly known in legal terms as rape (RAINN, n.d.). Implications for sexuality and intimacy include challenges forming intimate relationships, damage to a person's self-concept as a sexual being, and sexual dysfunction (Hall & Hall, 2011).

---

[4] *Gender nonconforming* is an umbrella term that describes people who do not follow gender stereotypes or who broaden ideas of gender expression or gender identity.

[5] *Gender-diverse* refers to people whose gender identity and/or gender expression differ from the cultural norms prescribed for people in a particular context, time, and place. The term includes those who exist beyond the male–female binary, and it may be less stigmatizing than the term *gender noncomforming*.

Victim Blaming

Victim blaming, a phenomenon that commonly occurs with sexual violence, refers to the ways in which people and society attribute the reason for the victim's sexual harm to the victim's behavioral or moral choices (Canadian Resource Centre for Victims of Crime [CRCVC], 2009). Examples of victim blaming include those relating to the choice of the victim to consume alcohol and therefore place themselves in a "vulnerable" position to be assaulted, their choice of clothing, or their presence at a certain event or choice to be alone with the person who harmed them.

Victim blaming can further amplify trauma because it inherently places the burden of blame on the person who was sexually harmed rather than the person who did the harming (CRCVC, 2009). Implications for sexuality and intimacy include feelings of self-blame, guilt, and shame, all of which potentially affect not only the healing process but also desire, arousal, or sexual pleasure.

Rape Culture

Another facet that can contribute to trauma is ***rape culture,*** commonly defined as a set of beliefs that give implied or explicit social permission to objectify or inflict violence toward marginalized people, typically women and minorities (Harding, 2015; Olfman, 2009). Examples of rape culture include the forms of advertising that objectify and stereotype already marginalized people; the violence and degradation seen in portrayals of sexual relationships in the media; and the ways in which women are often morally judged for the ways in which they choose to dress and behave, which can lead to victim blaming in relation to sexual violence (Olfman, 2009).

Rape culture fosters domestic and intimate partner violence. For example, an estimated 1 in 4 women and 1 in 10 men experience sexual violence, physical violence, or stalking by an intimate partner during their lifetime with consequences that include fear for one's safety, PTSD symptoms, injury, or needing victim services (National Coalition Against Domestic Violence, 2020). Implications for sexuality and intimacy include internalizing messages of sexual objectification, which can affect one's self-concept of sexuality and potentially autonomy and pleasure during sex and intimacy.

Purity Culture

Purity culture, as it is in known in many faith-based communities, is a set of values or beliefs that pertain to preserving the virginity, honor, and reputation of a girl or woman—and her family—through a set of commonly agreed on actions and beliefs by a certain community (Klein, 2019). Although being empowered to abstain from sex as an individual values-based decision is an example of being sex positive, purity culture's morally hindered messaging can lead to shame around sex by attempting to control a person's behaviors.

For example, purity culture overemphasizes the dangers and sinfulness of sex before marriage using fear-based approaches; associates dress, behavior, and conduct with moral frameworks of a woman's reputation and honor; and reduces sex to a physical act. It subordinates a woman's desire and pleasure to that of her male partner. The implications of purity culture messaging on sexuality include future dissatisfaction with sex, sexual dysfunction, rape culture, and shame related to receiving pleasure (Klein, 2019).

Slut Shaming and Blaming

In addition to purity culture, other forms of sexual trauma can have a great effect on sexuality and sexual self-view. A concept known as ***slut shaming and blaming*** is a form of bullying in which girls are targeted either in person or on social media and are bullied through degradation or humiliation for their sexuality. A form of this bullying is ***body shaming,*** when people (especially girls) are ridiculed for the way they look, the way they dress, and their presumed level of sexual activity.

The National Women's Law Center (2019) conducted a study in Washington, DC, schools and found that Black girls, especially curvier students, were disproportionately targeted. The message sent to girls in these situations reinforces that they must change their behaviors to avoid "distracting" their male classmates—or to avoid being sexually harassed. The implications for sexuality can include discomfort with one's own sexuality, sexual feelings, or body image. What could be more confusing to one's sexual self-view and body image than the experience of being praised or flattered for one's curvy hips but also harassed and made to feel unsafe because of the same curvy hips? For occupational therapy practitioners providing TIC, it is critical to explore with clients the impact of body shaming on self-worth and sexual identity.

Unplanned Pregnancy

Teens and young adults can also experience trauma as a result of unplanned pregnancy and the consequential decision making that may ensue. The experience of being pregnant itself, as well as the response of one's family, community, medical system, and partner, has the potential to be traumatic. In addition to pregnancy, the contraction of or risk of contracting sexually transmitted infections (STIs) may lead to various forms of trauma. For example, someone may experience hypervigilance and anxiety toward intimate occupations as a result of having contracted an STI, or they may experience shame toward their sexuality, leading to difficulty with seeking professional support and services.

Vicarious Trauma

Occupational therapy practitioners themselves are not immune from experiencing trauma as a result of working with clients who have experienced sexual trauma. Known as *vicarious trauma* among service providers and others in the realm of the helping professions (Pearlman & Saakvitne, 1995), this phenomenon, sometimes called "compassion fatigue," is generally associated with the "cost" of caring for others (Figley, 1982). Other terms used for compassion fatigue are *secondary traumatic stress* (American Counseling Association, n.d.) and *secondary victimization* (Figley, 1982). It is believed that professionals working with trauma survivors experience vicarious trauma because of the work they do.

Vicarious trauma is the emotional residue of exposure that professionals have from working with people as they hear their trauma stories and become witnesses to the pain, fear, and terror that trauma survivors have endured. Despite being clinicians dedicated to providing services to others, occupational therapy practitioners are still human and have their own experiences of trauma. They may experience triggers while engaging with clients who share their traumatic stories. For practitioners, implications for sexuality and intimacy include regression and revisiting their own trauma that has affected their personal relationships and interactions. In addition, hearing traumatic stories could possibly invoke a stress response, even if the practitioner has no history of trauma, and result in difficulties with intimate and sexual relationships.

It is important not to confuse vicarious trauma with "burnout." *Burnout* is generally something that happens over time. As it builds, a change, such as time off or a new and sometimes different job, can take care of burnout or improve it. Vicarious trauma, however, is a state of tension and preoccupation with the stories or trauma experiences described by clients (American Counseling Association, n.d.).

From Trauma Informed to Actionable

The ACE research was the catalyst highlighting the need for a values-oriented approach to address the needs of those who experience traumatic events (Leitch, 2017). As a result, TIC emerged, pivoting the pathological view of trauma to emphasizing respect and empathy for the people experiencing it. Applying the principles of TIC involves the four approaches of (1) realizing, (2) recognizing, (3) responding, and (4) resisting retraumatization described earlier in this chapter's "Being Trauma Informed" section (SAMHSA, 2014).

As occupational therapy practitioners, being trauma responsive and implementing a strengths-based approach aligns with the profession's scope of practice. TIC can lead to unintended consequences, such as labeling the person with their trauma (Leitch, 2017). The approach suggests moving from "What's wrong with you?" to "What happened to you?" Being responsive goes further because it recommends exploration of "How can I help you?" and identification of client-centered goals.

Although it is crucial to be trauma informed, occupational therapy practitioners must take actionable steps to address the effects of trauma on quality of life and occupational participation. Hence, ***ACTION-from-trauma*** provides a framework emphasizing a holistic approach that goes beyond talk therapy:

- *A*cknowledge and be *A*ware of trauma;
- *C*reate growth from trauma;

- *T*each neuroeducation and steps toward growth;
- Address *I*ntergenerational factors;
- Identify strategies to change policies and provide opportunities within *O*rganizations and systems to avoid retraumatization; and
- Set the stage for a call to action, recognizing that *N*ow is the time to take *ACTION* to create growth from trauma (Gibbs & Harley, 2021).

Before introducing these concepts of a trauma-responsive approach, however, it is crucial that practitioners assess their own readiness to do so using self-assessment tools, such as the Practitioner Readiness for Trauma Care Checklist (Cook et al., 2014). This step is key before assessing clients and families because practitioners can be triggered by personal experiences, be susceptible to vicarious trauma, and may require additional skills training.

Assessment

Both qualitative and quantitative assessment measures should be part of the evaluation process to initiate occupational therapy services, and the occupational therapist should use TIC approaches regardless of whether there is a known history of trauma. Although targeted TIC strategies are critical when discussing highly sensitive topics such as sex and intimacy, even if sexual and intimate occupations are not explicitly discussed at evaluation, many "routine" aspects of occupational therapy practice may be considered intimate and carry risk of retraumatization. For example, clients who have experienced forms of sexual trauma may be triggered by routine occupational therapy assessments for undressing, bathing, and grooming. This makes it essential for occupational therapy practitioners in all settings to embed TIC precautions into their practices (for in-depth content, see *Trauma, Occupation, and Participation: Foundations and Population Considerations in Occupational Therapy* [Lynch et al., 2021]).

During the intake interview and history taking, avoid requesting specific details of known traumatic events. For example, an intake dialogue might look like this:

> THERAPIST: Have you experienced trauma? *[If yes, people often will offer more explanation without being prompted to do so.]*

> THERAPIST: Okay, thanks for sharing that. *[Then add one of the following.]*
> 1. Do you feel comfortable elaborating a little bit? It is completely okay if you don't. Remember: You're the one driving this session.
>
>   *Or*
> 2. Just know those traumatic experiences can play a role in sexual activity and intimacy. Trauma might come up during our treatments, and it's okay to talk about it or not—you're the one in control of that conversation.

In addition, the *Occupational Therapy Practice Framework: Domain and Process* (4th ed.; *OTPF–4;* American Occupational Therapy Association [AOTA], 2020) emphasizes the importance of initiating services with proper evaluation. When recognizing trauma, occupational therapy practitioners must have procedures in place to ensure proper treatment intervention. This response may include interprofessional referrals and identification of proper assessment tools to develop a treatment plan. In addition to the Occupational Therapy Profile (AOTA, 2021), the assessment tools listed in Exhibit 9.1 can assist in determining the needs of clients who are seeking occupational therapy services and as part of the continuation of care. Before implementing such tools, the occupational therapist must explain to the client or caregiver how they intend to use the information generated (Gibbs & Harley, 2021).

The tools in Exhibit 9.1 are screening tools and assessments to identify possible trauma experienced by the client. For example, the ACE Questionnaire (Maciel & Basto-Pereira, 2020) could reveal a client history of childhood sexual abuse. This knowledge is vital in providing interventions that will allow the client to feel safe and mitigate triggers. For example, the occupational therapy practitioner should offer self-performed activities rather than impose sensory input or touch. When determining methods to support a client in exploring their sexuality or intimacy, understanding the client's ACE history allows for client-centered goal setting, treatment planning, and proper referrals, as needed.

Although some screening or assessment outcomes may reveal sexuality or intimacy-based trauma, the occupational therapist should consider additional outcomes, because the information gained can provide indirect factors to consider when supporting sexual and intimate occupations. For example, an occupational therapy practitioner working with a veteran with a high reactivity score on the PTSD symptom scale could explore this further and discover specific triggers for the client, such as hearing loud noises, being in crowds, sitting with their back to an entryway, and experiencing unexpected touch. With this understanding, the practitioner can work with the client on self-advocating with intimate partners on choosing date activities that reduce risk of those triggers (e.g., having meals earlier than the "dinner rush," reserving tables that face the entryway) as well as strategies to support the client if triggered (e.g., grounding strategies if the client is triggered during a fireworks display, approaching from where the client can see the partner before touching them).

EXHIBIT 9.1

Tools for Assessing Trauma and Client Area of Strength

- Adverse Childhood Experiences Questionnaire (ACE Questionnaire; Felitti et al., 1988)
- Child and Adolescent Needs and Strengths (CANS; Lyons et al., 1999)
- Childhood Trauma Questionnaire (CTQ; Bernstein et al., 1994)
- Clinician-Administered PTSD Scale (CAPS; Weathers et al., 2018)
- Mini-Mental State Examination (MMSE; Folstein et al., 1975)
- Pediatric Emotional Distress Scale (PEDS; Saylor et al., 1999)
- PTSD Symptom Scale Interview for *DSM–5* (PSSI-5; Foa et al., 2018)

Although discovering the client's history of trauma is beneficial, it is also important to unveil the client's strengths to properly implement a trauma-responsive approach. Tools like the VIA Character Strengths Survey (Peterson & Seligman, 2004) highlight character strengths that, in partnership with the client, the occupational therapy practitioner can target in treatment planning. If a client has a strength in creativity, perhaps a suggested strategy for intimacy would be a couple's date in which the pair creates sensual artwork together rather than focus on challenges, such as intimate touch.

Screening and assessment tools help initiate occupational therapy service provision, but they are just one aspect to consider. After assessment, the findings must be included in a formal evaluation to determine a proper plan of care. The case example provided in this chapter maps out what an occupational therapy plan of care may look like. As with any evaluation, the occupational therapist must implement the occupational therapy process based on the *OTPF–4* (AOTA, 2020). The process may require use of additional assessment measures, such as observation. In the presence of trauma related to sexuality or intimacy, the occupational therapy practitioner must recognize how the use of those assessment measures may retraumatize clients and therefore must incorporate strategies that allow the client to feel safe. And to ensure trust with the client, it is vital that the practitioner fully explain the use and purpose of the evaluation.

In addition, throughout the evaluation process, the occupational therapy practitioner must consider the environment, such as where the practitioner is positioned in relation to the client, as well as how the practitioner presents—for example, their dress, smells (e.g., perfumes, colognes), and tone of voice. Many things could be triggers. Clinicians also need to carefully consider any tactile or somatosensory interventions. Although environmental modifications may help prevent certain triggers from arising, others can be inadvertent, requiring the practitioner to support the client in the moment. For example, the practitioner may guide a client experiencing a trigger through diaphragmatic breathing techniques and to self-regulate with simple cues to identify what the client can touch, see, and hear in the moment. Finally, the clinician needs to remember that client permission is essential with any presented plan of care.

Goal Writing

After a holistic quantitative and qualitative evaluation with the client, the occupational therapist's clinical reasoning will lead to identification of trauma-related functional effects on a client's meaningful participation in sex and intimacy. Because trauma often results in certain triggered responses during sex and intimacy occupations, the therapist may believe it is important to focus solely on the mitigation of these triggers (i.e., stress, anxiety, fight–flight response) as a means to attain greater participation with sex and intimacy occupations. However, it is important to distinguish between short-term performance component goals of mitigating trauma responses and long-term goals for enthusiastic, pleasurable, and meaningful sex and intimacy (Exhibit 9.2). Case Example 9.1 describes an occupational therapy intervention with a client experiencing challenges with sex and intimacy.

EXHIBIT 9.2
Short- and Long-Term Goals for a Client Who Is Triggered During Physical Contact With a Partner

Trauma-informed care for sex and intimacy occupations includes short-term and long-term goals.

- *Short-term goals* (mitigate trauma responses and address the performance component of feeling grounded, safe, and self-regulated during sex and intimacy)
  - Client will participate in sexual intimacy, without aversion, 80% of the time during daily somatic, sensory-based self-regulation strategies (e.g., diaphragmatic breathing, deep pressure hugs, firm strokes), alone and with their partner.
  - Client will independently complete 5 minutes of visualization (e.g., sexual fantasizing) techniques to enhance their sexual desire before being intimate with their partner.
- *Long-term goals* (address desired outcome of enthusiastic, pleasurable, and meaningful sex and intimacy)
  - Client will report an increase in satisfaction with sexual activity, as measured by the Occupational Performance Inventory of Sexuality and Intimacy (Walker et al., 2020).
  - Client will self-report greater physiological arousal and pleasure during intimacy.

CASE EXAMPLE 9.1. KAREEM: TRAUMA AND CHALLENGES WITH SEX AND INTIMACY

Kareem is a 25-year-old African American transgender man with a history of trauma secondary to childhood physical and sexual abuse. He currently receives outpatient psychotherapy. His psychologist referred him to occupational therapy to further explore intervention strategies to address his challenges with sex and intimacy needs since the recent ending of his relationship with his partner. Kareem reported that the relationship ended secondary to personal factors and challenges with intimacy. Currently, he lives with roommates and attends a graduate program.

In a screening performed during his initial occupational therapy visit, Kareem expressed challenges with organizing his day-to-day activities and properly caring for himself (i.e., ADLs, IADLs, social participation). He shared his challenges with time management, lack of motivation, and distrust of others. As a result, his intimate relationships often end abruptly. Kareem also shared discomfort with sexual intercourse secondary to anxiety and being unable to relax or be present to experience pleasure.

(Continued)

CASE EXAMPLE 9.1. KAREEM: TRAUMA AND CHALLENGES WITH SEX AND INTIMACY *(Cont.)*

Although Kareem feels accepted by those in his circle, he is often anxious and nervous when interacting with his classmates and meeting new people. At times, he feels embarrassed secondary to poor personal hygiene, which is typically a result of having to rush to get to class lectures on time. Most important, he finds himself uncomfortable with the microaggressions and biases presented by his classmates and instructors. Kareem has a hard time determining whether the behaviors are from their discomfort with his gender identity or race. He feels powerless and lonely. When asked about his goals for therapy, Kareem shared that he wants to experience greater self-confidence and readiness for intimate relationships and, ultimately, feelings of pleasure during sex and intimacy.

The occupational therapist considered the following occupational therapy treatment approaches based on the *OTPF–4*.

Occupations

- *ADLs:* Establish habits, routines, and strategies to address numbness and a sense of not caring. Improve hygiene and self-care to enhance sexual intimacy.
- *Health management:* Identify goals and resources to address health and well-being and needed support systems to enhance confidence in building intimate relationships and to decrease anxiety during dating and sexual encounters.
- *Education/work:*
    - Focus on establishing healthy relationships and setting boundaries.
    - Provide strategies for self-advocacy and long-term goal development (e.g., educational or career goals).
- *Play/leisure:*
    - Implement sensory-based approaches to address self-regulation.
    - Provide strategies for self-advocacy during interaction with others (e.g., explore sensory preferences for pleasure during sexual play).
    - Identify sensory input that can be noxious versus arousing (e.g., feathers, soft touch, firm touch, erogenous zones).
- *Social participation:*
    - Support and provide approaches to address occupational justice.
    - Provide strategies for self-advocacy during interaction with others.
    - Identify methods for trust building.

(Continued)

CASE EXAMPLE 9.1. KAREEM: TRAUMA AND CHALLENGES WITH SEX AND INTIMACY *(Cont.)*

- Practice making small talk with new people.
- Identify potential conversation starters with classmates the client is interested in connecting with.

Contexts

- *Environmental factors:*
  - Identify supports and resources to address the client's environmental needs (e.g., safe travel routes or transportation services).
  - Help the client identify environmental triggers, such as sight, smells, or sounds.
  - Recognize the practitioner's opportunity to suggest training for faculty, staff, students, and members of campus organizations.
- *Personal factors:* Identify preferences and resources to allow the client to feel comfortable during sexual intercourse (e.g., lighting, surrounding smells, music preferences).

Performance skills

Social interaction skills: Apply trauma-responsive approaches to address social skills and engagement in posttrauma exposure.

Client factors

- *Body structures/body functions:*
  - Address chronic stress with self-regulation and mindfulness techniques.
  - Decrease hypersensitivity with sensory–motor strategies to decrease hyperresponsiveness during sexual and intimate acts.
- *Values, beliefs, and spirituality:*
  - Acknowledge the client's values, beliefs, and spiritual practices.
  - Gain clinician knowledge and training on antiracism and antigenderism approaches to care.

Intervention: An Opportunity to Show Occupational Therapy's Unique Value: Beyond Trauma-Informed Care

In this chapter, our review of the sensory and physical implications for trauma make it clear that intervention must address the autonomic nervous system response. The ACTION-from-trauma approach recommends activities including grounding, check-ins, body mapping, and contextual sensory investigation (Gibbs & Harley, 2021).

Grounding Activities

Grounding techniques assist clients in reorienting to the "here and now" and feeling safe; the technique can decrease dissociative symptoms and bring awareness to the present moment. Although the following activities may prepare the client by addressing the flight–fight reactions secondary to trauma, occupational therapy practitioners must ensure that they use an occupation-based approach. Hence, connecting such activities to treatment goals is vital:

- Breathwork, including diaphragmatic breathing, can allow the client to decrease hyperarousal in preparation for sexual activity.
- Guided meditation can allow the client to visualize intimate experiences and gain a sense of comfort with exploring sensuality.

Checking In

Within the session or throughout the day, depending on the setting in which the occupational therapy practitioner works, be intentional about checking in with the client. ***Checking in*** brings attention to the client's personal needs and recognizes the need for personal breaks and sensory strategies. This method also can serve as modeling for the client to learn how to better engage with partners by checking in with their feelings and experiences during sexual interactions.

Body Mapping

Body mapping is a technique that involves having the client shift their attention to the various regions of their body to acknowledge sensations, discomfort, and any areas of tension. Body mapping can assist in releasing internal stressors and help the client develop a personal awareness of their body's function to help them recognize desires and personal needs.

Contextual Sensory Investigation

In a ***contextual sensory investigation,*** the occupational therapy practitioner considers possible changes to the various settings that the client frequents (e.g., lighting, flooring, seating, smells) to decrease unnecessary stimuli. It is also crucial to address positioning and placement, such as allowing the client to see the exits and anyone entering into the space to avoid triggers. Recommendations can guide the client to setting up their environment and context to support their desires and avoid triggering stimuli. An example is teaching them methods to share with their partner about what they prefer and what they want to avoid during intimacy and sex.

Summary

Trauma is unique to the individual and requires a multidimensional approach to treatment. Clients do not require an official diagnosis of PTSD to require care and support related to adverse life experiences. It is necessary that occupational therapy practitioners acknowledge the existence of trauma and its effect on health, well-being, and sexuality. To decrease the likelihood of retraumatization for the client, practitioners must participate in TIC practices and implicit bias training, use antiracism practices, and prioritize cultural humility.

The ACTION-from-trauma approach is a good fit for occupational therapy. It is, however, crucial to incorporate interprofessional collaboration to allow for best practice when addressing the complexities of trauma. It is also essential to maintain boundaries around the occupational therapy process and scope of practice as well as to work collaboratively with other disciplines to enhance positive outcomes.

Finally, occupational therapy practitioners must recognize their own personal triggers. Conversations around trauma-related content can be intense as clients share traumatic experiences. To this end, it is crucial that every practitioner engage in self-care and self-reflection. This practice may provide solace for burnout and compassion fatigue.

Varleisha D. Gibbs, PhD, OTD, OTR/L, ASDCS, FAOTA, is an occupational therapist and expert, author, and speaker with more than 20 years of experience working with children and adolescents diagnosed with autism spectrum disorder, sensory processing disorders, and neurological disorders. She is the vice president of practice engagement and capacity building at the American Occupational Therapy Association. Gibbs is the former scientific programs officer at the American Occupational Therapy Foundation. She also served as the inaugural chair and director of Delaware's first master's programs in occupational therapy at Wesley College in Dover, Delaware, where she was a tenured associate professor. Prior to joining Wesley, she was the director of the doctoral programs in occupational therapy at the University of the Sciences in Philadelphia.

Sameera Qureshi, MS, OTR, has spent her career at the intersections of sexual and mental health with minority populations. She is the founder of Olive Tree Consulting LLC and works with clients internationally. Her expertise includes trauma-informed care, sexuality education, and culturally responsive approaches.

References

American Counseling Association. (n.d.). *Vicarious trauma* (Fact sheet no. 9). https://www.counseling.org/docs/default-source/trauma-disaster/fact-sheet-9---vicarious-trauma.pdf?sfvrsn=f0f03a27_5

American Occupational Therapy Association. (2020). Occupational therapy practice framework: Domain and process (4th ed.). *American Journal of Occupational Therapy, 74*(Suppl. 2), 7412410010. https://doi.org/10.5014/ajot.2020.74S2001

American Occupational Therapy Association. (2021). Improve your documentation and quality of care with AOTA's updated occupational profile template. *American Journal of Occupational Therapy, 75*(Suppl. 2), 7502420010. https://doi.org/10.5014/ajot.2021.752001

American Psychiatric Association. (1994). *Diagnostic and statistical manual of mental disorders* (4th ed.).

American Psychiatric Association. (2013). *Diagnostic and statistical manual of mental disorders* (5th ed.). https://doi.org/10.1176/appi.books.9780890425596

American Psychological Association. (2017, August). *Facts about women and trauma.* https://www.apa.org/advocacy/interpersonal-violence/women-trauma

American Psychological Association. (2023). Acute stress disorder. In *APA dictionary of psychology.* https://dictionary.apa.org/acute-stress-disorder

Barbash, E. (2017, March 13). Different types of trauma: Small "t" versus large "T." *Psychology Today.* https://www.psychologytoday.com/us/blog/trauma-and-hope/201703/different-types-trauma-small-t-versus-large-t

Bernstein, D. P., Fink, L., Handelsman, L., & Foote, J. (1994). *Childhood Trauma Questionnaire (CTQ)* [Database record]. APA PsycTests. https://doi.org/10.1037/t02080-000

Bowers, M. E., & Yehuda, R. (2016). Intergenerational transmission of stress in humans. *Neuropsychopharmacology, 41,* 232–244. https://doi.org/10.1038/npp.2015.247

Canadian Resource Centre for Victims of Crime. (2009, August). *Victim blaming.* https://crcvc.ca/docs/victim_blaming.pdf

Center for Substance Abuse Treatment. (2014). *Trauma-informed care in behavioral health services* (Report No. [SMA] 14-4816). Substance Abuse and Mental Health Services Administration. https://www.ncbi.nlm.nih.gov/books/NBK207201

Centers for Disease Control and Prevention. (2021). *About the CDC–Kaiser ACE Study.* https://www.cdc.gov/violenceprevention/aces/about.html

Cook, J. M., & Newman, E., The New Haven Trauma Competency Group. (2014). A consensus statement on trauma mental health: The New Haven Competency Conference process and major findings. *Psychological Trauma: Theory, Research, Practice, and Policy, 6,* 300–307. https://doi.org/10.1037/a0036747

Felitti, V. J., Anda, R. F., Nordenberg, D., Williamson, D. F., Spitz, A. M., Edwards, V., . . . Marks, J. S. (1998). Relationship of childhood abuse and household dysfunction to many of the leading causes of death in adults: The Adverse Childhood Experiences (ACE) Study. *American Journal of Preventive Medicine, 14,* 245–258. https://doi.org/10.1016/S0749-3797(98)00017-8

Figley, C. R. (1982). Catastrophes—An overview of family reactions. In C. R. Figley & H. I. McCubbin (Eds.), *Stress and the family, Volume I: Coping with catastrophes* (pp. 3–20). Brunner/Mazel.

Foa, E., Asnaani, S., Zang, Y., Capaldi, S., & Yeh, R. (2018). Psychometrics of the Child PTSD Symptom Scale for *DSM–5* for trauma-exposed children and adolescents. *Journal of Clinical Child and Adolescent Psychology, 47,* 38–46. https://doi.org/10.1080/15374416.2017.1350962

Folstein, M. F., Folstein, S. E., & McHugh, P. R. (1975). "Mini-Mental State": A practical method for grading the cognitive state of patients for the clinician. *Journal of Psychiatric Research, 12,* 189–198. https://doi.org/10.1016/0022-3956(75)90026-6

Gibbs, V. D., & Harley, N. (2021). *Trauma treatment in action: Over 85 activities to move clients toward healing, growth and improved functioning.* PESI Publishing.

Gorman, K. W., & Hatkevich, B. A. (2016). Role of occupational therapy in combating human trafficking. *American Journal of Occupational Therapy, 70,* 7006360010. https://doi.org/10.5014/ajot.2016.016782

Hall, M., & Hall, J. (2011). The long-term effects of childhood sexual abuse: Counseling implications. *Vistas Online.* https://www.counseling.org/docs/disaster-and-trauma_sexual-abuse/long-term-effects-of-childhood-sexual-abuse.pdf?sfvrsn=2
Harding, K. (2015). *Asking for it: The alarming rise of rape culture—And what we can do it about it.* Da Capo Press.
Kellermann, N. P. F. (2013). Epigenetic transmission of Holocaust trauma: Can nightmares be inherited? *Israel Journal of Psychiatry and Related Sciences, 50,* 33–39.
Kellie, D. J., Blake, K. R., & Brooks, R. C. (2019). What drives female objectification? An investigation of appearance-based interpersonal perceptions and the objectification of women. *PloS ONE, 14,* e0221388. https://doi.org/10.1371/journal.pone.0221388
Klein, L. K. (2019). *Pure: Inside the evangelical movement that shamed a generation of young women and how I broke free.* Atria.
Krugers, H. J., Lucassen, P., Karst, H., & Joëls, M. (2010). Chronic stress effects on hippocampal structure and synaptic function: Relevance for depression and normalization by anti-glucocorticoid treatment. *Frontiers in Synaptic Neuroscience, 2,* 24. https://doi.org/10.3389/fnsyn.2010.00024
Kutcher, S. (n.d.). *Mental health 101* [PowerPoint slides]. MentalHealthLiteracy.org. http://teenmentalhealth.org/schoolmhl/wp-content/uploads/2018/02/mental-health-101.pdf
Lawrence, E., Yoon, J., Langer, A., & Ro, E. (2009). Is psychological aggression as detrimental as physical aggression? The independent effects of psychological aggression on depression and anxiety symptoms. *Violence and Victims, 24,* 20. https://doi.org/10.1891/0886-6708.24.1.20
Leitch, L. (2017). Action steps using ACEs and trauma-informed care: A resilience model. *Health and Justice, 5,* 5. https://doi.org/10.1186/s40352-017-0050-5
Lynch, A., Aschraft, A., & Tekell, L. (Eds.). (2021). *Trauma, occupation, and participation: Foundations and population considerations in occupational therapy.* AOTA Press.
Lyons, J. S., Griffin, E., Fazio, M., & Lyons, M. B. (1999). *Child and adolescent needs and strengths: An information integration tool for children and adolescents with mental health challenges (CANS-MH), Manual.* Buddin Praed Foundation.
Maciel, L., & Basto-Pereira, M. (2020). Child sexual abuse: The detrimental impact of its specific features. *Child Indicators Research, 13,* 2117–2133. https://doi.org/10.1007/s12187-020-09730-y
Maren, S. (2014). Fear of the unexpected: Hippocampus mediates novelty-induced return of extinguished fear in rats. *Neurobiology of Learning and Memory, 108,* 88–95. https://doi.org/10.1016/j.nlm.2013.06.004
Merriam-Webster. (n.d.-a). Objectification. In *Merriam-Webster.com dictionary.* https://www.merriam-webster.com/dictionary/objectification
Merriam-Webster. (n.d.-b). Sexualize. In *Merriam-Webster.com dictionary.* https://www.merriam-webster.com/dictionary/sexualize#medicalDictionary
National Child Traumatic Stress Network. (2016). *Complex trauma in urban African-American children, youth, and families.* National Center for Child Traumatic Stress.
National Coalition Against Domestic Violence. (2020). *Domestic violence.* https://assets.speakcdn.com/assets/2497/domestic_violence-2020080709350855.pdf?1596811079991
National Network to End Domestic Violence. (2017). *Understanding the importance of trauma-informed care.* https://nnedv.org/spotlight_on/understanding-importance-trauma-informed-care
National Women's Law Center. (2019, April 24). *Dress coded: Black girls, bodies, and bias in D.C. schools.* https://nwlc.org/resource/dresscoded/

Neumann, N., Neu, D., & Ungco, J. C. (2021). Addressing LGBTQIA+ trauma: Your role and your responsibility. In A. Lynch, R. Ashcraft, & L. Tekell (Eds.), *Trauma, occupation, and participation: Foundations and population considerations in occupational therapy* (pp. 195–221). AOTA Press.

Olfman, S. (2009). The sexualization of childhood: Growing older younger, growing younger older. In S. Olfman (Ed), *The sexualization of childhood* (p. 5). Praeger.

Pearlman, L. A., & Saakvitne, K. W. (1995). *Trauma and the therapist: Countertransference and vicarious traumatization in psychotherapy with incest survivors.* W. W. Norton & Co.

Pelt, A. C. (2011). *Glucocorticoids: Effects, action mechanisms, and therapeutic uses.* Nova Science.

Perryman, K., Blisard, P., & Moss, R. (2019). Using creative arts in trauma therapy: The neuroscience of healing. *Journal of Mental Health Counseling, 41,* 80–94. https://psycnet.apa.org/doi/10.17744/mehc.41.1.07

Peterson, C., & Seligman, M. E. P. (2004). *Character strengths and virtues: A handbook and classification.* Oxford University Press and American Psychological Association.

Rape, Abuse & Incest National Network. (n.d.). *Types of sexual violence.* https://www.rainn.org/types-sexual-violence

Saylor, C. F., Swenson, C. C., Reynolds, S. S., & Taylor, M. (1999). The Pediatric Emotional Distress Scale: A brief screening measure for young children exposed to traumatic events. *Journal of Clinical Child Psychology, 28,* 70–81. https://doi.org/10.1207/s15374424jccp2801_6

Schechter, D. S., Willheim, E., McCaw, J., Turner, J. B., Myers, M. M., & Zeanah, C. H. (2011). The relationship of violent fathers, posttraumatically stressed mothers and symptomatic children in a preschool-age inner-city pediatrics clinic sample. *Journal of Interpersonal Violence, 26,* 3699–3719. https://doi.org/10.1177/0886260511403747

Sibrava, N. J., Bjornsson, A. S., Pérez Benítez, A., Moitra, E., Weisberg, R. B., & Keller, M. B. (2019). Posttraumatic stress disorder in African American and Latinx adults: Clinical course and the role of racial and ethnic discrimination. *American Psychologist, 74,* 101–116. https://doi.org/10.1037/amp0000339

Substance Abuse and Mental Health Services Administration. (2014). *SAMHSA's concept of trauma and guidance for a trauma-informed approach* (HHS Publication No. [SMA] 14-4884). https://store.samhsa.gov/sites/default/files/d7/priv/sma14-4884.pdf

van der Kolk, B. A. (2014). *The body keeps the score: Brain, mind, and body in the healing of trauma.* Viking.

Walker, B., Otte, K., LeMond, K., Hess, P., Kaizer, K., Faulkner, T., & Christy, D. (2020). Developmental of the Occupational Performance Inventory of Sexuality and Intimacy (OPISI): Phase one. *The Open Journal of Occupational Therapy, 8*(2). https://doi.org/10.15453/2168-6408.1694

Weathers, F. W., Bovin, M. J., Lee, D. J., Sloan, D. M., Schnurr, P. P., Kaloupek, D. G., . . . Marx, B. P. (2018). The Clinician-Administered PTSD Scale for *DSM–5* (CAPS–5): Development and initial psychometric evaluation in military veterans. *Psychological Assessment, 30,* 383–395. https://doi.org/10.1037/pas0000486

World Health Organization. (2020, June 17). *Mental health: Strengthening our response.* https://www.who.int/news-room/fact-sheets/detail/mental-health-strengthening-our-response

Yehuda, R., Lehrner, A. M. Y., & Rosenbaum, T. Y. (2015). PTSD and sexual dysfunction in men and women. *Journal of Sexual Medicine, 12,* 1107–1119. https://doi.org/10.1111/jsm.12856

10

Personal Narratives of Sex, Intimacy, and Meaning

Kathryn Ellis, *OTD, OTR/L, AASECT–SC;* **Joseph Christian Ungco,** *OTD, OTR/L;* **Dev Neu,** *MS, OTR/L;* **Emily Sherman,** *OTD, OTR/L, DPAM;* **Sakshi Tickoo,** *BOTh, CPC;* **Andrew Gurza; Jenn Soros,** *PhD, OTR/L;* **Karla D. Reese,** *DHSc, OTR/L; and* **M. Nicole Horsley,** *PhD*

> *The erotic is a measure between the beginnings of our sense of self and the chaos of our strongest feelings. It is an internal sense of satisfaction to which, once we have experienced it, we know we can aspire. For having experienced the fullness of this depth of feeling and recognizing its power, in honor and self-respect we can require no less of ourselves.*
>
> —Audre Lorde, "Uses of the Erotic: The Erotic as Power" (1984, as cited in brown, 2019, pp. 28–29)

This chapter provides five personal narratives for readers to reflect on the erotic human experience. These vignettes offer a deep and raw look at sexual and intimate experiences and the meaning made possible through them. Readers may experience a sense of voyeurism as they read. They are encouraged to be thoughtful and respectful of these stories by considering the following:

- Using as a guide the Audre Lorde (1984) quote that opens this chapter, reflect on how each narrator experiences an "internal sense of satisfaction" and how that influences the narrators' aspirations for future experiences.
- How can you relate to each of these stories? When have you had an experience or feelings similar to those of the narrators?
- Are you uncomfortable while reading these accounts? Why or why not? See Chapter 3, "Guided Self-Reflection of Self as a Sexual Being," and Chapter 4, "Sexuality, Bias, and Impact: Preventing Clinician Harm," for guidance.
- What can you learn about how occupation, context, and meaning interact from these narratives and how this interaction affects the narrators' participation in sexual and intimate occupations?

Each narrative is structured according to the narrators' preferences. The power of narrative has been used throughout occupational therapy's history to support practitioners in understanding meaning and experiences of people as occupational beings. Any one of these narratives could be a story that a client would share with an occupational therapy practitioner. A client could share the details of a traumatic event, their experience having sex for the first time, or why they find emotional intimacy so important.

Occupational therapy practitioners are equipped with the skills to use interviews and personal stories to obtain occupational information, build an understanding of the client as a whole person, develop the occupational profile, and identify client-centered intervention (American Occupational Therapy Association [AOTA], 2020). Practitioners also employ therapeutic use of self to establish trust and facilitate conversations with clients. Formal and informal conversations provide information about the client. As you read the narratives, think about whether you would be learning this kind of information when conducting an occupational profile in your current practice. In addition, consider how the narratives might influence the questions you would ask your client, the goals you and the client would co-create, and the interventions you would choose.

Each narrative is preceded by a content warning. The reader is given agency as to whether to read the story or to read them using some of the strategies in Chapter 3, "Guided Self-Reflection of Self as a Sexual Being," to help navigate discomfort.

"The Great Pleasure"

By Dev Neu, OTR/L

(*Content warning:* hostility toward LGBTQIA+[1] people, sexual assault and trauma, child abuse, physical assault)

The following is an interview with Dev Neu with questions from Kathryn Ellis and Joseph Christian Ungco.

Dev Neu (DN): There are so many life experiences that queer folks or gender-diverse folks experience that we don't talk about. In my journey as an occupational therapy advocate and educator on topics related to sexuality, LGBTQIA+ issues, and social justice, I share negative things that happen to me that I've come to view as normal. However, sometimes people are shocked. Their initial reaction is, "Wow, I'm so sorry that happened to you," and I realize most people have no idea about experiences shared among queer folks.

[1] The term *LGBTQIA+* refers to the diverse and unique communities formed by lesbian, gay, bisexual, transgender, queer, intersex, asexual, and additional sexual and gender minoritized people. As greater awareness, social acceptance, and safety improve for these individuals and communities, new terms may emerge as language evolves to describe identities that exist outside of societal recognition and acceptance.

Coming Out

DN: The pressure of "coming out" in high school, like actual heaviness, truly impacted my mental wellness. The only thing I knew about coming out was what I saw in the movies: this monumental, big, dramatic thing, and the kid gets kicked out of the house. I never saw images or references to queer joy; I only saw the negative consequences that will inevitably accompany and follow you throughout life when you finally express yourself authentically as a queer person.

Now, I don't use the phrase "coming out"; I use the phrase "letting others in." The reason I don't like "coming out" is because it implies people expect some information. Saying "letting others in" shifts the power to the person to decide when they want to let others share their experience and who they want to do this with. In high school, I didn't have that thought process, so back then, I was "coming out." If you are a straight cisgender person, you do not have to think about telling people you're straight. A straight 17-year-old kid doesn't feel pressure to make a Facebook status update that says, "In case you were wondering, I am, in fact, straight. I know you've been assuming it for years." It frustrates me that coming out was something I felt I needed to do and that queer people still need to do this now.

Prior to coming out, I had a lot of concerns that weighed on me. And I was only 17! I thought, "What if I tell my mom and she tells me to leave?" I decided to pack a bag before coming out. I had to think about what friend's house I was going to. What if I was not safe? What if it got physical? I had to have a disaster plan to deal with the impact of living my truth. It is a crappy experience, and I was doing this on top of all of the pressures of becoming an emerging adult.

Sex Education

DN: Kids at 17 are trying to figure a lot out: fitting in, dating, sex, and getting into college. Oh, and God forbid you had not had sex prior to going to college. You're supposed to learn about sex and safe sex practices as teenagers, but you're not going raise your hand and say to the sex ed teacher,

> That's great that you have all of these pictures of penises and vaginas, but what about anuses? What does it look like for an anus and penis to be together versus a vagina and a penis? What do you do with a vagina when there isn't a penis?

If you're "out" and asking these questions, the teacher probably doesn't know the answer, and you're setting yourself up for social ridicule. If you're not out, then you can't ask those questions.

The outcome of all of this is that queer folks don't have the education we need to engage in the things that bring us pleasure. I want cisgender straight folks to recognize that this is what it can feel like for some folks. I hope readers can empathize because, as health care providers, they will be working with marginalized folks, and that marginalization affects their quality of life, how they engage in occupation, and how they will respond to your clinical decisions and therapeutic use of self.

Fitting In and Sexual Assault

DN: How I engage in intimate activities and sexual activities is influenced significantly by my identities. I have to really think critically about whether I am safe. Am I am a target? Do I need to code switch (i.e., reflect the majority culture)?

Kathryn Ellis (KE): *Do you think having to think about how people will react to you and whether or not you're safe creates stress around sexuality and being sexual? Does this negativity creep into the bedroom?*
DN: Oh, yes. There's the normal stress: "Okay, I'm a 16-year-old, I've got these funny feelings going on with my body, and I want to get jiggy with someone." Add being naked with someone and then add how we figure out how to do things. Most folks my age were meeting other queer people on dating apps, which can be sketchy. Remember: Learning how to navigate safe dating was not included in our sex ed classes. Then you have the stress of maybe not finding a partner or needing to be discreet to get and hide sex toys. Sex was something I just wanted to get done. There was so much anxiety wrapped up in it that it really wasn't special. Additionally, within the queer community, there's a lot of pressure for sex to be this pornographic, perfect thing. But I thought, "No one told me how to do this, I don't know where to go to get experience in doing it, and I don't know who to ask because of fear of either ridicule or harm from straight people and looking inexperienced from queer people."

I just wanted to check it off the list. I was really worried about my first time. I was worried about not knowing what I was doing or having something embarrassing happen like passing gas. So, I wanted my first time to be with a random person, not someone I felt was really special. Maybe this isn't unique to queerness, but I'm not sure since so much of our sex ed wasn't accessible to me. It's even harder to answer the question about whether sex was—or is—stressful, because when I was younger, I experienced sexual assault. The idea of sex wasn't something I could even think about for a long time. For me, trauma was another complexity I had to navigate when having sex for the first time.

Joseph Christian Ungco (JCU): *Could you talk a bit more about why you thought your only option was to just "get it done" regarding losing your virginity?*
DN: Having sex for the first time was something I just had to "get done," probably as a result of existing in heteronormativity. Everyone was doing it, but I wasn't. I always felt a lot of extra pressure to be "normal" and do what was expected of me to avoid abuse, which was something I had experienced as a child. Additionally, I didn't have tons of opportunities to fit into what I perceived as a normal childhood or adolescence, and I thought having sex was one of the ways I could. I really wanted to have sex before I went to college, which was something everyone talked about or wanted to do.

I had partners and boyfriends in high school, but because of the trauma associated with my sexual assault, it was harder for my body to respond when I was sexual with them. The person who assaulted me was someone I was close with, so when I was younger and hooking up with my boyfriends, I couldn't do it with someone I was close with. My body did not respond in a sexual way. Instead, my body would shake, and I'd have panic attacks. So, most of my early sexual experiences were with people I didn't know or care about. I thought I just needed to get it done, so I could say I am like everyone else. At the time, I thought it would be therapeutic for me to have a sexual encounter that wasn't emotional, so I could see that I could do it. I liked the idea of having control over sex. After my assault, I thought sex could be a way I could reclaim my body, making a choice to be sexual versus during my assault, when I had no choice.

JCU: *And was it therapeutic?*
DN: No. The first time I had sex, I had a sense of relief. Just like, "Okay, this is done and over with, and my body did it." I remember the person kept asking me if I was okay. I can only imagine my face. It was probably panicked. Having sex didn't achieve what I wanted it to, but it did start me on the path of the real work and the real therapy that got me to where I needed to be in my body today.

Sexual Assault and Trauma

JCU: *I'm kind of curious whether you ever feel like a statistic.*
DN: My sexual assault 100% feels like a statistic. It was done by someone I knew who was close with my parents. I didn't report the assault, and that person knew I wouldn't be able to. Nothing was ever done about it. I didn't get justice, and that person had the reinforcement that the behavior was something they could do. I fall into the category of "acquaintance rape": underreported and unresolved.

This year, someone tried to run me over with their car for wearing a rainbow jacket while going on a run. I tried to report it to the police; the police told me that my jacket was provocative. That was crushing because that's what I told myself when I was assaulted—that it was my fault, and I brought it on. This caused a lot more trauma than just the incident itself. It validated the storyline I told myself when I was younger—that I must have been provocative—and that was infuriating. I was doing something normal. I was working out, and this happened to me.

To think I can't exist in this world while doing normal mundane things without being harmed is incredibly distressing. With the sexual assault, I was doing something normal. I was at my parents' friend's house. One of my parents left to go do something, and that's when it happened. He was a family friend—it was somewhat normal to be at this person's house. This situation isn't unique to queerness, but the queerness added an extra layer because even when you're screaming, it feels like people hear you even less. In terms of the statistics, what's missing is the whole sentence. The statistic is the period at the end of the sentence, and you're missing the whole sentence of what led up to that.

Queer Joy

KE: *There is so much focus on pathology, statistics, and caution in sexual health research. Let's talk about what's missing. What's the other side? What is queer joy?*

DN: When I think about queer joy, I think of the first time I went to a coffee shop in Rochester, New York. It's a coffee shop for queer people, and I remember the sheer joy I experienced to just be around openly queer people. I saw all sorts of people: young gay people, people gender bending, cool people wearing nail polish. And I remember thinking, "Okay, I can come here and do work, and it's fine. I can be who I am and feel like there is a place for me." The joy didn't come from social interaction or confirmed acceptance. No one spoke to me. I just got to exist and enjoy a sense of normalcy. It was a space where those parts of me that had always been tokenized, different, or just didn't make me feel special could just exist. I loved the coffee shop for that. It was my first experience with a dedicated queer space; I'd had no idea something like that existed.

The Great Pleasure

JCU: *I'll use the phrase "the great pleasure." When was your first experience with pleasure?*
DN: I don't think the first great pleasure happened until I acknowledged my gender diversity. Before I acknowledged my gender, sex felt different identifying "as a man," because I didn't feel like all of me was present. I had to hide parts of myself during sex to be masculine. I did things I thought my partners would expect when having sex with a man. I didn't have *great* pleasure from sex until I found great pleasure being in my body, as it is. After I arrived at a place of "any and all of Dev is fine," I started really being able to enjoy myself during sex. Sex had felt good because there are just things biologically that feel good, but I didn't feel good in my body doing it, but once I allowed the expansiveness of my gender diversity to show during sex, then I began to truly feel great pleasure.

I don't think I would have arrived here without my current partner. He has helped me arrive at a place of comfort where I could actually work through the last couple of things that previous trauma caused. Only recently have I felt whole; I didn't realize I wasn't until I arrived here. When I think about the question asked earlier about whether the one-night stands achieved what I wanted to, in terms of physical sensation in my body, they did. But sensation in my soul? I didn't gain any wholeness from them. If anything, they made me feel more empty. When I was holding true to myself, that's when the big pleasure happened.

KE: *Can you give us a concrete example of something you had to work through during sex to have sex true to yourself?*
DN: What was holding me back was this need to be overly masculine during sex. Especially with men who have sex with men, there's a lot of pressure on masculinity. But for me, I've never been a fully masculine person. I enjoy gender bending, I enjoy being masculine and feminine. I am a feminine person, and I love those parts of me, but during sex, I was having to think a lot about not being feminine, and it was very cerebral. During sex, I thought about having to sound a certain way and position my body in a certain way to be more masculine and not feminine. It was exhausting and took away from the pleasure. I was held back from truly letting loose in my body and actually having true sensation, spiritually and also physically.

But when I felt I could be intimately connected to my partners and respected for who I was, I could make the sounds I made, move my body in a way that prioritized pleasure over masculinity, then it really allowed me to deeply connect to myself, my body, and also my partner. I don't think of masculinity or femininity in terms of sex anymore. For me, it's a deeper process with those things stripped away. Now I wouldn't be with a partner where masculine or feminine matters during sex.

KE: *I wonder if some readers will wonder, "Do I think too much, if at all, about masculinity or femininity during sex"?*
DN: I had some self-awareness. I remember during sex thinking, "Should I be thinking this much? I'm really in my head about this." This habit or defense mechanism that's just ingrained in you is like code switching[2] during sex. For people who have to code switch throughout their daily life, code switching during sex is probably subconscious and secondhand.

JCU: *How would you describe yourself as a sexual and intimate being today?*
DN: It is queer joy. It is freeing. My partner and I have navigated what is enjoyable for us, but I don't have expectations for myself or how I look. When I say "freeing," I mean that sex and intimacy for me is something I feel I can do now without having to be self-conscious and cerebral about it. I can just be with someone, and that's magical in itself. There aren't expectations to be, sound, or perform a certain way. It's freeing to me that sex can look different each time, and we can do what feels right in the moment. It's the great pleasure. It's magical.

Desire

KE: *What are the occupations you do by yourself or with your partner that get you in the mood or build your want for sex?*

JCU: *I think what she's trying to ask is, "What turns you on, Dev?!"*
DN: Oh! One thing that was incredibly helpful was pleasure mapping. It helped me work out some of the trauma because I had so much agency and choice while exploring where in my body I feel pleasure. Spending time touching myself or being touched by my partner and identifying what felt good, what felt really good, what didn't feel good, and what specific technique felt good was really helpful. It was freeing to learn about my body and to view parts of my body as sexual not because socially I'm told this area of my body is sexual, but because I actually felt

[2] *Code switching* is a sociolinguistic concept referring to when a person switches between two or more languages or language varieties in a single conversation or interaction. This term can also be used to describe ways that marginalized communities may adapt their presentation, mannerisms, and behavior to appeal to dominant social groups. In this case, Dev is referring to having a habit of code switching for personal safety as an LGBTQIA+ person who has repeatedly dealt with a hostile cisnormative and heteronormative environment. They describe code switching to act as and present themselves as a "man" during sex because of concerns for their safety and acceptance during sexual interactions.

pleasure in it when touched. It was equally as empowering to think, "Okay, I don't like that sort of touch, or I don't like to be touched in that area."

Pleasure mapping also taught me how my anxiety affects how I feel pleasure and the differences I feel depending on whether I am anxious or not. When I am anxious or coming off of being really anxious, I have found that my body is hypersensitive. So, stimulation that would have been usually very pleasurable, for example nipple stimulation, varies dramatically from the stimulation I crave when I am more anxious. When I am anxious, I don't want light touch, I want a really firm, heavy, weighted, squeezy touch.

KE: *You're really describing a very somatic way to build desire.*
DN: Totally. It seems obvious because sex can be so touch based, but were any of us taught how to explore this for ourselves and communicate this to a partner? Turn the lights off, have no noise, so you can really home in on the tactile sensory. It can be really powerful.

KE: *No one teaches this. Not in literature, in movies, and certainly not in sex ed. But I always think whenever there are experiences of trauma or even reinforcing messages that critique our bodies and what we do with them, I think it can be very hard for people to then go and feel pleasure in their bodies. We think we should just feel sex in our penis and our vagina. Yet, our body is the biggest sex organ, so exploring all of the body, all the parts, especially the parts that get critiqued or experience the trauma, having those parts be the vessel of pleasure can be really powerful.*
DN: Retweet.

Occupational Therapy's Role in Queer Sex Ed

JCU: *How could sex ed serve queer people better, and how do occupational therapy practitioners fit into this? I know straight people also have to figure out their pleasure, but I'd imagine there are more models presented for them to figure this out.*
DN: We have to look at the roots of the problem and the background many practitioners have: They are likely to be sexual people and probably went through really crappy sex ed. Sex ed is such an important class, and we suck at it. I wish it could include concepts such as different relationship dynamics or even just what healthy relationships look like. Or that you don't have to be gay to talk about anal play. I was left googling this information. At least the straight folks got pictures showing how to put a penis in a vagina. I knew nothing about hygiene related to anal play or preexposure prophylaxis. This lack of information adds to the anxiety queer people have about not being sure how things work or how to protect themselves.

KE: *Right, like even the basic hygiene of "pee after sex." This is a common message I heard throughout my life in school from doctors, family, friends. And pee after sex is hygiene education for heterosexual people. This is the bare minimum, but at least we straight people got it.*

JCU: *I also feel like I heard the message of peeing after sex, but because of the lack of representation in sexual health conversations, it left me wondering, "Oh, is that what I need to do?" My assumption was it's for heterosexual sex, so part of my brain was already off. The sex talked about in my sex ed class wasn't the sex I was having. To "pee after sex" was never directly explained to me or people who have the sex I have, so I questioned whether this hygiene instruction was even for me.*

When I would be sexual with someone who seemed to know more than me, I'd follow their lead and do what they suggested without really exploring or figuring out what I liked. I never knew there were infinite ways sex could look and pleasure could be felt, so I assumed there was one way it was supposed to be, and I fit myself into that.

Lack of sex ed is really problematic both in accessing pleasure and putting people at risk. But some occupational therapy practitioners might read this and say, "Well, I'm not a health education teacher, so I don't need to worry about this." What are your thoughts on that?

DN: Look, as occupational therapy practitioners, we claim a lot of things as within our scope of practice, and then we don't always deliver on things we'd prefer not to discuss. We, as humans, even people who are asexual and aromantic, are sexual and intimate beings in some capacity.[3] Practitioners need to have the knowledge to address sexuality with clients, even when it's far outside of their comfort zone.

When you signed up to be a health care provider, you committed to treat all people equally, so you don't get to start excluding queer people because you are uncomfortable. I am tasked with presenting information relative to straightness to straight folks all the time, but I'm not a sex educator. This is the expectation of me as an occupational therapist working with heteronormative populations. I have to do heterosexual things all day. If you have a queer person come in, then you have to do queer stuff for your 30-minute treatment session. That's okay. Look, if I can play straight for a few hours, you can play queer for a few hours with your clients.

Occupational Therapy Application

1. In the first portion of the narrative, Dev describes coming out, sex education, and experiences with sexual assault. As you reflect on Dev's story, consider the *Occupational Therapy Practice Framework: Domain and Process* (4th ed.; *OTPF–4;* AOTA, 2020) domains of context, occupations, performance patterns, and person factors. How did the social environment shape Dev's occupational experiences around sex and intimacy? How is this reflected in their occupations, performance patterns (i.e., roles and habits), and client factors (e.g., sexual self-view)?

---

[3] Many people who are asexual and/or aromantic may or may not label themselves as "sexual and intimate" beings. Dev's point here is to highlight how sexuality and intimacy are aspects of humanity like any other aspect. Social expectations around sex and intimacy are part of everyone's context, including those who may be excluded from social contexts because they are asexual and/or aromantic. For further definition, please review Chapter 2, "Understanding Sexual Identity."

2. Imagine working with a client who experiences anxiety during sex. Anxiety can often make it difficult for people to focus on pleasurable sensations they are receiving in their body. The occupational therapy practitioner can suggest mindfulness, grounding into the body, and somatic exercises to bring people's awareness back into their body. Sensory-based approaches could be helpful for this client; however, part of their anxiety is rooted in not expressing their self authentically during sex. How could an occupational therapy practitioner downgrade the activity of engaging in sex to help the client express their authentic gender?
3. Dev says, "Look. As practitioners, we claim a lot of things as within our scope of practice, and then we don't always deliver on things we'd prefer not to discuss." What are some areas within a practitioner's scope of practice that you could deliver on better? How can you start improving in that area?

"It's Only Weird if You Make it Weird"

By Emily Sherman, OTD, OTR/L, DPAM

(*Content warning:* description of domineering parental behaviors)

"Another day, another empty referral page," quipped one of my colleagues as the all-too-familiar slap of a manila folder hit my desk. I opened it reflexively, but I already knew what it said: "OT recommended—eval and treat as per protocol." I read what little information I had: age, diagnosis, and a brief intake assessment making broad (and likely inaccurate) recommendations about possible interventions and adaptive equipment. However, nothing—not my years in occupational therapy school, not my months of fieldwork, and certainly not my brief time as a new practitioner—could have prepared me for when my 11 a.m. evaluation appointment arrived that same day.

Andrea was a 26-year-old with a quick wit and even quicker smile. Much to my surprise, she arrived at her first occupational therapy appointment with an older woman, who never met my gaze but who stood up and entered the doors to the outpatient therapy gym before Andrea even had the time to wake her power wheelchair from sleep mode.

Caught off guard, I reluctantly guided our little trio to a therapy mat and table in the far and slightly quieter corner of the gym, my preferred spot for a new evaluation. I introduced myself, asked Andrea and her apparent chaperone to do the same, and gave my occupational therapist elevator speech. I was careful to keep my eyes on Andrea, who unfortunately kept her eyes on the person she introduced as "my shadow." This was Andrea's mother, Alma. To hear them both tell the story, the role of shadow had been Alma's role since Andrea was first diagnosed with a chronic and progressive condition in her late elementary school years. Since then, Alma had assumed the role of 24/7 caregiver—whether Andrea needed this level of care or not.

And so began an unsuccessful battle of wills as I urged Andrea to walk me through a typical day in her life and to tell me her prior and current level of satisfaction and participation in her routine. To my dismay, Alma answered each of my questions and most of my redirections. After minutes that felt like years hearing about *Alma's* routine with Andrea's positioning and pressure relief, BADLs, IADLs, leisure, and community mobility, finally we got to the heart of the issue: "So, *Andrea,* what brings you in today?"

Andrea had recently enrolled in courses at a local community college that would have her spending 3–4 hours away from home and the watchful eye of her mother for 4 days a week. I felt my skin get hot as I realized this was my chance to make Andrea the focus in our work the way she deserved to be. Not trusting my own clinical reasoning and for fear of damaging what seemed like an already delicate rapport, I waited. I instead switched gears to more formal assessments: numeric pain scale, range of motion, manual muscle testing, sensation, coordination, and, finally, her goals. Andrea reported that she wanted to be more independent with managing her new school schedule and workload; wanted to learn how to navigate her power wheelchair on a college campus with small classrooms, narrow hallways, and especially with regard to public restrooms; and learn strategies to use when her fatigue, muscle weakness, or pain got in the way of her paying attention and taking notes in class or doing her homework.

When asked why she was enrolling in classes, Alma answered first: "She wants a degree, so she can get a job and be more independent." I looked at Andrea, but her face was blank with a vague tinge of resignation. When asked what courses and degrees of study interested her, Andrea was not certain yet. "I want to try a few classes and just see what's out there." I then inquired about Andrea's long-term plans for herself. Again, Alma answered, "She doesn't need to think about that. You're the expert; you set the goals and she'll do it." I tried to explain that for the goals to not only be achievable and realistic but also worthwhile, Andrea would need to start the ball rolling. "Well," said Andrea, "it's probably not possible, but I'd really like to be able to live alone one day . . . or with 'my Geoffrey.'"

Before I could follow up, Alma clutched at her chest. "Not again with this!" she exclaimed. When I inquired as to who "my Geoffrey" was, Alma insisted I move on with the evaluation. Andrea deflated—her eyes downcast, her smile gone. And so it was that I had already failed my client. Not knowing what else to do, I went back to my elevator speech. I explained that sex and intimacy are considered BADLs, and perfectly safe to talk about at any point in our sessions. The family resemblance between the two of them was never more apparent than when they both wrinkled their nose at me and fell quiet.

I circled back to her goals. Andrea's response seemed reflexive, "Whatever my mom thinks is safest. I don't care." She was unemotional in her reply, giving every impression that this was the sort of pragmatism the two of them came to embrace in the years since Alma became Andrea's so-called shadow. At the end of the first session, the evaluation was *technically* complete: All necessary areas of documentation were filled out, and all required assessment scores were gathered. However, the most important aspects—the things most important to Andrea—were clearly missing. The mystery of Andrea's Geoffrey would have to be solved in the next session.

However, the next few sessions came and went without any answers. Andrea still made progress. She was learning and applying strategies of energy conservation and work simplification to her daily routine, she began keeping a pain journal to help identify her triggers and remedies, she made daily and weekly schedules for herself to use at school and at home, and she tried a few different mobile arm supports to assist with various school- and home-related tabletop tasks. Once Andrea mastered her first bathroom transfer, a deal was struck with Alma: "If Andrea were to truly prepare for time at school away from home, then it would serve us best to have Andrea and me work in close partnership and collaboration—just the two of us." Alma reluctantly agreed, and I only ever saw her in the waiting room.

It was an otherwise unremarkable day when Andrea arrived at her session with a plan to put all of her new skills and strategies into practice: We would mount her newly acquired mobile arm support to her power wheelchair and perform a community college simulation. Andrea would enter the therapy gym; navigate to and from the ADA[4]-accessible mock bathroom and the various cone-demarcated areas for hallways, classrooms, and a bookstore/restaurant; retrieve and replace all necessary items from her bag and tray table; and participate in various school-related tasks. The activity went off without a hitch! Weeks of Andrea learning to do more for herself were successfully undoing the years of Alma jumping in prematurely. Andrea was learning she no longer needed her mother to do *everything*—or really anything—for her. In fact, there was much she could do for herself. Admittedly, this left more time in the session than I had planned for, so I resorted to my usual backup: "So, what questions do you have for me?"

Andrea paused to think. She asked about setting up her mobile arm support in new configurations—not just to write, type, or eat. She now wanted to learn how to set it up to help hold a game controller when her hands got tired, how to help her style her hair, et cetera. Finally, she asked, "What if I meet someone, and I want to shake their hand?" I helped reconfigure the device, and we tried it out. "What if I want to just *hold* someone's hand?" Again, I reconfigured the device, and we tried it out. "This is perfect!" Andrea beamed, "I just wish this wasn't all I could do." I asked what she meant.

Finally, I would learn about her Geoffrey. They met online 8 months ago playing *League of Legends,* their favorite game. He was a skilled piano player but only played for relatives and close friends (Andrea included), and he studied graphic design at the same community college where she had enrolled. Andrea explained

[4] Americans With Disabilities Act of 1990.

that, from her perspective, she referred to Geoffrey simply as "hers" because she did not have a good noun to place after that.

"Well, he's not my *friend* because we're in love. But he's not my *boyfriend*, because we obviously can't have sex or anything."

"What do you mean by that?" I asked.

She blinked at me. "Am I allowed to talk to you about this? I mean . . . can we really work on this in OT?"

"We can. In OT, we can talk about anything and everything that *occupies* your time. But only if you want to. This is *your* OT session—not mine, not Geoffrey's, and not your mother's."

She let out a laugh that sounded like a sigh. Then the real work started, and as it did, I realized the blatant gap in our plan of care: sex and intimacy. The next several sessions consisted of discussing Andrea's interpersonal relationships, the sociocultural values she was raised to espouse, and her personal beliefs. This included her sexual and romantic life. She said she identified as "something close to heterosexual, but I've never really thought about it—I didn't think I was allowed to!" With Andrea's permission and avid contribution, I amended her goals and our focus in therapy. Her goal to increase her safety and independence during BADLs included not only toileting and grooming, but also sexual activity. Her goals for promoting independence with positioning, pressure relief, skin integrity, energy conservation, and the safe use of adaptive equipment and devices were all explicitly discussed, if not formally rewritten, to include a focus on sex and intimacy.

Conversations ensued about the breadth and depth of her sexual identity and experiences, which, in turn, led to a series of activity analyses. Because of Andrea's specific personal performance capabilities and constraints, I then recommended she use imagination, adaptive devices, and giving direction as a way to be sexual, which for Andrea included thinking about different fantasies of how she wanted to touch Geoffrey, how she wanted Geoffrey to touch her, and what she wanted to watch Geoffrey do to himself. We again performed an activity analysis for each one. For example, I made suggestions on where Geoffrey could commonly stand so that Andrea could reach out for his hand when she wanted to.

As our sessions progressed, Andrea made the transition to community college without much ordeal—a few strategies were needed here and there, and a letter of medical necessity or two was written. But in our last few weeks of working together, sex and intimacy became the last bastion of Andrea's transition to independence. In each session, she would report back with questions on how to troubleshoot various issues, and I would respond matter-of-factly with regard to positioning, optimal body mechanics, adaptive equipment options and uses, communication, and safety. "I'm so used to this being weird! Isn't this weird?" she asked during one of our sessions.[5] To use her own terminology, I first explained that "it's only *weird* if *we* make it weird. If it's not weird to make you independent with going to the bathroom and managing your clothing, then it's not weird to make you independent

[5] Many clients and clinicians report that it "feels weird" or "awkward" to talk about sex in clinical settings. Please see Chapters 3 and 4 for strategies on working through this initial challenge.

with loving Geoffrey." She accepted this logic. However, I was careful not to take this for granted. ("Never forget: the P in PLISSIT [(Annon, 1976)] is for Permission!" I could almost hear my mentor's voice in my head.)

Regardless of her interest at the start of our conversations or at the end of our previous session, I always asked, "So what would you like to work on today?" Sometimes it was about sex and intimacy, sometimes not. Sometimes it was about Geoffrey, sometimes not. I will never forget how startled I felt when Andrea arrived at one of our sessions and announced, "Because of you, I saw my mother cry for the first time!" She was practically gleeful, but I was terrified. Outwardly calm but inwardly thinking about what sort of apology I owed to Alma, I asked what happened. Andrea launched into her story:

> She was upset about something—I honestly don't even remember what anymore. I think it was something about my aunt and the holidays. Anyway, she was getting all worked up, and I was trying to interrupt her, but she wouldn't listen, and so I used my mobile arm support to reach out and touch her arm. I really wasn't thinking about it at the time, I swear, I just wanted to touch her like she does to me when I'm upset. But I guess I've never done that before. Like, *ever*. So, we both just stopped and stared at my hand on top of her hand. And then before I knew it, we were both crying! It was *awesome*!

I never ended up needing that hastily drafted mental apology to Alma. She never came to another session, and to hear Andrea talk about her, Alma certainly did not find all of our occupational therapy session topics to be equally "awesome." I told Andrea she was welcome to bring Alma, or Geoffrey, or anyone else she wanted to our sessions. My only rule was that Andrea remained the priority in our work. She never took me up on that offer to include others in our sessions. But I still made sure to remind her of all of her options and of her power as the head of her own treatment team—whether that was working with me or working with any of the other peer-led or professional resources that myself and a couple of colleagues put together over hurried lunch breaks and outside of work hours after encountering entirely too many clients like Andrea, and none of us feeling equipped to help.

In the end, Andrea embraced the following as her own active and satisfying participation in the act of sex: independently setting up and directing Geoffrey in the setup of sex toys she could use to pleasure herself; instructing Geoffrey in how to digitally stimulate her nipples, clitoris, and labia solo, and/or in tandem with his own masturbation; and lots and lots of hugging, kissing, and cuddling. At the end of our last session, she presented me with a sticker that Geoffrey had designed according to her instructions. In big, bold letters it read: "It's only weird if you make it weird."

Occupational Therapy Application

1. Consider doing an activity analysis on holding someone's hand while seated in a wheelchair. The occupational therapy practitioner assesses range of

motion and watches the movement attempted. Based on the findings, what might be some intervention strategies to advance toward this goal?

Now consider the activity analysis of directing another person to use a sex toy on themself. What would you assess to give you the necessary information to establish goals and intervention?

2. Emily describes her clinical reasoning process throughout working with Andrea. Many occupational therapy practitioners describe internal and interpersonal barriers to providing sexuality- and intimacy-focused occupational therapy, such as the internal barrier of assuming that if a client cannot have penetrative sex, then they are not interested in sexual activities. A common interpersonal barrier is fear that discussing sexual activity in a therapy session is "unprofessional" or "inappropriate."

   What barriers, internal or interpersonal, are described in this case? What tools or strategies does Emily use to effectively meet the client's goals?

"My Martinis, Sexuality, and Mental Health: All With a Twist"

By Sakshi Tickoo, BOTh, CPC

(*Content warning:* internalized ableism, fat phobia, deaths from COVID-19, grief)

I'm a 24-year-old, Kashmiri Hindu Pandit, cisgender, queer woman who has been diagnosed with multiple conditions over 13 years. I have a list of diagnoses. I sincerely believed my body failed to live up to my standards of normal or society's standard of normal. For everyone else around me, my sickness seemed normal based on my diagnosis; they expected it. I was an outcast that made people curious about my *diagnosis,* not about *me.* To others, I wasn't amicable, not smart, not talented, not sexy, just sick.

Initially, I was too young to understand internalized ableism but not young enough not to experience it. I felt alienated in my body. My body limited me, and I hid that. But I wasn't okay. I wasn't physically okay because I couldn't do what I loved. I wasn't mentally okay because I had to act in a calculated way, to pretend. It was exhausting. And I never made friends I could be vulnerable with.

Ableism is horrible. It creates this constant feeling of discomfort that I don't belong; it's unsettling. Instead of feeling like I could reach out for help, I developed unhealthy ways of coping, like being an extremely opinionated and harsh person socially but loathing myself when I returned home. When hiding my pain was no longer an option, I finally came out to my friends and told them about my diagnoses, limitations, and vulnerabilities. I felt that if I had to pretend one more day, I would die. I have had several "coming-outs" since then, but I remember the first time I did so and how liberating it felt. My friends had so many questions about how certain conditions affected my body and what they could do to make me feel better. While some tried to remain close, others kept their distance. Some wanted to know if I'm disabled. In all fairness, I had never given it a thought. Teen me had bigger problems at hand: "How do I get accepted?" Because it feels like I am not.

I was too young to wrap my head around my diagnoses, and they just kept coming: more surgeries, more doctor visits, more pain. Despite investing so many years into my health care, the only diagnosis that shocked my parents was generalized anxiety disorder, moderate depression with borderline OCD [obsessive-compulsive disorder], and an eating disorder. My parents could not fathom that their cheerful 5-year-old who "endured it all" could have depression when she could live an *almost* normal life. But how could this *not* impact my mental health? Not once during my journey has anyone asked me if I feel alienated in my body. Not once has anyone cared to address how I feel emotionally. Not once has anyone asked me if I'm having mental health symptoms. Not once has anyone paid attention to my lack of desirability as a friend, partner, and sexual being. Not once have I been told to acknowledge and embrace my lows. Not once has anyone cared if I adapted the occupations I loved the most. Experiencing pleasure in my body seemed unattainable to me. No one asked me about this, which validated my assumptions that pleasure was not something I could, should, or would feel.

I'm thoroughly disappointed to know that I didn't belong in Indian society because I couldn't participant in "conventional" ways of living. Deviating from traditional norms is not accepted; sharing my identities and struggles was discouraged because everyone was expected to have the same identities and struggles. Sharing my experiences and identities required vulnerability, and it would have been great to have had some practice with sharing my vulnerabilities for when I was seeking romantic relationships.

Having autonomy and being assertive in relationships was uncharted territory for me. I sucked so bad at it! This made it difficult to learn what I want in a partner and make decisions based off of those wants. The same goes for pleasure. Because of the pain I experienced in my body, I needed to explore and learn how I best received pleasure. But I never felt I could do this because I didn't have an autonomous relationship with my body, and experiencing pleasure in a way that was different from what "everyone else did" reinforced how my pleasure was not "conventional."

Mainstream media and entertainment do a horrible job of showing disabilities, illnesses, and sexuality. I remember movie dialogues that covertly meant people with disabilities are flawed and it was okay to assume that people with disabilities and illnesses will have a difficult time finding a partner(s) for themselves. Movies and media portray that being disabled or limited is a benchmark against which people will weigh your value or worthiness of being loved in relationships or marriage. You see fat girls eating chips and being mocked for being fat and reminded that they are not marriage material. How can I forget fairness cream[6] ads

[6] A "fairness cream" is a cosmetic product that claims to "lighten" one's skin tone. Such products are frequently marketed toward darker-skinned individuals, relying on stigma toward being dark skinned and emphasizing White-centered notions of beauty.

and no-hair legs being waxed that made these models look unrealistically beautiful, while I kept wondering why am I brown and gaining weight when my diet was moderated?

I was "informed" that too much exercise or dance meant more blood clots and pain for weeks. I have spent hours debating with myself if it was the recommendations from doctors or my mind that was responsible for making me fat and losing a leisure occupation—dancing—that made me feel beautiful. The occupation of dancing was never modified; the doctors just said, "Don't do it." But dance grounded me and made me feel good about myself. When I stopped, nothing grounded me against the negative messages from the media and pathetic advice from friends. I wondered, "How do I fit into this world as a worthy match? Am I sexy? Am I too fat? Are my stretch marks repulsive? Can I wear dresses? What will be people think of my legs?"

I gave myself a pep talk a few years ago that inspired me to reclaim my identity. Why is "fat" as a term considered derogatory? Why can't I just say I'm fat and move on? I was still living a healthy lifestyle by doing everything in my physical capacity. Reclaiming the words helped me change my narrative. All that had changed was my perception of me and the world I'm living in; this didn't mean I had stopped caring about external validation. But now, I wasn't waiting around to be validated, live up to unrealistic beauty or body standards, and be loved. Am I saying self-love and claiming my identity fixes everything? No. I have felt heartbroken and helpless, changed the narrative, stood up for myself, challenged the norms, failed again, felt heartbroken, and watched the cycle continue. Changing the narrative has been a powerful tool to return to my desired occupations, be it dancing, finding love, wearing dresses that flaunt my curves, or having sex.

During my transition to young adulthood, I thought my body stopped me from experiencing sex the way I wanted to. Then I stopped feeling the desire to have sex or self-pleasure. Was my first guess that my genitals were broken? Yes, absolutely! The idea of having sex did nothing to me. It didn't make my vagina skip a beat like it used to, nor did I have a mini-orgasm when [actor] Chris Evans did a squat. And that's outrageous in my world!

It took a breakup for me to understand that it was not my genitals or my partner that was the problem. It was lower desire and mourning the loss of how I used to feel sexual arousal. At the time, however, it was easier for me to project my irritation at my partner and highlight his inabilities to justify why I didn't desire sex. I mistook low desire for sex as a loss of spark then. I had not considered the domino effect of living with multiple chronic illnesses and the long-lasting impact they had on my body. SSRIs [selective serotonin reuptake inhibitors] were working just fine for my brain, but the medication took away the way I experienced sensations, pleasure, and desire in the conventional ways I was taught. In previous days, when my genitals worked, I could rely consistently on sexual arousal, lubrication, and orgasm. I felt an overwhelming sense of loss and grief at having a body that does not always do what I want it to do.

The sex nerd in me is never at rest, so I explored whether people have similar experiences. Instagram and blogs have been a true blessing. Although others' disabilities differed from mine, our experiences did not. The voices of disabled people taught me more than any institution ever could! I felt heard, validated, and truly represented. Joanne Summers of *Sex Machine Reviews* taught me the benefit of doing something fun or pleasurable despite being in constant pain. Andrew Gurza's[7] tweets are a reminder of how I can challenge internalized ableism on a daily basis and why "clicking nudes" can be therapeutic. Soumita Basu (2018), on the *Skin Stories* blog, said,

> I am writing a story about my life in which I am at the centre, and my disabilities are sketching bits of the background. It is a story of bold moves. It is a story of gentle swaying. It is mine. (Para. 21)

This quote roused me to transform my internal narratives as my liminal spaces change.

These few years of exploration have made me realize how mind and body go hand in hand. Does this mean my genitals are fixed now? Well, actually, they were never broken! However, the way my body and mind attune to each other fluctuates, as do my pleasure needs and practices. Pleasure and pain are two sides of a coin and two essential aspects of the disabled and invisible illness experience. Experiencing pleasure while also being in pain is liberating. Knowing that, despite the limitations, our bodies have the potential of controlling and creating powerful sensations, is an indescribable feeling. I have learned to experience sex beyond penetration, which is probably why I value sex and pleasure so much. Touch, movement, breath, and communication are essential to my sexual life. On the days when I know my body cannot sustain vigorous movements, my sex life does not need to stop.

Having known the effects of my medications and mental health on desire and arousal, I started creating more mindful pleasure practices and daily routines to infuse pleasure throughout my day instead of just during sex. Taking pleasure inspiration from disabled stories around the world, I customized pleasure, ranging from self-care to nurturing. Self care included infusing pleasure into daily tasks. This could mean taking 5 minutes extra in the shower; putting on mascara; or setting intentions, journaling, twerking, or putting on a face mask while I meditate.

Over the past 2 years, my pleasure practices took a 180-degree turn. I lost eight people in 7 months to COVID-19 and cancer, my father being one of them. Grief and trauma have a weird way of staying with you. You may forget about it, but your body remembers.[8] My relationship with pleasure tanked. My capacity to love others romantically was nil. The old strategies didn't work anymore, but to my delight, I knew I wasn't inevitably relegated to just surviving in the status quo. Because of my strong pleasure practice, I had the skill sets to adapt. I just had to think of new strategies to move from surviving to thriving. I added a few tricks in my ever-expanding sexual experience bubble. I learned some fun tantric techniques and

[7] To learn more about Andrew Gurza, visit http://www.andrewgurza.com/ and https://twitter.com/andgurza.

[8] See *The Body Keeps the Score* (van der Kolk, 2015) for more information on healing from trauma using advances in brain science, attachment research, and body awareness.

included them in my pleasure practice to keep myself grounded when my anxiety peaks, while still enhancing the ways I experience pleasure sexually. One of the crucial experiences I live with is not assuming anything about my body, thoughts, or people. This has been a key to my pleasure practices so far: to stay curious and keep learning about my illness, love, pleasure, pain, sex, and life.

Occupational Therapy Application

1. How people experience pleasure is specific and unique to each person. The variety of sexual pleasure is rarely represented in mainstream media, and people rarely have sexual health education that explains this concept. Further, Sakshi shares that not experiencing pleasure the "conventional ways" has made her even more hesitant to explore her pleasure.

   Using a graded approach to work toward the end goal of communicating one's preferences to a partner through building sexual knowledge, an occupational therapy practitioner could consider the following steps:

   a. Provide education on the nuances of the client's pleasure preferences;
   b. Encourage the client to give self-permission to explore the client's body;
   c. Ask the client to practice mindful and curious awareness of sensations without judgment;
   d. Categorize and organize what the client learned from self-exploration; and
   e. Script how to communicate this information to a partner.

   With a classmate, script exactly how you would practice directing the preceding intervention. List some intervention strategies for each step.

2. Activity analyses require the occupational therapy practitioner to consider how the activity demands interact with client factors, performance patterns, and the environment. Sakshi mentions that she is still sexual even on days when her "body cannot sustain vigorous movements." Through activity analysis, practitioners can consider energy conservation strategies; for example, they can suggest changing the pace of movement during oral sex or the depth of thrusting during penetrative sex. Sakshi also mentions integrating pleasure practices into her daily routines to help reinforce her body's capacity to feel pleasure. What are some environmental modifications that could help a similar client navigate pain or build desire?

"My Story"

By Andrew Gurza, as told to Jenn Soros, PhD, OTR/L, and Karla Reese, DHSc, OTR/L

The following is Andrew's story told through interview responses. The interview questions have been removed to center Andrew's voice and perspective.

(*Content warning:* ableism, medical trauma)

About Andrew

My name is Andrew Gurza. I'm 36 and a half right now. I live in Toronto, Canada, with spastic quadriplegic cerebral palsy. I'm a power wheelchair user. I am queer. I have a master of arts in legal studies and disability. I have two brothers and one sister.

I saw a speech therapist when I was a little boy because I had a really bad stutter. I have seen physical therapists and occupational therapists throughout my life. I've seen doctors for things like spinal fusion surgery, hip surgery, and tendon-lengthening surgery. I've seen occupational therapy practitioners for wheelchair fittings, and physical therapists for exercises they made me do as a kid. Those are my experiences of backgrounds with any kind of medical workers. Then, I have personal support workers who help me with my day-to-day. I'm in a weird place because I'm living in a quasi-medical environment all the time. I see personal support workers all the time.

On Sexuality

I'm queer. I would say I'm masculine presenting. I would say that I'm cis. I would say that I sometimes use "they" and "them" pronouns, particularly around gay male spaces, where gay men don't see me as sexually viable. I like to use "they" because then I don't have to conform to some standard of masculinity and male sexuality that I can't meet because of my disability. I'm queer, as in, I like to play with men.

COVID-19 has affected my sexuality and intimacy a lot. With the pandemic, I haven't been able to access my sexuality in any way that is shared with another person, and I really miss it. Sex and disability are really important to me because I've fought so hard for it as a disabled person. It's an experience that I didn't think I'd ever get to have as a disabled person. I predominantly have sex with sex workers right now to have my needs met as somebody with a disability. I take great pride in that because trying to meet somebody in conventional ways wasn't working for me. I found that sex work gave me an avenue to explore my sexuality in a way that was really safe and comfortable.

[The topic of] *sex and disability* is something that I talk about a lot in my work because it's something we in the disability community discuss. To me, sex and disability means connection, means friendship, means possibility. Intimacy is something that I don't get very often. I get touched primarily by my caregivers, like a bunch of times per day, but that's very medicalized and very regimented. It has a routine. During the pandemic, I couldn't have any kind of intimate touch in the way that I wanted, which greatly affected my mental health, comfort level, and body dysmorphia. Sex and intimacy are so much more than just the physical act; it's all the emotional and interpersonal pieces, and how do you how do you fit disability into all those pieces? That's why I really love doing this work, because it's like putting a puzzle together every time you talk about it.

On Dating

I don't date much anymore. I've never gone on a second date with somebody, because people are afraid of disability. They don't know how to navigate it. Dating is very rare for me, which is why, about 4 years ago, I decided to turn to sex work and hire sex workers because I was not getting what I needed. I wasn't able to meet somebody the conventional way. I also realized that because of the social assistance that I that I receive from the government here in Canada, if I was to be with somebody long term, I might lose my benefits because of the way the system is set up. As much as I wanted a long-term relationship and dating, I learned very quickly that it might not be something that I could access easily.

With the privileges of the work I do and the little bit of money that I make, I realized that I could have enough money to engage with a sex worker. While not a typical relationship, I realized I could still build a relationship with a person that I trusted, have a good time with them, and enjoy myself. So, my experiences of intimacy really have been informed by relationships with sex workers over the last 3 to 4 years, and that's an experience that I wouldn't trade for anything. I speak about sex work all the time in my work as a disability advocate because it's something that I was really ashamed about at first—I was scared to admit that I hired sex workers. But it's not like the scary back-alley thing we're all taught that it is. It's actually a really beautiful, powerful experience with another person.

Experiences in Health Care

In my 20s, I was living in my first apartment in Ottawa, Ontario, in the university dorms, and I had needed to see an occupational therapist, and I hadn't seen one in a while. (In Ontario at that time, you were allowed four visits with an occupational therapist per year.) You tell them what you want the occupational therapist for, and they'll set up a schedule.

After the fourth visit with the occupational therapist—who was young, hip, and cool, and we got along well—I said to her, "I have question for you. I want to learn how to have better sex with a partner, and I'd like to learn how to do different sexual positions. Could I talk to you about it?" She got red in the face and started giggling. She gathered her stuff and said, "I can't help you with that" and turned around and walked away. I never saw her again. I felt ashamed. I was kind of in shock, and at that point, I didn't call another occupational therapist to talk about my sexual health, and I haven't spoken to an occupational therapist—other than you guys[9]—about my sexual health since that moment.

With the company that my sister and I are working with, Handi, and our goal of creating the first line of sex toys for people with disabilities, we have had the opportunity and the luck to speak with a lot of occupational therapy practitioners out of Australia who are very eager to work with clients to bridge the gap between sex intimacy and disability. Although my personal experience was different, on a professional level,

---

[9] Here, Andrew is speaking directly to his interviewers, Jenn Soros and Karla Reese.

we're finding that many occupational therapists are really excited by this area because they talk to clients all the time—but it never gets talked about publicly.

A couple years ago, I woke up with what I thought were flulike symptoms, and I lost the ability to pee. I ended up not being able to pee for about 24 hours. I freaked out and went to my doctor, and she referred me to a specialist at the hospital. An indwelling catheter was put in for a couple of weeks. Then weeks turned into a few months. After a few months, I finally went to see the urologist. I was trying to muster the courage to ask this guy, "Can I take the catheter out so I can have sex again?" But I was so nervous because he was an old White guy who probably didn't want to talk to his disabled client about sex. When I finally asked, the doctor said, "Oh, we'll just leave it in. It'll be easier for you—don't worry about it."

He dismissed me and walked out of the room. I chased him down the hall and said, "No, no, no, doc. I need you to look at me for a minute. I want to have sex again. I'm a queer man, and I want to have sex again." I had waited 2 hours for the doctor to come in, and he was going to dismiss me within about 2 minutes. So, I said to him, "I want to take this thing out. Can we look into other options?"

The doctor said, "Yeah, I guess we could. But it would be hard." And I was like, "I don't care—what are the options?" The doctor laid out the options for me and said, "Yeah, I guess we'll do that, no problem." Then he dismissed me and walked away, but all I could think about was that if I hadn't had the balls to speak up for myself and say that I don't want it this way, he would have simply left in the catheter. I am very grateful that I spoke up, but I'm also appalled that the medical doctor wasn't being like, "Hey, what's your sex life like? Have you been able to get around this?" I just thought about how dismissive he was about what I was telling him. If an able-bodied man had walked into his office and had the same issue, he would have fought really hard for him to have his dick back. But for me, he didn't seem to care. He saw me as not having sexual needs and tried to deter and dismiss me by saying something that was "no problem" would be "hard."

Advice for Occupational Therapy Practitioners

My advice to occupational therapy practitioners is to address your own ableism. Figure out what your biases are, own them, and work through them before you get into the room with another disabled person so that by the time you get in there, no matter what they throw at you, you have an answer that helps them feel seen and feel like they matter. So many people in occupational therapy school, or going to school to work with disabled people, they do it out of the goodness of their heart and they want to make a difference. That's all very nice, but they are failing to address their biases and their own discomfort.

I think occupational therapy practitioners think there has to be a boundary—a very, very clear boundary—and the minute I say the word "sex," that boundary is somehow broken. If I want to talk to my occupational therapist about sex, it doesn't mean I want to have sex with my occupational therapist. It means I want to talk to my occupational therapist about sex. A client being inappropriate is obviously very different, and a boundary needs to be set. But if the client is just asking questions about sex, why wouldn't you answer? And if you don't have the answer, go find out. An occupational therapy practitioner is often the person a client will see the most often, one of the people who touches their bodies the most. So, when it comes to sex, why wouldn't the client want to go to you for guidance? You're the one who can help them with their ADLs. Why can't you help them have better sex? It is a privilege when somebody with a disability asks you for help. It's a real privilege because you have the chance to help them have a better life.

Disability, just like sexuality, is a spectrum, and it's okay if your sex changes because of disability. Occupational therapy practitioners: It's okay if you don't know something. It's okay if you have stuff to learn. Work through your ableism. Be comfortable with not knowing and be comfortable in your discomfort around sex and disability.

Occupational Therapy Application

1. Advocating for the sexual rights of occupational therapy clients includes educating other professionals. This narrative introduces us to an occupational therapist who giggles when her client, Andrew, brings up the topic of sex. Occupational therapy practitioners are likely to experience a scenario in which they learn of another practitioner feeling uncomfortable or making jokes in the office about a client who has brought up sex with them. Sex-positive occupational therapy practitioners can consider sharing what they learned in Chapter 3. They can encourage the practitioner who made jokes to explore why they thought it was funny and consider their biases about people with disabilities who are interested in having sex. Together, they can identify what questions they need to ask the client to address their positioning needs. Consider: What questions and/or assessments does the practitioner need to ask to do activity analysis for sex?
2. What could an occupational therapy practitioner do to establish change clinic-wide to improve how the practitioners at their clinic address sexuality?

"Big Black Clit Energy"

By M. Nicole Horsley, PhD

(*Content warning:* medical trauma experienced by Black people, reinforcing historical views of Black people's genitalia,[10] anti-Blackness, internalized anti-Blackness)

[10]During Colonialism, the European medical community began to view the genitalia of Africans as both an oddity and enticing or exciting. The imagined view of the Black body was both sexualized and exposed by Europeans in the 18th century, and these views persist today (Friar, 2021). The exhibition of Sara Baartman, a South African Khoikhoi woman, at European freak shows in the early 1800s is one of the earliest examples of European obsessing and degrading of Black female bodies (Friar, 2021). To learn more, see "Understanding Sexual Identity: Difference and Intersectionality" and "The Black Female Body: Representation of the Erotic in Contemporary Visual Art in Africa" (both in Friar, 2021).

One finger at a time, he shoved his hands into each latex glove, letting the gloves snap. Looking both hands once over, he inspected the fit of the gloves. Introducing himself as doctor "so and so," he quickly read from the chart my reason for the visit. Setting the chart down with one gloved hand, he flung off the small white sheet draped over my legs as he pushed my legs wide open, instructing me to place both feet in the stirrups.

Shivering as the cold air touched the tiny hairs on my arms, rubbing against the whole of my skin, the cold crept between my toes, tingled my hairless thighs, and moved against each fold and crease of skin as he pulled and pushed back and to the side to better see my vulva. His touch, cold and invasive. Without warning, he grabbed folds of skin, wrestling with the fleshiness of the labia as his fingers and eyes marveled at the strangeness I found in his "hmm." He used his gloved fingers to pull back my clitoral hood for a closer look. I felt cold air swoosh between the folds of my vulva at the same time the doctor practically flew back in his wheeled stool. The doctor quickly left the room, returning with a nurse who, glasses on the brim of her nose as she recorded each measurement, joined him to stare between my legs in awe. They began talking about me as if I wasn't in the room, using medical terms that were unrecognizable to me.

The word "abnormal" slapped me, as if the doctor's tongue had wrapped itself around the word and whipped it across the room as he said it. I lay stunned as he continued speaking with no explanation given. He sat down on the stool and scooted closer to marvel at the size of my clit. I found the doctor's preoccupation with the appearance and feel of my genitals embarrassing. I had never seen another woman's clitoris. I had nothing to compare mine to and no reason to think about it. I could now only assume that my clitoris was an oddity.

I was 18 years old and experiencing my first gynecology appointment, and I was unaware of the enslaved children, women, and men on whom doctors such as J. Marion Sims had experimented. Today, I imagine my experience as something far milder and less gruesome than the fear, humiliation, and excruciating pain they endured but also a continuation of the medical trauma experienced by Black people.[11]

"Are you a diabetic?" The question brought me back to the present. "No," I replied. He continued to examine my vulva, calling for a nurse to bring the urine results. "I am sorry to tell you, but you are a diabetic. Your blood sugar levels are over 300. What you are experiencing is a yeast infestation as a result of your body trying to rid itself of the excess." He continued to lift and pull back the fleshiness of the labia minora. With a sigh of relief, I asked if this was why my clitoris was "abnormal." Hesitantly, I asked if my butt was abnormal too. I had always wondered why it was not big and round like my mother's. But the doctor, completely focused on my genitals, ignored my questions, making a comment to the nurse regarding the size of my clitoris and suggesting further tests be performed for polycystic ovary syndrome.

[11] See Washington (2006).

His preoccupation with the size of my clitoris as an oddity or freak of nature concerned me. Without any additional diagnosis or information into the condition or cause of this abnormality, I was left to think maybe it was a deformity. I had no idea what constituted an abnormal clit—or a normal one, for that matter. I left unsure what this revelation meant. Would I be seen as grotesque? Was it abnormal because of its size, or was its size related to me being Black? Did all Black women have "abnormal" genitalia? It would take a few more years, and my first relationship with a woman, before I would reconsider the abnormality of my clitoris and come to understand that a big Black clit was something to be desired.

Big Black Clit Energy: It's a Vibe

I had long since developed a dislike for my body. I was often teased about how my body wasn't "Black" enough. I was compared to the other girls and found wanting. I felt like an outsider. My ass was too small, and my breasts, too big. I longed for a body like my mother's: smaller breasts, tiny waist, curvy thighs, and a large tabletop booty. She occupied her brick-house body seemingly flawlessly, wearing tiny tank tops with tight jeans painted onto her thick thighs and belts to accentuate her waist. When she walked down the street nonchalantly, it was music playing. I can recall walking behind her, watching men's eyes dance across her body. Unsure what to take in first, they would stop and stare. I had seen men slapped by their partners for looking at her ass as she flowed by gracefully, ass sitting on her back, perfectly round and tight. She had the type of big Black ass that inspired men and women to stop and stare. An ass that is the object of many songs. My mother's ass was an entire album.

As a child, I had no idea my butt was considered flat, of course, but I recognized that my body was different from my mother's and the other women around me. As my body developed, it became clear that large breasts and a smaller butt would be my plight to bear. No one ever rapped about smaller booties as an object of desire; Black men desired a big, fleshy butt. I saw my flat ass as a sign of something disgusting. But my mother and aunt gushed over my body: "Look at her booty. Don't you wish you could wear jeans like that?" They would tell me how lucky I was to have a "White girl's booty." Complaining about how hard it was to find jeans that would fit their big asses, they presented sophisticated reasoning as to the advantages of a small or no-ass-at-all type of booty. Think of the designer jeans made for flat asses! My aunt would say, "Boy, I wish I had her 'White girl shape.'" And then she would get up to dance, imagining what she would wear and what she could do with a body unlike her own.

I always wondered how they could not enjoy the epitome of blackness, the Black ass. Much like the big Black cock, it exists in our imaginations beyond its pathology.[12] My curiosity would lead me into the unknown, to explore the spectacle and pleasures of possessing a big Black clit. In grad school, I began to seek the origins

[12]See Pilgrim (2002/edited 2012) for more information on myths and stereotypes about Black bodies and their roots in racism.

of these mythical bodies, locating them in archives and medical journals, and learning that descriptions of abnormal genitalia, especially when associated with the Black or homosexual body, was an indication of sexual deviance.[13]

Big Black Clit Energy: A Manifesto

I have chosen the memory of the violence of a Black girl's first gynecological visit scripted by the memory of trauma; feelings of distrust; and the experience of being a spectacle, oddity, and medical fascination due to the doctor's perception of difference. I was determined to define "big Black clit energy" informed by these experiences and the multiple histories and stories I've researched in my academic work. In doing so, I give some legacy back to the lifeless bodies of the unrememberable, dismembered, and disposable bodies of Black medical subjects. People left out of history books and health care curriculums and whose disturbing omission continues to haunt medicine, health, sex and sexuality, gender, and racial liberation.

Things started to change when I met my then partner, Latoya. A Black woman from a predominantly White community, she was the Black friend from the other side of the tracks in graduate school. We started dating a year prior to her 30th birthday; I was her first Black girlfriend. Often, she'd say, "Gosh, you are so Black." It wasn't a compliment. Most often, it was an insult or judgment. Her internalized anti-Blackness was her lens to see my personality and body. She didn't appreciate my "Black girl attitude," but she did enjoy our sexual escapades and my body. I enjoyed this, too. The relationship taught me the joy and pleasure in having a big Black clitoris.

The first and every time she saw and touched my body, she did so with love and admiration. Sitting face-to-face with my clit, much like the doctor some years earlier, a deep sigh escaped her lips at the sight of my clitoris peeking out beyond the labia majora. "Wow it's big. You even have a Black girl clit." She moved in closer until I could feel her warm breath, and I felt wetness flood my vagina in anticipation. "Your piercing is beautiful," she breathed, kissing it lightly. "Your clit is beautiful. It even smells Black, like shea butter and rose petals." She taught me to love my clitoris. I have explored the fullness of having a larger clit, with the help of some big Black clit porn, and I'm not hiding it anymore. It isn't abnormal. My big Black clit is beautiful.

[13] "The portrayal of Black women as lascivious by nature is an enduring stereotype. The descriptive words associated with this stereotype are singular in their focus: seductive, alluring, worldly, beguiling, tempting, and lewd. Historically, White women, as a category, were portrayed as models of self-respect, self-control, and modesty—even sexual purity, but Black women were often portrayed as innately promiscuous, even predatory" (Pilgrim, 2002/edited 2012). See also Friar (2021) and Washington (2006) for more on White supremacy and patriarchal views of femininity and sexuality.

Big Black Clit Energy: Noun

Confidence. A bit cocky: bold and brazenly self-assured. When I walk, I understand the magic of having a big Black clit. My energy.

Occupational Therapy Application

Many clients come to occupational therapy with a history of invalidation and trauma from medical providers. Nicole shares her story of how the trauma of her first gynecological visit influenced her sexual self-view. Through her 20s and 30s, she shifts her self-view and empowers herself and her body by redefining herself as too big, too small, not enough, and too much, to refusing to consider any aspect of her body as an oddity or abnormal; instead, these aspects of her body are beautiful because they are authentically her. She also shares that experiencing pleasure in her body helped her feel more positively about her desirability and sexual self-view. The sensory experience of pain or discomfort reinforced a confusing and negative self-view, and the sensory experience of pleasure helped reinforced positive thoughts.

Consider an occupational therapy practitioner who is working in an outpatient mental health center and is running a psychosocial group that focuses on skills for participation in valued occupations for people who have experienced physical trauma. The topic for the group is "Engaging in Sexual Occupations."

1. Using what you learned in Nicole's and Sakshi's narratives, script how you would explain the benefits of using pleasure as way to heal from trauma.
2. Using a graded approach, consider what pleasurable occupations you might suggest to the group for people who find it difficult to pay attention to the sensations in their body.

Summary

Sexual and intimate occupations are powerful, meaningful and, yet, often hidden. The narrators of this chapter have written truthfully of the strangeness, fear, joy, weirdness, beauty, empowerment, pain, pleasure, relief, discomfort, love, admiration, humor, affirmation, and empowerment as part of their sexual and intimate experiences. Occupational therapy practitioners will hear stories during assessment and treatment similar to those that these narrators shared.

The purpose of these narratives is to challenge readers' assumptions and biases and provide opportunity for readers to practice curiosity versus judgment. Occupational therapy practitioners are encouraged to understand how clinician curiosity and nonjudgment are essential to effective intervention. The "Occupational Therapy Application" sections for each narrative guide practitioners to consider how they navigate their own biases, educate other providers, conduct activity analysis, and determine interventions.

Kathryn Ellis, OTD, OTR/L, AASECT–SC (she/her), developed the Occupational Therapy Sexuality and Intimacy Clinic at Walter Reed National Military Medical Center (Bethesda, MD) and is the co-author of *Sex and Intimacy for Wounded Veterans: A Guide to Embracing Change* (Sager Group, 2015). She is the founder/CEO of a continuing education company, the Institute for Sex, Intimacy & Occupational Therapy and an American Association of Sexuality Educators, Counselors, and Therapists Certified Sexuality Counselor. Her private practice, Dr. Kathryn Ellis Sexual Wellness Counseling, is based in Delaware.

Joseph Christian Ungco, OTD, OTR/L (they/them), is the associate director for diversity, equity, and inclusion (DEI) education, client services, and data analytics for the Fred Hutchinson Cancer Center in Seattle. They lead several organization-wide DEI initiatives, including the bias mitigation education program and gender-inclusive and accessible spaces initiative. They also continue to serve in DEI roles in occupational therapy, including serving as co-chair of the national Network for LGBTQIA+ Concerns in Occupational Therapy and sitting on the executive council for the Occupational Therapy Multicultural, Diversity and Inclusion National Network. Dr. Ungco's work is centered on amplifying the voices of those most affected by systems of oppression and actualizing structural change.

Devlynn "Dev" Neu, MS, OTR/L (he/him/they/them), is a queer and gender-fluid occupational therapist living in Rochester, New York. They obtained their combined bachelor's and master's degrees in Human Occupation and Occupational Therapy from D'Youville College in Buffalo, where they fiercely advocated for diversity, equity, and inclusion within and outside of the occupational therapy profession. Dev is passionate about amplifying the voices of LGBTQIA+ individuals, educating others on the diverse needs of members of the LGBTQIA+ community on social media as The Rainbow OT, serving on the leadership team of the Network for LGBTQIA+ Concerns in Occupational Therapy, and facilitating action regarding change for improving equity, inclusion, and quality of life for those within the LGBTQIA+ community. Dev recently joined the Ithaca College Occupational Therapy Department as a part-time professor.

Emily Sherman, OTD, OTR/L, DPAM (she/her), is a traveling occupational therapist experienced in hospital and community settings from California to Kentucky. She is a staunch advocate of the LGBTQIA+ community and strongly committed to helping people reach their highest level of independence by collaborating with clients and their communities.

Sakshi Tickoo, BOTh, CPC (she/her), is a Mumbai, India–based occupational therapist and sexuality counselor. She is the founder of Sex, Love, and OT, an occupational therapy practice providing sexuality and mental health rehabilitation across the lifespan. She is also the author of *SexCare—A Self-Help Guide to Sexual Wellness,* which that focuses on techniques to incorporate pleasure through self-care.

Andrew Gurza (he/they), is a disability awareness consultant. He has presented all across North America on sex and disability as a self-described Queer Crippled Man. He hosts the *Disability After Dark* podcast and is the cofounder of Handi, a company that develops sex toys for people with disabilities. More on his work is at https://www.andrewgurza.com/.

Karla D. Reese, DHSc, OTR/L (she/her), is a clinical assistant professor at Cleveland State University in the Department of Occupational Therapy in Cleveland, Ohio. She is the co-creator and co-host of *OT After Dark,* a podcast focusing on sexuality and intimacy for individuals with disabilities.

Jenn Soros, PhD, OTR/L (she/her/hers), is an assistant professor at Cleveland State University in the Department of Occupational Therapy in Cleveland, Ohio. Dr. Soros's area of research focuses on sexuality and intimacy from an occupational perspective.

M. Nicole Horsley, PhD, is an assistant professor of African diaspora studies and affiliate faculty in Women's, Gender, and Sexuality Studies and Screen Cultures at Ithaca College (New York). Her work interrogates the discourse on Black women bodies, disease, organs, and sexual pleasure.

References

American Occupational Therapy Association. (2020). Occupational therapy practice framework: Domain and process (4th ed.). *American Journal of Occupational Therapy, 74*(Suppl. 2), 7412410010. https://doi.org/10.5014/ajot.2020.74S2001

Americans With Disabilities Act of 1990, Pub. L. 101–336, 42 U.S.C. §§ 12101–12213 (2000).

Annon, J. S. (1976). The PLISSIT model: A proposed conceptual scheme for the behavioural treatment of sexual problems. *Journal of Sex Education and Therapy, 2*(1), 1–15. https://doi.org/10.1080/01614576.1976.11074483

Basu, S. (2018, December 18). *Can we ever have a conversation about desire without centering my disability?* [Blog post]. https://medium.com/skin-stories/by-soumita-basu-64274f2bcd62

brown, A. M. (2019). *Pleasure activism: The politics of feeling good.* AK Press.

Friar, T. (2021). The black female body: Representation of the erotic in contemporary visual art in Africa. *E-REA: Revue Électronique d'Études sur le Monde Anglophone, 19*(1). https://doi.org/10.4000/erea.13034

Lorde, A. (1984). *Sister outsider: Essays and speeches.* Crossing Press.

Pilgrim, D. (2002/edited 2012). *The Jezebel stereotype* [Exhibit]. Jim Crow Museum, Ferris State University, Big Rapids, MI. https://www.ferris.edu/HTMLS/news/jimcrow/jezebel/index.htm

van der Kolk, B. A. (2015). *The body keeps the score: Brain, mind, and body in the healing of trauma.* Penguin Books.

Washington, H. A. (2006). *Medical apartheid: The dark history of medical experimentation on Black Americans from Colonial times to the present.* Doubleday.

11

Interventions for Sexual and Intimate Occupations

Kathryn Ellis, *OTD, OTR/L, AASECT–SC;* **Carla Wilson Walker,** *OTD, OTR/L, ATP; and* **Elizabeth K. Schmidt,** *PhD, OTR/L*

CHAPTER HIGHLIGHTS

- Cognitive interventions
- Interventions for emotional wellness
- Physical considerations
- Sensory considerations
- Working with others to support clients
- Accessibility considerations

KEY TERMS AND CONCEPTS

Cognitive interventions
Emotional regulation
Friendships and Dating Program
Intimacy with self
Occupational Therapy Sexual Assessment Framework
Program for the Education and Enrichment of Relational Skills
Self-awareness
Self-compassion
Self-love
Sensate focus
Sexual self-advocacy
Sexual self-expression
Sexual self-view
Social skills groups
Social Stories™

The *Occupational Therapy Sexual Assessment Framework* (Walker et al., 2020) provides a structure through which occupational therapy practitioners can better serve their clients who experience challenges or dissatisfaction with sexual and intimate occupations. People are sexual beings[1] from "womb to

[1] An asexual person may or may not identify with the language "individuals are sexual beings." Our use is intended to consider how all people have an orientation—asexual included—as sexual beings. Some people are asexual or demisexual, among other sexual orientations that experience no or limited sexual attraction. This is distinct from *celibacy*, which is a choice to abstain from sexual behaviors regardless of sexual attraction.

tomb," and clients with or without a specific pathology can benefit from occupational therapy interventions focused on enabling participation in sexual and intimate occupations. Sexual and intimate occupations have activity demands that require processing, social, and motor skills. As discussed in previous chapters, a thorough, client-centered evaluation is required before launching into potential interventions. Many activity demands can be accommodated with interventions focused on environmental modifications, adaptive strategies, changes to habits and routines, and changes to context. This chapter focuses on the activity demands and skills required for engagement in sexual activity through holistic consideration of cognitive, emotional, and physical requirements.

Having occupation-focused interventions might seem confusing for an occupational therapy practitioner, because one might think it means having their clients engage in the sexual occupations during treatment. In most scenarios, that is not what is suggested. Instead, intervention can include scripting out communication, verbalizing a specific sequence, modeling behavior, practicing positioning with clothes on, and simulating touch on areas of the body that do not elicit a sexual response. Although it might be unlikely that a client would become aroused or "turned on" during a treatment session, it would not be inherently wrong or inappropriate. The practitioner can normalize this response for the client, provide education on the physiological reactions that can automatically occur without regard for context, and consider using compassion or humor. It is important to recognize that what we are referring to here is the practitioner having a discussion about a client's reactions to consensual conversations and treatment. In the next section, we provide suggestions for how the practitioner can respond to inappropriate touching, harassment, or flirting.

Cognitive Interventions

Occupational therapy practitioners can help their clients effectively apply knowledge, adapt performance, and understand their sexual self-view. ***Cognitive interventions*** may be beneficial for a variety of clients, depending on their abilities and life stage. For example, the practitioner may implement cognitive interventions for adolescent or older adult clients who have intellectual disability, traumatic brain injury (TBI), cognitive impairments poststroke, or Alzheimer's disease or dementia.

Occupational therapy practitioners may encounter situations in which the client flirts with or makes inappropriate advances toward the clinician. These situations could happen in any therapeutic interaction, whether or not sex and intimacy are being discussed, and they can be distressing for the practitioner. It is possible that flirting is the client's way of practicing social skills related to acquiring an intimate partner or that the client considers a health care setting a realistic place to meet a potential partner. In response, the practitioner can set a boundary that the therapeutic relationship is strictly clinical and use the flirtation as a segue to discuss the client's goals related to intimacy and partnership. If a practitioner experiences harassment or inappropriate touching, they can consider terminating the treatment session, verbalizing the boundary, or referring to legal or human resources. In some cases, the behavior can be a catalyst for a goal and intervention that focus on sexual behavior appropriate for various social interactions and contexts.

Applying Knowledge

Clients with new disabilities may require information to safely engage in occupations associated with sexuality and intimacy. For example, clients with a TBI may require education and cognitive interventions to facilitate safe and appropriate participation in sexuality and intimacy following the onset of their injury or disability. Clients with childhood-onset disabilities, in contrast, may have never received sexuality education (Barnard-Brak et al., 2014) or may not have received information that was accessible to them. Further, they may have missed valuable experiences in adolescence that provide them with the skills necessary for healthy relationships and sexuality (Swango-Wilson, 2011).

For example, many people with intellectual or developmental disabilities demonstrate low levels of sexual health knowledge (Schaafsma et al., 2017). Sexual health knowledge is important for everyone because it can help prepare them to recognize signs of unhealthy relationships or potential abuse, advocate for themselves and their rights, and report potential abuse or assault (Swango-Wilson, 2011). Therefore, occupational therapy practitioners should support their clients by facilitating understanding of sexual health, to include providing information on healthy relationships, consent, information about sexual activities, prevention of sexually transmitted infections, or family planning.

Occupational therapy practitioners should use best practice recommendations for providing accessible sexual health information, including the use of didactic teaching with clear instructions, discussion, and structured routines for education provision (Schaafsma et al., 2015; Schmidt et al., 2020). They may also consider using illustrations (e.g., pictures, videos) that match their clients' self-identity (e.g., Brown, disabled, queer), visual schedules or reminders, and universal design for learning when providing information about specific content (Ferrante & Oak, 2020; Grove et al., 2018; Roden et al., 2020; Sala et al., 2019; Schaafsma et al., 2015; Schmidt et al., 2020).

The more sexual health knowledge a person has, the more equipped they will be to manage their own sexual health and advocate for their rights. Occupational therapy practitioners can support their clients by educating them on what they should expect at annual appointments (e.g., what is and is not appropriate for health care providers to ask or do with the client, instruments providers may use during the appointment), accommodations clients can advocate for that may facilitate the ease of that appointment (e.g., positioning for gynecological exams for individuals with spasticity), and considerations or modifications related to engaging in healthy behaviors. For example, if someone is interested in using contraception, there are additional considerations that the prescribing physician may not consider, such as fine motor skills required to insert a vaginal ring or memory strategies that enable remembering daily oral contraceptives.

Occupational therapy practitioners can also assist their clients in establishing and maintaining intimate relationships throughout various stages by applying knowledge of social skills. Specifically, the practitioner may address verbal and nonverbal communication skills that are involved in sexual health management and that support intimate partnerships (e.g., establishment of relationships, maintenance of relationships, negotiation of consent, sexual self-advocacy). Social skills have been shown to predict the ability of individuals with disabilities, specifically autism spectrum disorder (ASD), to form romantic partnerships (Stokes et al., 2007); such skills have been identified as important areas in which people with various disabilities need support (Exell et al., 2020). Practitioners can intervene and support their clients to apply knowledge of social skills needed for intimate partnerships through social skills groups and Social Stories.™

Social Skills Groups

A variety of ***social skills groups*** are available for adolescents and adults with specific diagnoses, such as ASD, intellectual disability, and schizophrenia (Exell et al., 2020; Gantman et al., 2012; Laugeson et al., 2012, 2014, 2015; Park et al., 2011; Plavnick et al., 2015). These group interventions typically incorporate didactic instruction, role playing, demonstration or modeling, feedback, and "homework" (Gantman et al., 2012; Laugeson et al., 2012, 2014, 2015), whereas others use innovative techniques, such as video-modeling and virtual reality interventions (Park et al., 2011; Plavnick et al., 2015). One of the best studied programs currently available is designed for autistic youths and adults: the ***Program for the Education and Enrichment of Relational Skills*** (PEERS®). PEERS uses a variety of didactic lessons focused on communication, how to find friends, dating etiquette, and how to handle peer pressure and arguments with friends or partners. This program has been shown to reduce loneliness, improve social skills knowledge, and increase frequency of hosted and invited get-togethers with peers (Gantman et al., 2012; Laugeson et al., 2012, 2014, 2015). Teachers also have reported improved social responsiveness, social communication, social motivation, social awareness, and non–statistically significant improvements in social cognition (Laugeson et al., 2012, 2014). Parents have reported that the PEERS program has improved their young adult's overall social skills, social responsiveness, empathy, and frequency of get-togethers with peers (Gantman et al., 2012).

A few programs are explicitly designed to support people with dating, such as the ***Friendships and Dating Program*** (FDP) for people with intellectual and developmental disabilities (Ward et al., 2013). The FDP focuses on protecting oneself and creating opportunities to experience sexuality; it uses some of the same intervention techniques as other general social skills interventions (e.g., instructions, modeling, role play). The FDP has demonstrated improvements in social networks and decreased instances of interpersonal violence (Ward et al., 2013). Occupational therapy practitioners can use these intervention techniques to address areas of need for their clients and support them in engaging in healthy intimate partnerships.

Social Stories

Social Stories can be used to support clients in engaging in a variety of occupations associated with sexual health, including preparing children for the changes they are going to experience during puberty, increasing independence with menstrual management, and decreasing inappropriate masturbatory behaviors. To obtain best effects, Social Stories should use recommendations provided by Gray (n.d.). Specifically, the story should have a clearly defined goal and topic area, an illustration of a body that includes relevant details, and a summary or concluding statement (Gray, n.d.). Social Stories often consist of 5 to 10 pages, with one sentence per page and images on each page. Images should look realistic and be similar to the client for whom they are being used. Social Stories have been found to be effective with autistic children for generalizing skills for menstruation management (Ballan & Freyer, 2017; Klett & Turan, 2012) and for decreasing inappropriate sexual behaviors (e.g., masturbating in public; Banerjee et al., 2013).

Adapting Performance

To generalize information learned in other contexts, people need an opportunity to practice and apply the information. It is critical that occupational therapy practitioners consider the specific nature of the goal, intervention, and outcome that they are using with each client and the appropriateness of individual versus group intervention. For example, if the practitioner is providing recommendations for the client to engage in sexual activities, a group setting may not be the best place. However, if the practitioner is working on applying social skills associated with flirting and dating, group intervention may be a great setting in which to practice generalizing these skills.

As occupational therapy practitioners, we might start working with our clients on a one-on-one basis. As clients develop certain skills, we might then transition our interventions to group, community, or natural environment settings so that clients have an opportunity to practice and apply their new skills in a variety of contexts or with other people.

If no opportunity for group or community-based skill practice for a client is available, the practitioner can instead use role playing to help clients practice skills in a way similar to what would occur with others or in other settings. Role playing is considered an evidence-based intervention to support the application of both sexual health knowledge and other skills (e.g., social skills; Exell et al., 2020; Gantman et al., 2012; Laugeson et al., 2012, 2014, 2015; Sala et al., 2019; Schaafsma et al., 2015). An alternative to role playing is to provide home programming, or "homework," which is another commonly used social skills intervention technique (Gantman et al., 2012). The client can work on homework with someone else outside of therapy and then journal about the process, audio record their immediate reflections, or wait to reflect with the practitioner in the next therapy session about how their home practice went.

Self-Awareness

Self-awareness includes an awareness of one's sexual self-view. ***Sexual self-view*** is "how a person views [themself] as a sexual being and includes aspects of sexual identity, gender identity and body image" (Walker et al., 2020, p. 10). Some people may need assistance understanding their sexual self-view. For example, people with intellectual and developmental disabilities have spoken out about the need for more support in receiving didactic information about gender identity and sexual orientation (Schmidt et al., 2021). In this case, the occupational therapy practitioner can work with the client to build self-awareness by asking, "How do you want to feel?" and "Who is someone you feel inspired by?" The practitioner can then support the client with exploring different clothing styles, hair accessories, grooming techniques, and mannerisms that they might feel good, sexy, or confident wearing or doing.

Sexual Self-Advocacy

Occupational therapy practitioners can support their clients by developing sexual self-advocacy skills. ***Sexual self-advocacy*** is the process by which a person speaks up, gets the information they need, and makes informed decisions when participating in the occupations of sexuality and intimacy (Friedman et al., 2014). Practitioners can engage in sexual self-advocacy training by first ensuring that their clients have the education they need to make informed choices about their sexuality and sexual health. This process might include providing accessible sexuality education. In addition, practitioners can educate clients on how to use assertive and effective communication to relay their specific needs and interests so that they can successfully advocate for themselves and access reproductive health care.

For example, when working with a client with a spinal cord injury (SCI), the occupational therapy practitioner can provide education around engaging in sexual activity with a catheter, including the positive and negative features of each catheter type as they relate to the client. If the client expresses a preference for suprapubic catheters over indwelling catheters, the practitioner can support the client by engaging in assertive communication training and role play so that the client can effectively communicate their interests to their physician.

Occupational therapy practitioners working with clients who use mobility devices or adaptive equipment or who may need support during sexual activities can also educate clients on how to engage in sexual activities with these devices or with the assistance of their partner(s). Practitioners can inform clients about disability educators and advocates, such as Andrew Gurza (https://www.andrewgurza.com) and Eva Sweeney (https://www.crippingupsexwitheva.com), who draw attention to how equipment and effective communication that guides partners to support them may be incorporated into sexual activities. Again, practitioners can provide education and assertive communication training as well as engage the client in role play so that the client can effectively communicate their needs during sexual activities with their partner(s).

Interventions for Emotional Wellness

An important area for occupational therapy practitioners to address is emotional wellness, a topic that spans ages and populations. Regardless of age, ability, and mental health status, many people experience challenges with emotional wellness in relation to their engagement in intimate partnerships and sexual activities. In the sections that follow, we offer recommendations for addressing anxiety, loss or limited desire, shame, and insecurities as well as recommendations for fostering coping skills, emotional connection, and emotional regulation.

Occupational therapy interventions should be occupation focused and aim to enhance occupational engagement as the end goal as well as address emotional wellness as a barrier to that engagement. Occupational therapy practitioners might consider collaborating with a licensed mental health professional or complementary or alternative health therapist (e.g., movement therapist, art therapist) to address shared goals using combined approaches.

Addressing Anxiety

A person can experience generalized anxiety that influences sexual activity and intimate social participation, or they can experience anxiety specific to participation in sexual activity and intimate partnerships. Interventions focused on reducing anxiety and developing coping skills (e.g., cognitive reframing, reality checking) can be helpful when the client knows the thoughts that cause unsettled emotions. For example, a client might state, "I am worried I won't be able to maintain my erection, and then sex will just be over," or "I think I'd look so awkward." The occupational therapy practitioner can guide the client to think more broadly about sexual participation and reframe the client's understanding of what they need to be sexual. As an example of cognitive reframing, the practitioner might ask, "Can you think of ways you could be sexual without having the pressure of needing an erect penis? This might make you feel more relaxed and could actually help your body sustain an erection." For reality checking, the practitioner could, for example, call into awareness that sex is a practice and that people can naturally look or feel awkward.[2]

Occupational therapy practitioners can introduce graded approaches to engaging or reengaging in sexual activity if clients have anxiety about certain sexual

[2] Later in the chapter, we offer suggestions for attaining and sustaining erections. However, somatic or physical strategies to facilitate an erection often pair nicely with emotional regulation strategies to reduce pressure to have an erection.

activities that they have set as goals to do. Often, clients can feel that when they are reengaging in being sexual, they have to do everything they "used to do" in that first encounter. For example, a client who experienced a sexual trauma might feel anxious about being sexual again but have a goal of being able to participate in all of their previous activities. Using a graded approach, the practitioner can guide the client to identify which sexual activities would be easiest or the most comfortable and help the client script how they might explain to a partner or partners the sexual activities they want to do and—perhaps most important—which ones they do not want to do. The practitioner can work with the client to develop an incremental plan to slowly engage in a variety of sexual activities. Another example is someone who feels anxious about masturbating but knows that doing so would help them understand their body. This client can start with sensually and mindfully touching their body in nongenital areas with the intent of upgrading to the genital areas.

Once a graded approach is understood and implemented, clients can then work on communicating their limits—what they want to do and what they do not want to do—with potential partners through assertive communication training. Assertiveness training should include opportunities to practice asserting the client's best interest to others. It can be practiced via scripting and role playing with the occupational therapy practitioner, with others in a group setting, or on community outings (Speed et al., 2018). Practitioners can empower their clients by helping them understand that grading, limit setting, and assertive communication are components of healthy sexual behaviors, not necessarily something they have to do because they are anxious. The practitioner can bring awareness to the client that they can communicate and set limits in a way that is flirtatious, sexual, or playful—if that is what the client wants.

Embodiment practices, which center cognitive awareness on the sensations of the body (e.g., mindfulness), should always be considered when working with clients who have anxiety, especially with sexual activities related to the body's prominent role in receiving pleasure. For example, posttraumatic stress disorder and anxiety can often lead to the client's focusing on their fears and worries as well as centering on the body's sympathetic responses to this anxiety through increased heart rate, freezing, or emotionally checking out (Rosebrock & Carroll, 2017). Occupational therapy practitioners can educate the client that sexual pleasure, arousal, response, and satisfaction occur when the parasympathetic nervous system is activated, and they can teach mindfulness techniques to counter the anxiety and increase the pleasure (Brotto & Goldmeier, 2015). Chapter 9, "Trauma-Informed Care," offers information on working with clients with anxiety.

Addressing Loss of or Limited Desire

Occupational therapy practitioners should be prepared to provide psychoeducation on the factors that fuel and stifle desire as well as to engage the client in a conversation about what factors they think limit their desire. Many factors, such as stress, fatigue, busy schedules, partner satisfaction, and insecurities, moderate desire and should be addressed in treatment. Factors such as hormonal changes might be best addressed with clinical education; the practitioner should encourage the client to discuss the matter further with their primary care doctor or gynecologist (Carvalho & Nobre, 2010, 2011; Dosch et al., 2016; Nimbi et al., 2019; Parish & Hahn, 2016; Thorpe et al., 2021). Low desire can often be a source of anxiety for clients because they may feel that their desire should immediately match that of their partner at the time their partner initiates sex. These clients typically benefit from education about ways to build desire and to give themselves permission to slowly become interested in sex—at their own pace—instead of (1) consenting to sex and emotionally checking out or feeling anxious throughout because they are not taking the time to become interested and aroused or (2) declining sex.

Working on increasing desire itself can be a significant focus of occupational therapy intervention because of the inherent influence of the environment on doing and on interacting with others that can either fuel or stifle desire. This understanding mirrors the specific education occupational therapy practitioners receive about person, occupation, and environment. Once the client has an understanding that desire can be facilitated through engagement and environmental context versus an expectation to be constantly present, they can begin to explore what they could do to increase their desire (Nagoski, 2015). To facilitate this exploration and awareness, the occupational therapy practitioner can offer open-ended questions, such as the following:

- "What do you feel you need in order to be sexual? What do you want?"
- "What would make you feel relaxed or excited about being sexual?"
- "How do you want your partner to initiate with you?"
- "Are there certain smells you enjoy? Music you find sensual?"
- "What is your favorite way to be flirted with?"
- "When do you feel is the best time for you to have sex?"

As clients verbally share their answers and reflections, the clinician should engage in active listening and look for patterns to suggest a sequence or list of activities. A clinician might make suggestions as in the following examples:

- "Well, it sounds like your desire could be stimulated by your partner cleaning the kitchen after dinner so you have time to take a hot shower, followed by 5 minutes of alone time, and receiving text messages from your partner with positive affirmations or flirtations during the day when you are apart."
- "It sounds like music, a cedar candle, and wearing clothing that affirms you as a man really helps you unwind and feel more in the mood for sex. Could you plan to do these things in preparation for sexy time with your partner?"

- "It sounds you need space away from your children to transition into a more erotic headspace. Perhaps you can ask your partner not to initiate sex immediately after you put the kids to bed. And since you're both early risers, do you think the morning would be a better time for you?"

Occupational therapy practitioners are uniquely suited to analyzing the person, environment, and occupation in alignment with concepts that promote sexual self-advocacy. For example, a practitioner can work with a client to script how to assert their desire patterns to their partner(s), organize their daily activities, and modify their environment so they have a routine that supports facilitating desire.

Use of pelvic floor exercises, muscle relaxation, mindfulness interventions, physical exercise, cognitive–behavioral therapy, and couples therapy may promote positive sexual health (Günzler & Berner, 2012; Male et al., 2016). Günzler and Berner (2012) found that cognitive–behavioral therapy and pelvic biofeedback for low sexual desire are helpful strategies, and Guess et al. (2017) found that vibratory stimulation improved sexual function, satisfaction, and sensation and reduced distress. Strategies for confidence building with people with physical disabilities (PwPD) include addressing emotional issues, such as depression and anxiety (Fritz et al., 2015; Hess & Hough, 2012).

People can enjoy the sex they have and yet still have low desire for it. Consider this a challenge with facilitating desire, or transitioning to a sexual context when starting out in a nonsexual context; the preceding strategies can help in those cases. Sometimes low desire can be a result of not enjoying the sex, and sometimes it is a combination of the two. Clients who report limited enjoyment of sex might think they do not like sex, which can certainly be the case. However, through questioning, the occupational therapy practitioner and client can collaborate and build awareness around whether the client does not enjoy sex or does not enjoy the sex they typically have. The practitioner can ask questions such as the following:

- "Do you enjoy the sex you have?"
- "What is your favorite part about sex or your favorite thing to do? And do you do that often?"
- "Think of a time you really enjoyed sex. Is that typically what you do with your partner?"

Focusing on technique and sequence

When clients want to enjoy sex more but do not typically engage in the sex that they enjoy, the occupational therapy practitioner can implement a few strategies. For instance, they can educate the client that everyone has unique preferences for how they want their body to be touched and when they want certain body parts to be touched. Someone might, for example, enjoy clitoral stimulation in a circular motion but only after kissing, neck touches, and breast play because otherwise they do not feel "ready" to have their clitoris stimulated, and it just does not feel the same.

Unlearning and relearning

Clients sometimes report a rigid pattern of how they are sexually with their partners; ultimately, that pattern is hard to change, even when it is not effective for them. Activities or sequencing suggestions that get clients to try something different to break a typical pattern can be powerful. ***Sensate focus*** is a prescribed and intentional touch exercise in which touching and kissing are the role of the "giver," and receiving the touch is the role of the "receiver." The giver touches the way they would like to, and the receiver simply receives. The couple then switches roles, and afterward, they discuss what they learned, what they liked, and what they would like to carry forward into their sexual patterns. Sensate focus can also be helpful for other people—for example, those with strong sensory preferences or those who are reprocessing touch after sexual trauma. For more information on sensate focus, see *Sensate Focus in Sex Therapy: The Illustrated Manual* (Weiner & Avery-Clark, 2017).

Addressing Insecurities

Insecurities can limit engagement and satisfaction with sexual activity and intimate partnerships. Cultural messaging steeped in ableism, sexism, fatphobia, a strict standard of beauty, body shaming, and sex negativity, among others, can be powerful influencers of people's beliefs around who is desirable and who is expected to be sexual (Collins et al., 2017; Mathias & Harcourt, 2014; see Chapter 4, "Sexuality, Bias, and Impact: Preventing Clinician Harm"). Low self-esteem can often lead people to feel embarrassed about their bodies or inadequate as a sexual person. Mindfulness has been shown to mitigate sexual insecurities and enhance sexual satisfaction (Dunkley et al., 2015). Teaching clients to engage in mindful awareness and focus on the body sensations of pleasure can help them focus on the physical pleasure and not the cognitive insecurities.

Both self-love and self-compassion center on acceptance of self and one's own insecurities (Lorde, 2020; Marshall et al., 2015). Occupational therapy practitioners can instruct clients to practice ***self-love*** by acknowledging their uniqueness and attaching positive affirmation to that uniqueness, by setting limits that serve their overall quality of life, and by engaging in pleasure-oriented activities and self-care activities (Lorde, 2020). Conversely, ***self-compassion*** can be practiced by acknowledging the universal nature of insecurities as a source of suffering; clients can begin to reality check and normalize their feelings (Marshall et al., 2015). A study of a body image intervention that involved writing exercises to acknowledge body functions that PwPD *can* perform—as well as creative endeavors, self-care, and communication—found that depression decreased and body image improved (Alleva et al., 2018).

Fostering Coping Skills

Sexual activity and intimate social participation can enhance quality of life, but they can also create significant stressors in people's lives. Discussing and normalizing feelings around frustration, insecurities, loss, and rejection are imperative to a holistic approach to sexual interventions. Occupational therapy practitioners can work with clients to help them develop a strong sense of the coping skills that work for them and use those coping strategies when necessary.

In addition, because rejection is inevitable and a normal part of sexual and intimate engagements, occupational therapy practitioners can work with their clients to normalize rejection and to develop a "rejection plan" for taking care of themselves and practicing self-love and self-compassion. This can be particularly helpful when working with clients who are starting to date or are reengaging in dating.

Fostering Emotional Connection

Occupational therapy practitioners can guide clients through considering what occupations can build ***intimacy with self*** and partners. Intimacy with another person can be defined as a close, personal, trusting relationship where love, affection, respect, and nonjudgment is shared. Intimacy with oneself is much the same, but the love, affection, and respect, along with the curiosity and nonjudgment, are turned inward to build self-awareness. Encourage the client to think about occupations that result in new information about themselves or their partner(s), facilitate feelings of closeness and bonding, or generate curiosity.

Some ideas for intimacy with self might be journaling, engaging in pleasure-oriented self-care, taking oneself out on a date, engaging in self-pleasure, or learning a new skill as a hobby. Ideas for building intimacy with others include engaging in a mutually enjoyed activity, asking each other questions, playing a game, doing an eye-contact exercise, or making each other laugh (Herrick, 2018). Support the client by establishing a plan to incorporate these occupations into their daily routine, habits, and rituals. In addition, clients might need support to control their sensory environment to optimally engage in these activities.

Focusing intervention on the couple rather than the individual can have beneficial effects. A 6-week psychoeducational group intervention for couples in which one or both partners had cancer provided information on enhancing communication, reducing anxiety, and improving body image along with foundational lessons on sexual anatomy, sexual attitudes and behaviors, menopause, and sexual function and enhancement. Although pain and comfort were not affected by the program, the participants reported improvements in sexual satisfaction and emotional connection (Rowland et al., 2009).

Fostering Emotional Regulation

Emotional regulation requires building awareness of one's internal emotional state and sensations from interoception as well as developing strategies to participate in activities within an optimal zone of emotional arousal or state. For example, managing conflict with intimate partners requires strategies to promote emotional regulation. Clinicians can educate clients on the importance of building awareness of their internal emotional states and to consider implementing coping strategies if their emotional state is not ideal for difficult conversations that require calm communication. Occupational therapy practitioners can teach clients to request time-outs and space from conversations if they feel they are becoming overwhelmed by a conversation.

In addition, occupational therapy practitioners can educate clients on controlling the environment to support their internal emotional state when engaging in difficult conversations (e.g., turning off the television, scheduling the conversation for a time they feel less fatigued, using a pen and paper to write down what their partner is saying to make processing the information easier). Further, practitioners can consider cognitive reappraisal and mindfulness approaches to help the client develop strategies for emotional regulation (Erkan et al., 2021; St-Louis et al., 2021).

Physical Considerations

Common diagnoses that occupational therapy practitioners may need to consider when addressing physical skills include SCI, multiple sclerosis (MS), Parkinson's disease, amputations, stroke, and cerebral palsy. Rowen et al. (2015) reported that people who have experienced their physical impairment for a longer period have significantly more positive feelings about their sexuality, indicating that change is possible and is therefore worthwhile to pursue if clients' needs are not currently being met. Although many of the conditions discussed in this section may also have psychological, emotional, or cognitive aspects, the section focuses on some of the common physical considerations and evidence-based occupational therapy interventions.

Occupational therapy practitioners and other health professionals may use a variety of strategies to enable their clients to manage primary and secondary conditions to promote safe, satisfying sexual and intimate relations. Specifically, clients may need strategies to assist with vaginal lubrication and erectile responses, pain management and joint protection, cardiac considerations, bowel and bladder function, spasticity management, autonomic dysreflexia, and range of motion (ROM) interventions. Practitioners may also consider physical aspects associated with sexual self-expression (e.g., clothing management) and medication management to engage in occupations of sexuality and intimacy, which are described later in the chapter.

Vaginal Lubrication and Erectile Response

Decreased vaginal lubrication and erectile response are controlled by neural pathways often affected by SCI, MS, and other diagnoses, but they can be accommodated. Strategies to address vaginal dryness include promoting lubrication through focusing on what that person finds pleasurable, finessing the specific technique for stimulation, or enabling pleasure with adaptive equipment, such as universally cuffed vibrators; providing graded support from significant others; using over-the-counter or prescription lubrication; taking pain medication 20 to 30 minutes before sexual activity; stretching pelvic musculature; and using massage, a hot bath, or a vibrator for sore muscles (Kautz & Van Horn, 2017).

Clients who experience erectile dysfunction can benefit from *pleasure mapping,* an exercise to build more awareness of where and how the genitals receive pleasurable sensations. This exercise helps the person get clearer on the techniques, pacing, pressure, and penetrative positions that provide pleasure for them or work for them. Clients also can benefit from increasing stimulations from assistive devices, planning sex for a time they are most rested or interested in sex, engaging in psychoeducation regarding the central nervous system's role in sexual response (see Chapter 7, "Intimate Partnerships"), and using relaxation strategies.

In addition, clients can be referred to a urologist and may expect interventions ranging from medication to noninvasive vacuum-assistive devices to a penile prosthesis (Foley & Beier, 2006). Ideally, clients will consider the least invasive options first as well as adaptive strategies in combination with these approaches. Sexual activities that do not require an erect penis should be discussed (de Almeida et al., 2015). For decreases in libido, hormonal replacement of testosterone or estrogen has been used with some success; however, tackling conditions, such as pain, fatigue, bowel and bladder function, depression, and anxiety, may more readily address client goals and lead to greater satisfaction with sexual health (Basson et al., 2010; Lew-Starowicz & Gianotten, 2015).

Pain Management and Joint Protection

Occupational therapy practitioners are well suited to address secondary conditions, in particular, as part of a team of professionals working with PwPD. Energy conservation to manage fatigue and pain has long been credited for success in occupations ranging from ADLs to community engagement. Applying self-management strategies, such as postponing sexual activity until after a flare has passed, along with traditional pain and fatigue management, such as stretching and the use of more passive positions, can assist clients in improving sexual satisfaction (Helland et al., 2011).

Roditi and Robinson (2011) described relaxation training, graded exposure to sexual activity, and scheduling of pain medication as effective strategies for some couples. Hill (2016) described the role of occupational therapy in pain management as assisting clients to manage sexual activity through the use of activity analysis, skill development, activity adaptation, problem solving, prioritizing, planning, pacing, ergonomic application, stress management, communication skills training, relaxation training, environmental modifications, and social support. For example, Rosenbaum (2010) suggested promoting neutral wrist positioning and using pillows to support larger joints—helpful joint protection methods that can translate to sexual activity—as well as mapping or charting symptoms, cognitive reframing, and therapeutic exercise for the purposes of increasing ROM, strength, or endurance.

Endurance for Cardiac Considerations

For clients experiencing cardiovascular incidents, Steinke et al. (2013) suggested the following: Involve partners in communication and medication management; provide information through verbal, written, visual, seminar discussion, or practical training methods; encourage use of a comfortable or cool space as well as positions that require less energy expenditure; provide a graded progression of intimacy; and use supplemental oxygen during sexual activity, if prescribed.

Occupational therapy practitioners should ask the doctor about contraindications to participation in sexual activity and if there is a time frame to not engage after surgery. Instructions from surgeons can be vague—for example, what does "No sex for 3 to 4 weeks after surgery" actually mean? Is masturbation permitted? What activities are prohibited? Practitioners can help customize the physician's recommendation to each client. Precautions can be for heart rate and endurance reasons or musculoskeletal reasons, such as sternal precautions or hip precautions. Practitioners can apply this information to their knowledge of their client's sexual activities and develop appropriate recommendations for maintaining sexual engagement.

Bowel and Bladder Function

In addition to addressing the common conditions of pain and fatigue, occupational therapy practitioners can promote improved sexual health through the management of bowel and bladder function. Examples include adoption of strategies such as voiding before sexual activity, using a condom over a catheter, positioning in ways that avoid pressure on the bladder of the PwPD, and engaging in communication management with new or existing partners on what to expect when intimate. Some couples find it helpful to have sexual activity in a shower or bathtub so that fluid leaving the body is less noticeable and easier to clean. However, it is important that the surface be nonslippery, safe, and comfortable for all partners (Hess & Hough, 2012). If the PwPD uses an indwelling catheter, the catheter may be removed before intercourse or taped to the side in a slack position to allow for penile entry. Suprapubic catheters are often preferred over indwelling catheters because they result in less urethral trauma and are more conducive to sexual activity.

Spasticity Management

Spasticity is another common physical consideration for engaging in various sexual activities. Spasticity may cause hip and knee flexion that promotes the use of a wheelchair as a more supportive location for sexual activity, with the use of removable armrests to facilitate positioning of both partners. Using pump dispensers for decreased hand function to access lubricants, experimenting with new erogenous zones, and planning for sexual activity when pain is the lowest may also assist with managing spasticity (Rosenbaum et al., 2014).

Autonomic Dysreflexia

Autonomic dysreflexia is an abnormal sympathetic response to a stimulus, most commonly occurring in people with SCI. It is considered a medical emergency because it creates sudden increases in blood pressure. Ejaculation may be a trigger for autonomic dysreflexia. The PwPD's partner should be advised to place the person in an upright position to reduce blood pressure and ensure that all triggers are removed and pressure points alleviated (Alexander et al., 2017; Blackmore et al., 2011; Brotto & Goldmeier, 2015; Esmail et al., 2001; Fritz et al., 2015; Hess & Hough, 2012; Salomè et al., 2019).

Range of Motion

Decreased active ROM in hip extension, abduction, and external rotation may affect sexual activity. Making adjustments so that both partners are side-lying or using pillows or supports to lift the pelvis may be indicated. Slings may assist with thigh abduction if they do not cause pressure points or spasms (Hess & Hough, 2012). Positioning of devices such as vibrators with the use of straps when there is limited-to-no fine motor grasp or use of customized or universal splints to hold sexual aids may be beneficial (Guess et al., 2017).

Sexual Self-Expression

Sexual self-expression is one's "ability to express [oneself] as a sexual being" through "behaviors, mannerisms, preferences, appearance, pronouns, political engagement, acquired tendences, daily routines, symbolic actions or preferred roles" (Walker et al., 2020, p. 10). Similarly, someone with a new injury or disease may need assistance or modifications to engage in their sexual expression routines. For example, occupational therapy practitioners can support their transgender clients in gender-affirmative practices of sexual expression, such as safely binding, tucking, packing, or padding[3] (Neumann et al., 2021).

Expressing oneself as a sexual being can be an exciting and important part of intervention for clients. People may feel limited in expressing themselves because of external familial and social influences as well as whether they feel safe authentically expressing themselves—examples include a client exploring nonbinary ways of dressing or a client who has experienced sexual harassment throughout childhood desiring to wear an outfit that makes them feel sexy. A graded approach to trying out new ways of expressing oneself is by first wearing the style alone, then

---

[3] Tucking, packing, and padding are dressing ADLs that support one's desired appearance. By affirming a person's gender identity and expression, these dressing ADLs may enhance their sexual self-expression, depending on the meaning the person ascribes to the activity.

perhaps with a group of trusted friends or family, and then progressing to wearing the style out in public.

Clothing Management

Occupational therapy practitioners can assist clients in problem-solving clothing management challenges by providing resources on adaptive clothing, which is more easily donned and doffed through the use of hook-and-loop fasteners, snaps, and magnets, and ways to manage catheters and ensure that pressure relief is not compromised by ridges in clothing. Ensuring that clients are using clothing and apparel to express their identity and sexuality can aid in improving satisfaction with sexual expression. For example, it is common for lingerie to have many fasteners that can be difficult to manage for people with limited fine motor skills. "Sexy" clothing and undergarments can be adapted for ease of donning and doffing, or clients can seek out items that have more universal design (i.e., snaps versus ties).

Medication Management

Roditi and Robinson (2011) suggested improving satisfaction with sexual activity by scheduling the use of medication to limit pain coupled with graded exposure to sexual activity and relaxation training. Another aspect to consider regarding medication is that some medications, such as antidepressants, may interfere with sexual function. It is crucial, however, that clients consult with their physicians to discuss alternatives before discontinuing or changing the regimen of antidepressants or any other medication. Occupational therapy practitioners should always advise a discussion about alternatives and options with the client's physician, because some clients may not know to inquire.

Another medication management strategy Roditi and Robinson (2011) described is to take prescribed or over-the-counter pain medications 20 to 30 minutes before sexual activity, in addition to using lubricants and positioning strategies, to assist in managing any pain associated with sexual activity. Although occupational therapy practitioners may assist in medication management of prescribed and over-the-counter medication to manage pain, spasticity, mood, erectile dysfunction, and the like, they are not in the business of prescribing medication. Promoting the adaptive strategies of medication timing and communicating with the physician are within the scope of practice and may assist clients in improving their sexual health.

Assistive Devices

Clients can make choices about their medical equipment in a variety of ways to support their sexual expression and engagement. They may view their equipment as facilitating and enhancing their sexual experience—for example, grab bars assisting with balance while having sex with someone in a shower chair. They might view the equipment as erotic and sexualize the equipment as part of their own sexual expression and experience—for example, feeling that their wheelchair is a sex toy.

Conversely, some clients may view the medical equipment as nonerotic and a distraction from the sexual experience. For these clients, Taylor (2011) suggested arranging assistive devices at home in a way that compartmentalizes medical equipment from the sexual environment, such as storing medical equipment in a room other than the place where sexuality and intimacy take place. A variety of potentially helpful assistive devices are available to assist clients in achieving satisfying sexual encounters through increasing stimulation and sexually pleasing sensations. One resource that provides pictures and descriptions of sexual pleasure toys and ways to adapt them so PwPD can use them is *Sex and Intimacy for Wounded Veterans: A Guide to Embracing Change* (Ellis & Dennison, 2014).

Working With Others to Support Clients

Occupational therapy practitioners are likely to interact with and support families, parents or legal guardians, partners, and personal assistants when facilitating their clients' participation in occupations associated with sexuality and intimacy.

Working With Parents or Guardians

Some family members may have concerns with occupational therapy practitioners addressing occupations associated with sexuality and intimacy, depending on, for example, the client's age, diagnosis, gender, and family values related to religion and culture. Research demonstrates that people with intellectual and developmental disabilities are often infantilized and seen as needing protection instead of encouragement to engage in sexuality and intimacy occupations, yet they experience a higher risk of sexual assault, suggesting that efforts to protect are not effective (Brown & McCann, 2019). In accordance with the *Occupational Therapy Practice Framework: Domain and Process* (4th ed.; American Occupational Therapy Association, 2020), practitioners should support their client in achieving occupational justice, which may include advocating on behalf of the client to receive support in these occupations.

Occupational therapy practitioners can advocate for the need to address and support their clients in their sexual and intimate relationship goals, despite possible pushback from family members or guardians. One avenue of advocacy is to educate the family or guardians about guardianship—specifically, that guardianship in most states does not, in and of itself, remove the right to consent to relationships and sexual activities (Linder, 2018) and that everyone has the right to intimate partnerships and sexual expression (American Association on Intellectual and Developmental Disabilities, 2013). Practitioners should consult with their organizations and state policies for support when providing this education. Further, they may want to educate family or guardians about how sexual health education has been shown to decrease risky behaviors associated with sexual activity and does not encourage engagement in sexual activity (Kirby & The National Campaign to Prevent Teen and Unplanned Pregnancy, 2007).

Working With Partners

A large portion of therapy services may involve talking individually with clients or in conjunction with their partner(s). Many times, intimate partners also provide personal care assistance tasks, which can interfere with the promotion of intimacy if not managed well. Open communication and planning for intimacy are vital to managing personal care tasks. Blackmore et al. (2011) documented the importance of partner support in working with clients with MS. Women with SCI have reported concerns about caregiver burden as well as body image concerns when having to explain indwelling catheters and leg bags to potential partners (Beckwith & Yau, 2013).

Some clients may just want practical information on sensation, positioning, and knowing what other people with similar disabilities have experienced. Six months postdischarge for people experiencing injury has been found to be a critical time for sexual exploration (Beckwith & Yau, 2013). Timing of education is important: Occupational therapy practitioners must meet clients and their partners where they are and build from there. Promoting safety through open communication at the right time, as well as partnering with peers and other helpful supports, can promote positive sexual health.

Working With Personal Assistance Services

When a personal care attendant (PCA) is not an intimate partner, the PCA may assist in the preparatory setup as well as with managing bowel or bladder needs, medication management, setting up access to positioning items, and the like. Occupational therapy practitioners may play a role in educating PCAs about options for best supporting their clients with sexuality and intimacy. Practitioners can also provide training about advocacy and sexual rights to people with disabilities and the people working with them.

Accessibility Considerations

Occupational therapy practitioners should ensure that their clinic space is accessible to PwPD (Rowen et al., 2015). Practitioners should have assistive sexual devices, positioning aids, and mobility devices that are usable by or made specifically for people with disabilities, for example, the IntimateRider™ swing chair and Bump'n™ sex toys. In addition, practitioners should ensure that any educational materials are accessible to clients' cognitive and sensory needs and adapt the educational materials if they are not.

The incidence of violence against PwPD is higher than among people without disabilities (Rowen et al., 2015). As a result, care should be taken to ensure privacy when working with all clients and to provide opportunities for clients to speak freely without an attendant or partner present. If a client reports sexual abuse, pre-existing sexual dysfunction, or recent relationship problems, consider any immediate threats and how to partner with the appropriate team to refer the client to counseling. Also, explore cultural and religious needs when connecting clients with referral sources to ensure the best fit by explaining the reason for a referral, asking a client if they would be interested in the referral, or asking the client if there are any preferences the client might have for their ideal provider (Alexander et al., 2017).

Summary

This chapter was developed to bridge the gap between occupational therapy practitioners' resistance to addressing sexuality and intimacy in clinical practice and actualization of the holistic intent of occupational therapy to address the whole person. When considering sexuality and intimacy interventions, practitioners should think holistically and consider the multidimensional factors that influence performance. Before considering interventions, competent clinicians will have a consistent self-reflection practice and continue to seek out new information and experiences. They seek to broaden their view and understanding of the various ways of being sexual, expressing sexuality, and forming relationships. Practitioners need to be committed to getting to know their client, learning not just what is meaningful to the client but also the client's sexual goals and what challenges those goals. This approach will help practitioners determine which of the intervention strategies mentioned in this chapter can effectively support their individual clients as they participate in sexuality and intimacy occupations.

Kathryn Ellis, OTD, OTR/L, AASECT–SC (she/her/hers), developed the Occupational Therapy Sexuality and Intimacy Clinic at Walter Reed National Military Medical Center in Bethesda, Maryland, and is the co-author of *Sex and Intimacy for Wounded Veterans: A Guide to Embracing Change.* She is the founder and CEO of a continuing education company, the Institute for Sex, Intimacy & Occupational Therapy. She is an American Association of Sexuality Educators, Counselors, and Therapists Certified Sexuality Counselor and a consultant on sexuality and intimacy projects and initiatives. Her private practice, Dr. Kathryn Ellis Sexual Wellness Counseling, is based in Delaware.

Elizabeth K. Schmidt, PhD, OTR/L (she/her/hers), completed both her master's degree in occupational therapy and PhD in health and rehabilitation sciences at The Ohio State University. She completed her postdoctoral training at Boston University and is currently an assistant professor of occupational therapy at the DeBusk College of Osteopathic Medicine at Lincoln Memorial University in Knoxville. She has grant funding from the National Institutes of Disability, Independent Living and Rehabilitation Research to conduct a participatory approach research study alongside queer autistic researchers to better understand supports and barriers to community participation for queer autistic adults. Schmidt's research is primarily focused on accessibility of sexuality education for adolescents and adults with neurodevelopmental disabilities. She is passionate about occupational justice and sexual and reproductive health autonomy for people with neurodevelopmental disabilities.

Carla Wilson Walker, OTD, OTR/L, ATP (she/her/hers), serves as an instructor and advanced practice clinician through the Washington University Program in Occupational Therapy in St. Louis. She provides clinical interventions in the areas of parenting, wheelchair seating and positioning, sexuality and intimacy, and community participation to adults with disabilities. She is a Certified Assistive Technology Professional and provides adaptive equipment in the home, clinic, and community to promote independence.

References

Alexander, M. S., Aisen, C. M., Alexander, S. M., & Aisen, M. L. (2017). Sexual concerns after spinal cord injury: An update on management. *NeuroRehabilitation, 41,* 343–357. https://doi.org/10.3233/NRE-172202

Alleva, J. M., Diedrichs, P. C., Halliwell, E., Peters, M. L., Dures, E., Stuijfzand, B. G., & Rumsey, N. (2018). More than my RA: A randomized trial investigating body image improvement among women with rheumatoid arthritis using a functionality-focused intervention program. *Journal of Consulting and Clinical Psychology, 86,* 666–676. https://doi.org/10.1037/ccp0000317

American Association on Intellectual and Developmental Disabilities. (2013). *Sexuality: Joint Position Statement of AAIDD and the Arc.* https://aaidd.org/news-policy/policy/position-statements/sexuality

American Occupational Therapy Association. (2020). Occupational therapy practice framework: Domain and process (4th ed.). *American Journal of Occupational Therapy, 74*(Suppl. 2), 7412410010. https://doi.org/10.5014/ajot.2020.74S2001

Ballan, M. S., & Freyer, M. B. (2017). Autism spectrum disorder, adolescence, and sexuality education: Suggested interventions for mental health professionals. *Sexuality and Disability, 35,* 261–273. https://doi.org/10.1007/s11195-017-9477-9

Banerjee, M., Ray, P., & Panda, A. (2013). *Role of sex education on odd sexual and problem behavior: A study on adolescents with autism.* Community Psychology Association of India.

Barnard-Brak, L., Schmidt, M., Chesnut, S., Wei, T., & Richman, D. (2014). Predictors of access to sex education for children with intellectual disabilities in public schools. *Intellectual and Developmental Disabilities, 52,* 85–97. https://doi.org/10.1352/1934-9556-52.2.85

Basson, R., Rees, P., Wang, R., Montejo, A. L., & Incrocci, L. (2010). Sexual function in chronic illness. *Journal of Sexual Medicine,* 7(1, Part 2), 374–388. https://doi.org/10.1111/j.1743-6109.2009.01621.x

Beckwith, A., & Yau, M. K. S. (2013). Sexual recovery: Experiences of women with spinal injury reconstructing a positive sexual identity. *Sexuality and Disability, 31,* 313–324. https://doi.org/10.1007/s11195-013-9315-7

Blackmore, D. E., Hart, S. L., Albiani, J. J., & Mohr, D. C. (2011). Improvements in partner support predict sexual satisfaction among individuals with multiple sclerosis. *Rehabilitation Psychology, 56,* 117–122. https://doi.org/10.1037/a0023362

Brotto, L. A., & Goldmeier, D. (2015). Mindfulness interventions for treating sexual dysfunctions: The gentle science of finding focus in a multitask world. *The Journal of Sexual Medicine, 12,* 1687–1689. https://doi.org/10.1111/jsm.12941

Brown, M., & McCann, E. (2019). The views and experiences of families and direct care support workers regarding the expression of sexuality by adults with intellectual disabilities: A narrative review of the international research evidence. *Research in Developmental Disabilities, 90,* 80–91. https://doi.org/10.1016/j.ridd.2019.04.012

Carvalho, J., & Nobre, P. (2010). Predictors of women's sexual desire: The role of psychopathology, cognitive-emotional determinants, relationship dimensions, and medical factors. *The Journal of Sexual Medicine, 7,* 928–937. https://doi.org/10.1111/j.1743-6109.2009.01568.x

Carvalho, J., & Nobre, P. (2011). Predictors of men's sexual desire: The role of psychological, cognitive–emotional, relational, and medical factors. *The Journal of Sex Research, 48*(2–3), 254–262. https://doi.org/10.1080/00224491003605475

Collins, R. L., Strasburger, V. C., Brown, J. D., Donnerstein, E., Lenhart, A., & Ward, M. (2017). Sexual media and childhood well-being and health. *Pediatrics, 140,* S162–S166. https://doi.org/10.1542/peds.2016-1758X

de Almeida, P. H. T. Q., de Castro Ferreira, C., Kurizky, P. S., Muniz, L. F., & da Mota, L. M. H. (2015). How the rheumatologist can guide the patient with rheumatoid arthritis on sexual function. *Revista Brasileira de Reumatologia (English Edition), 55,* 458–463. https://doi.org/10.1016/j.rbr.2014.08.009

Dosch, A., Rochat, L., Ghisletta, P., Favez, N., & Van der Linden, M. (2016). Psychological factors involved in sexual desire, sexual activity, and sexual satisfaction: A multi-factorial perspective. *Archives of Sexual Behavior, 45,* 2029–2045. https://doi.org/10.1007/s10508-014-0467-z

Dunkley, C. R., Goldsmith, K. M., & Gorzalka, B. B. (2015). The potential role of mindfulness in protecting against sexual insecurities. *Canadian Journal of Human Sexuality, 24,* 92–103. https://doi.org/10.3138/cjhs.242-A7

Erkan, I., Kafesçioğlu, N., Cavdar, A., & Zeytinoğlu-Saydam, S. (2021). Romantic relationship experiences and emotion regulation strategies of regular mindfulness meditation practitioners: A qualitative study. *Journal of Marital and Family Therapy, 47,* 629–647. https://doi.org/10.1111/jmft.12462

Ellis, K., & Dennison, C. (2014). *Sex and intimacy for wounded veterans: A guide to embracing change.* Sager Group.

Esmail, S., Esmail, Y., & Munro, B. (2001). Sexuality and disability: The role of health care professionals in providing options and alternatives for couples. *Sexuality and Disability, 19,* 267–282. https://doi.org/10.1023/A:1017905425599

Exell, R., Hilari, K., & Behn, N. (2020). Interventions that support adults with brain injuries, learning disabilities and autistic spectrum disorders in dating or romantic relationships: A systematic review. *Disability and Rehabilitation, 44,* 2567–2580. https://doi.org/10.1080/09638288.2020.1845824

Ferrante, C. A., & Oak, E. (2020). "No sex please!" We have been labelled intellectually disabled. *Sex Education, 20,* 383–397. https://doi.org/10.1080/14681811.2020.1719479

Foley, F. W., & Beier, M. (2006). *Assessment and treatment of sexual dysfunction in multiple sclerosis.* National Multiple Sclerosis Society. https://www.nationalmssociety.org/NationalMSSociety/media/MSNationalFiles/Brochures/Clinical_Bulletin_Sexual-Dysfunction-in-MS.pdf

Friedman, C., Arnold, C. K., Owen, A. L., & Sandman, L. (2014). "Remember Our Voices are Our Tools": Sexual self-advocacy as defined by people with intellectual and developmental disabilities. *Sexuality and Disability, 32,* 515–532. https://doi.org/10.1007/s11195-014-9377-1

Fritz, H. A., Dillaway, H., & Lysack, C. L. (2015). "Don't think paralysis takes away your womanhood": Sexual intimacy after spinal cord injury. *American Journal of Occupational Therapy, 69,* 6902260030. https://doi.org/10.5014/ajot.2015.015040

Gantman, A., Kapp, S. K., Orenski, K., & Laugeson, E. A. (2012). Social skills training for young adults with high-functioning autism spectrum disorders: A randomized controlled pilot study. *Journal of Autism and Developmental Disorders, 42,* 1094–1103. https://doi.org/10.1007/s10803-011-1350-6

Gray, C. (n.d.). *Comparison of Social Stories™ 10.0–10.2 criteria.* https://carolgraysocialstories.com/wp-content/uploads/2015/09/Social-Stories-10.0-10.2-Comparison-Chart.pdf

Grove, L., Morrison-Beedy, D., Kirby, R., & Hess, J. (2018). The birds, bees, and special needs: Making evidence-based sex education accessible for adolescents with intellectual disabilities. *Sexuality and Disability, 36,* 313–329. https://doi.org/10.1007/s11195-018-9547-7

Guess, M. K., Connell, K. A., Chudnoff, S., Adekoya, O., Richmond, C., Nixon, K. E., . . . Melman, A. (2017). The effects of a genital vibratory stimulation device on sexual function and genital sensation. *Female Pelvic Medicine and Reconstructive Surgery, 23,* 256–262. https://doi.org/10.1097/SPV.0000000000000357

Günzler, C., & Berner, M. M. (2012). Efficacy of psychosocial interventions in men and women with sexual dysfunctions—A systematic review of controlled clinical trials. *The Journal of Sexual Medicine, 9*(12), 3108–3125. https://doi.org/10.1111/j.1743-6109.2012.02965.x

Helland, Y., Kjeken, I., Steen, E., Kvien, T. K., Hauge, M. I., & Dagfinrud, H. (2011). Rheumatic diseases and sexuality: Disease impact and self-management strategies. *Arthritis Care & Research, 63,* 743–750. https://doi.org/10.1002/acr.20424

Herrick, P. (2018). *The presence of playfulness in the context of couple relationship, relationship satisfaction and its associations with symptoms of depression* [Doctoral dissertation, University of Maryland, College Park]. Digital Repository at the University of Maryland. https://drum.lib.umd.edu/handle/1903/21022

Hess, M. J., & Hough, S. (2012). Impact of spinal cord injury on sexuality: Broad-based clinical practice intervention and practical application. *Journal of Spinal Cord Medicine, 35,* 211–218. https://doi.org/10.1179/2045772312Y.0000000025

Hill, W. (2016). The role of occupational therapy in pain management. *Anaesthesia and Intensive Care Medicine, 17,* 451–453. https://doi.org/10.1016/j.mpaic.2016.06.008

Kautz, D. D., & Van Horn, E. R. (2017). Sex and intimacy after stroke. *Rehabilitation Nursing, 42*(6), 333–340. https://doi.org/10.1002/rnj.296

Kirby, D., & The National Campaign to Prevent Teen and Unplanned Pregnancy (U.S.). (2007). *Emerging answers, 2007: Research findings on programs to reduce teen pregnancy and sexually transmitted diseases.* The National Campaign to Prevent Teen and Unplanned Pregnancy.

Klett, L. S., & Turan, Y. (2012). Generalized effects of social stories with task analysis for teaching menstrual care to three young girls with autism. *Sexuality and Disability, 30,* 319–336. https://doi.org/10.1007/s11195-011-9244-2

Laugeson, E. A., Ellingsen, R., Sanderson, J., Tucci, L., & Bates, S. (2014). The ABC's of teaching social skills to adolescents with autism spectrum disorder in the classroom: The UCLA *PEERS®* program. *Journal of Autism and Developmental Disorders, 44,* 2244–2256. https://doi.org/10.1007/s10803-014-2108-8

Laugeson, E. A., Frankel, F., Gantman, A., Dillon, A. R., & Mogil, C. (2012). Evidence-based social skills training for adolescents with autism spectrum disorders: The UCLA PEERS program. *Journal of Autism and Developmental Disorders, 42,* 1025–1036. https://doi.org/10.1007/s10803-011-1339-1

Laugeson, E. A., Gantman, A., Kapp, S. K., Orenski, K., & Ellingsen, R. (2015). A randomized controlled trial to improve social skills in young adults with autism spectrum disorder: The UCLA PEERS® program. *Journal of Autism and Developmental Disorders, 45,* 3978–3989. https://doi.org/10.1007/s10803-015-2504-8

Lew-Starowicz, M., & Gianotten, W. L. (2015). Sexual dysfunction in patients with multiple sclerosis. In D. B Vodušek & F. Boller (Eds.), *Handbook of clinical neurology: Vol. 130. Neurology of sexual and bladder disorders* (pp. 357–370). Elsevier. https://doi.org/10.1016/B978-0-444-63247-0.00020-1

Linder, A. (2018). Capacity to consent to sexual activity among those with developmental disabilities. *Stanford Intellectual and Developmental Disabilities Law and Policy Project (SIDDLAPP).* SLS Publications. https://law.stanford.edu/publications/capacity-to-consent-to-sexual-activity-among-those-with-developmental-disabilities/

Lorde, A. (2020). *Sister outsider: Essays and speeches.* Penguin Classics.

Male, D. A., Fergus, K. D., & Cullen, K. (2016). Sexual identity after breast cancer: Sexuality, body image, and relationship repercussions. *Current Opinion in Supportive and Palliative Care, 10,* 66–74. https://doi.org/10.1097/SPC.0000000000000184

Marshall, S. L., Parker, P. D., Ciarrochi, J., Sahdra, B., Jackson, C. J., & Heaven, P. C. (2015). Self-compassion protects against the negative effects of low self-esteem: A longitudinal study in a large adolescent sample. *Personality and Individual Differences, 74,* 116–121. https://doi.org/10.1016/j.paid.2014.09.013

Mathias, Z., & Harcourt, D. (2014). Dating and intimate relationships of women with below-knee amputation: An exploratory study. *Disability and Rehabilitation, 36,* 395–402. https://doi.org/10.3109/09638288.2013.797509

Nagoski, E. (2015). *Come as you are: The surprising new science that will transform your sex life.* Simon & Schuster.

Neumann, N., Neu, D., & Ungco, J. (2021). Addressing LGBTQIA+ trauma: Your role and your responsibility. In A. Lynch, R. Ashcraft, & L. Tekell (Eds.), *Trauma, occupation, and participation: Foundations and population considerations in occupational therapy* (pp. 195–222). AOTA Press.

Nimbi, F. M., Tripodi, F., Rossi, R., Michetti, P. M., & Simonelli, C. (2019). Which psychosocial variables affect drive the most? Analysis of sexual desire in a group of Italian men. *International Journal of Impotence Research, 31,* 410–423. https://doi.org/10.1038/s41443-018-0105-8

Parish, S. J., & Hahn, S. R. (2016). Hypoactive sexual desire disorder: A review of epidemiology, biopsychology, diagnosis, and treatment. *Sexual Medicine Reviews, 4,* 103–120. https://doi.org/10.1016/j.sxmr.2015.11.009

Park, K.-M., Ku, J., Choi, S.-H., Jang, H.-J., Park, J.-Y., Kim, S. I., & Kim, J.-J. (2011). A virtual reality application in role-plays of social skills training for schizophrenia: A randomized, controlled trial. *Psychiatry Research, 189,* 166–172. https://doi.org/10.1016/j.psychres.2011.04.003

Plavnick, J. B., Kaid, T., & MacFarland, M. C. (2015). Effects of a school-based social skills training program for adolescents with autism spectrum disorder and intellectual disability. *Journal of Autism and Developmental Disorders, 45,* 2674–2690. https://doi.org/10.1007/s10803-015-2434-5

Roden, R. C., Schmidt, E. K., & Holland-Hall, C. (2020). Sexual health education for adolescents and young adults with intellectual and developmental disabilities: Recommendations for accessible sexual and reproductive health information. *The Lancet: Child and Adolescent Health, 4,* 699–708. https://doi.org/10.1016/S2352-4642(20)30098-5

Roditi, D., & Robinson, M. E. (2011). The role of psychological interventions in the management of patients with chronic pain. *Psychology Research and Behavior Management, 4,* 41–49. https://doi.org/10.2147%2FPRBM.S15375

Rosebrock, L., & Carroll, R. (2017). Sexual function in female veterans: A review. *Journal of Sex and Marital Therapy, 43,* 228–245. https://doi.org/10.1080/0092623X.2016.1141822

Rosenbaum, T. Y. (2010). Musculoskeletal pain and sexual function in women. *Journal of Sexual Medicine, 7,* 645–653. https://doi.org/10.1111/j.1743-6109.2009.01490.x

Rosenbaum, T., Vadas, D., & Kalichman, L. (2014). Sexual function in post-stroke patients: Considerations for rehabilitation. *Journal of Sexual Medicine, 11,* 15–21. https://doi.org/10.1111/jsm.12343

Rowen, T. S., Stein, S., & Tepper, M. (2015). Sexual health care for people with physical disabilities. *Journal of Sexual Medicine, 12,* 584–589. https://doi.org/10.1111/jsm.12810

Rowland, J. H., Meyerowitz, B. E., Crespi, C. M., Leedham, B., Desmond, K., Belin, T. R., & Ganz, P. A. (2009). Addressing intimacy and partner communication after breast cancer: A randomized controlled group intervention. *Breast Cancer Research and Treatment, 118,* 99. https://doi.org/10.1007/s10549-009-0398-x

Sala, G., Hooley, M., Attwood, T., Mesibov, G. B., & Stokes, M. A. (2019). Autism and intellectual disability: A systematic review of sexuality and relationship education. *Sexuality and Disability, 37,* 353–382. https://doi.org/10.1007/s11195-019-09577-4

Salomè, A., Sasso D'Elia, T., Franchini, G., Santilli, V., & Paolucci, T. (2019). Occupational therapy in fatigue management in multiple sclerosis: An umbrella review. *Multiple Sclerosis International, 2019,* 2027947. https://doi.org/10.1155/2019/2027947

Schaafsma, D., Kok, G., Stoffelen, J. M. T., & Curfs, L. M. G. (2015). Identifying effective methods for teaching sex education to individuals with intellectual disabilities: A systematic review. *Journal of Sex Research, 52,* 412–432. https://doi.org/10.1080/00224499.2014.919373

Schaafsma, D., Kok, G., Stoffelen, J. M. T., & Curfs, L. M. G. (2017). People with intellectual disabilities talk about sexuality: Implications for the development of sex education. *Sexuality and Disability, 35,* 21–38. https://doi.org/10.1007/s11195-016-9466-4

Schmidt, E. K., Brown, C., & Darragh, A. (2020). Scoping review of sexual health education interventions for adolescents and young adults with intellectual or developmental disabilities. *Sexuality and Disability, 38,* 439–453. https://doi.org/10.1007/s11195-019-09593-4

Schmidt, E. K., Robek, N., Dougherty, M., Hand, B. N., Havercamp, S., Sommerich, C., . . . Darragh, A. (2021). Recommendations to improve accessibility of sexuality education for individuals with intellectual or developmental disabilities: A qualitative study. *American Journal of Sexuality Education, 16,* 38–56. https://doi.org/10.1080/15546128.2020.1860177

Speed, B. C., Goldstein, B. L., & Goldfried, M. R. (2018). Assertiveness training: A forgotten evidence-based treatment. *Clinical Psychology: Science and Practice, 25,* e12216. https://doi.org/10.1111/cpsp.12216

Steinke, E. E., Jaarsma, T., Barnason, S. A., Byrne, M., Doherty, S., Dougherty, C. M., . . . Moser, D. K. (2013). Sexual counseling for individuals with cardiovascular disease and their partners: A consensus document from the American Heart Association and the ESC Council on Cardiovascular Nursing and Allied Professions (CCNAP). *Circulation, 128,* 2075–2096. https://doi.org/10.1161/CIR.0b013e31829c2e53

St-Louis, A. C., Rapaport, M., Poirier, L. C., Vallerand, R. J., & Dandeneau, S. (2021). On emotion regulation strategies and well-being: The role of passion. *Journal of Happiness Studies, 22,* 1791–1818. https://doi.org/10.1007/s10902-020-00296-8

Stokes, M., Newton, N., & Kaur, A. (2007). Stalking, and social and romantic functioning among adolescents and adults with autism spectrum disorder. *Journal of Autism and Developmental Disorders, 37,* 1969–1986. https://doi.org/10.1007/s10803-006-0344-2

Swango-Wilson, A. (2011). Meaningful sex education programs for individuals with intellectual/developmental disabilities. *Sexuality and Disability, 29,* 113–118. https://doi.org/10.1007/s11195-010-9168-2

Taylor, B. (2011). The impact of assistive equipment on intimacy and sexual expression. *British Journal of Occupational Therapy, 74*(9), 435–442. https://doi.org/10.4276/030802211X13153015305637

Thorpe, S., Nichols, T. R., Tanner, A. E., Kuperberg, A., & Foh, E. P. (2021). Relational and partner-specific factors influencing Black heterosexual women's initiation of sexual intercourse and orgasm frequency. *Sexuality and Culture, 25,* 503–521. https://doi.org/10.1007/s12119-020-09780-y

Walker, B. A., Otte, K., LeMond, K., Hess, P., Kaizer, K., Faulkner, T., & Christy, D. (2020). Development of the Occupational Performance Inventory of Sexuality and Intimacy (OPISI): Phase one. *Open Journal of Occupational Therapy, 8,* 1–18. https://doi.org/10.15453/2168-6408.1694

Ward, K. M., Atkinson, J. P., Smith, C. A., & Windsor, R. (2013). A Friendships and Dating Program for adults with intellectual and developmental disabilities: A formative evaluation. *Intellectual and Developmental Disabilities, 51,* 22–32. https://doi.org/10.1352/1934-9556-51.01.022

Weiner, L., & Avery-Clark, C. (2017). *Sensate focus in sex therapy: The illustrated manual.* Routledge. https://doi.org/10.4324/9781315630038

Index

Note. Page numbers in *italics* refer to exhibits, figures, and tables. Page numbers followed by "n" refer to notes.

FSC
www.fsc.org
MIX
Papier | Fördert gute Waldnutzung
FSC® C083411

Kolibri 360 GmbH
Ferdinand-Jühlke-Straße 7
99095 Erfurt, Deutschland
produktsicherheit@kolibri360.de